Pathobiology of Soft Tissue Tumours

CURRENT PROBLEMS IN TUMOUR PATHOLOGY
THE PATHOBIOLOGY OF MALIGNANT DISEASE

Series Editors

Nicholas A. Wright MA, MD, PhD, FRCPath Professor and Director, Department of Histopathology, Royal Postgraduate Medical School, Hammersmith Hospital, London, UK

J.G. Azzopardi MD, FRCPath Professor of Oncology, Department of Histopathology, Royal Postgraduate Medical School, Hammersmith Hospital, London, UK

Published volumes in this Series

Pathobiology of Soft Tissue Tumours

C.D.M. Fletcher MB BS MRCPath
Senior Lecturer/Honorary Consultant in Histopathology and
Director of Soft Tissue Tumour Unit, United Medical and
Dental Schools (St Thomas's Hospital), London, UK

P.H. McKee MB Bch BaO FRCPath
Senior Lecturer/Honorary Consultant in Histopathology,
United Medical and Dental Schools (St. Thomas's Hospital),
London, UK

CHURCHILL LIVINGSTONE
EDINBURGH LONDON MELBOURNE AND NEW YORK 1990

CHURCHILL LIVINGSTONE
Medical Division of Longman Group UK Limited

Distributed in the United States of America by Churchill
Livinstone Inc., 1560 Broadway, New York, N.Y. 10036, and
by associated companies, branches and representatives
throughout the world.

First published 1990

ISBN 0-443-03790-6
ISSN 0266-9927

British Library Cataloguing in Publication Data

British Library Cataloguing in Publication Data
Pathobiology of soft tissue tumours.
  1. Man. Soft tissues. Tumours. Pathology
  I. Fletcher, C. D. M.   II. McKee, Phillip H.   III. Series
  616.992

Library of Congress Cataloging in Publication Data
Pathobiology of soft tissue tumours/[edited by] C.D.M. Fletcher,
  P.H. McKee
        p. cm. – (Current problems in tumour pathology)
    Includes index.
    ISBN 0-443-03790-6
    1. Tumours—Pathophysiology.   I. Fletcher, Christopher D. M.
  II. McKee, Phillip H.   III. Series.
    [DNLM: 1. Soft Tissue Neoplasms—pathology.   WD 375 P297]
  RC254.6.P37   1990
  616.99'2071—dc20
  DNLM/DLC
  for Library of Congress   90-2131
                                                                       CIP

Produced by Longman Singapore Publishers Pte Ltd
Printed in Singapore

Foreword

In the emergence of histopathology specialisation, that of the pathology of soft tissue tumours has perhaps been tardy: this probably reflects the fact that this has been a very difficult area. However, over the past 10 years, there has been a veritable explosion of interest and information, largely occasioned by advances in nosology and accurate delineation. Through these studies, diagnosis and prognostic forecasting has markedly improved and, recently, basic scientists have turned their attention to soft tissue tumours.

While the literature contains several excellent compendia on diagnostic aspects, this is the first work of synthesis on the *biology* of soft tissue tumours. Drs Fletcher and McKee have assembled a formidable team of experts who have addressed the major current problems in this field; we believe that the next few years will see signal advances in our ideas about the causation and nature of soft tissue tumours, and we feel that this volume very much sets the scene for this development.

1990   N.A.W.
                                                                     J.G.A.

Contributors

Anne C. Bayley OBE FRCS
Professor of Surgery, University Teaching Hospital, Lusaka, Zambia

Knud Bendix-Hansen MD
Senior Registrar, University Institute of Pathology, Aarhus, Denmark

E. B. Chung MD PhD
Professor of Pathology, Howard University; Director of Surgical Pathology, Howard University Hospital, Washington DC, USA

José Costa MD
Professor and Chairman, Institut de Pathologie, Centre Hospitalier Université Vaudois, Lausanne, Switzerland

William B. Dupree MD
Department of Pathology, Lehigh Valley Hospital Center, Allentown, Pennsylvania, USA

Frederick R. Eilber MD
Professor of Surgery, Division of Surgical Oncology, UCLA School of Medicine, University of California, Los Angeles, USA

Munemoto Enjoji MD
Professor of Pathology, Faculty of Medicine, Kyushu University, Fukuoka, Japan

Christopher D. M. Fletcher MB BS MRCPath
Senior Lecturer/Honorary Consultant in Histopathology and Director of Soft Tissue Tumour Unit, United Medical and Dental Schools, (St. Thomas's Hospital), London, UK

Giulio Gabbiani MD PhD
Professor of Pathology, Centre Medical Universitaire, Geneva, Switzerland

Michael R. Hendrickson MD
Associate Professor of Pathology; Associate Director, Laboratory of Surgical Pathology, Stanford University Medical Center, Stanford, California, USA

James F. Huth BS MD
Associate Professor of Surgery, Chief, Surgical Oncology Section,
Department of General Surgery, School of Medicine, University of North
Carolina at Chapel Hill, NC, USA

Hisami Iri MD
Professor, Central Laboratories, Keio University Hospital, Tokyo, Japan

Richard L. Kempson MD
Professor of Pathology; Co-Director Surgical Pathology, Laboratory of
Surgical Pathology, Stanford University Medical Center, Stanford,
California, USA

Sebastian Lucas MA BM BCh MRCP MRCPath
Senior Lecturer, Department of Histopathology, University College School
of Medicine, London, UK

Bruce Mackay MB ChB PhD
Professor of Pathology, University of Texas, MD Anderson Hospital and
Tumour Institute, Houston, Texas, USA

Phillip H. McKee MB BCh BaO FRCPath
Senior Lecturer/Honorary Consultant, Department of Histopathology, St
Thomas' Hospital Medical School, London, UL

Makio Mukai MD
Lecturer, Department of Pathology, Keio University School of Medicine,
Tokyo, Japan

O. Myhre-Jensen PhD, MD
Professor, University Institute of Pathology, Aarhus, Denmark

Omar Skalli PhD
Research Assistant, Department of Pathology, Centre Medical
Universitaire, Geneva, Switzerland

A. C. Templeton FRCP FRCPath
Professor of Pathology, Rush Medical College, Chicago, Illinois, USA

Chikao Torikata MD
Assistant Professor, Department of Pathology, Keio University Medical
School, Tokyo, Japan

M. Tsuneyoshi MD
Associate Professor, Department of Pathology, Faculty of Medicine,
Kyushu University, Fukuoka, Japan

Contents

1. Introduction

C. D. M. Fletcher

Despite the fact that this volume forms part of a series entitled *Current Problems in Tumour Pathology*, soft tissue tumours have been a great source of difficulty, and controversy, ever since Arthur Purdy Stout brought this group of neoplasms to general attention between 1930 and 1960. Furthermore, although Enzinger (and latterly Weiss) at the Armed Forces Institute of Pathology in Washington have been largely responsible for the truly enormous advances in our understanding of these lesions over the last 25 years, major problems are undoubtedly going to persist, both at the clinical and research levels, for the foreseeable future.

The root cause of these problems is the fact that accurate classification of a given lesion is often not easy, so much so that acknowledged international experts are still unable to pin a label on about 10% of sarcomas. Attempts by non-specialist surgical pathologists to classify these tumours are rendered even more hazardous by the constant recognition of new entities and alterations in the designation, or categorisation, of better known neoplasms as our understanding of them is modified or increased. The influence of this fairly ceaseless reclassification is underlined by changes that have occurred in the 'league' table of large series of sarcomas collated over the last 25 years (Table 1.1).

Some might argue that many of these 'new entities' represent valueless examples of subdivision or splitting. However, this is patently not the case, since most of the recently delineated lesions have distinctive, if not unique, histological features and a reasonably predictable clinical course, often very different from that of the lesion with which they may have been formerly classified. Striking examples are the spindle cell and pleomorphic lipomas, Shmookler & Enzinger 1981, Fletcher & Martin-Bates 1987) and cellular schwannomas (Woodruff et al 1981, Fletcher et al 1987), many of which had been inappropriately called sarcomas and treated as such in the past.

The rate at which new entities have been recognised and accurately described over the last 10 years is readily appreciated by examining Table 1.2. Many of the 'new' benign neoplasms were formerly misclassified as sarcomas. It is fairly self-evident that the reason for this phenomenon lies in the relative rarity of many types of soft tissue tumour. This has not only led to problems in collating large enough series of single entities to allow worthwhile

Table 1.1 Changes in the frequency distribution of the more common sarcomas over the last 25 years

Hare & Cerny (1963) 200 cases*		Russell et al (1977) 1215 cases		Hajdu (1979) 2489 cases		Enjoji & Hashimoto (1984) 752 cases		Material on file at St Thomas's Hospital (1989) 1095 cases	
Fibrosarcoma	43%	Fibrosarcoma	19%	Rhabdomyosarcoma	22%	MFH	26.7%	Liposarcoma	17%
Unclassifiable	28.5%	Rhabdomyosarcoma	19%	Liposarcoma	16.7%	Rhabdomyosarcoma	11.8%	Leiomyosarcoma	14%
Liposarcoma	11.5%	Liposarcoma	18%	MFH	15.7%	Liposarcoma	9.8%	Rhabdomyosarcoma	12%
Leiomyosarcoma	6.5%	MFH	10.5%	Fibrosarcoma	14.4%	Leimyosarcoma	8.8%	MFH	11%
Rhabdomyosarcoma	5%	Unclassifiable	10%	Angiosarcoma	8.5%	Unclassifiable	7.7%	Unclassifiable	10%
Dermatofibrosarcoma	3%	Synovial sarcoma	6.9%	Tendosynovial sarcoma	7.5%	Fibrosarcoma	7.2%	MPNST	9.5%
Synovial sarcoma	2.5%	Leiomyosarcoma	6.5 %	MPNST	5.7%	Synovial sarcoma	5.7%	Synovial sarcoma	6%
		MPNST	4.9%			MPNST	4.9%	Angiosarcoma	3%

MFH = malignant fibrous histiocytoma, MPNST = malignant peripheral nerve sheath tumour
* This is the only series which included dermatofibrosarcoma in the total.

Table 1.2 Soft tissue tumours which have been described or accurately delineated for the first time over the last 10 years.

Benign	
Fibroma of tendon sheath	Chung & Enzinger 1979
Intravenous pyogenic granuloma	Cooper et al 1979
Dermal nerve sheath myxoma	Gallager & Helwig 1980
Cranial fasciitis	Lauer & Enzinger 1980
Infantile myofibromatosis	Chung & Enzinger 1981
Intravascular fasciitis	Patchefsky & Enzinger 1981
Pleomorphic lipoma	Shmookler & Enzinger 1981
Cellular schwannoma	Woodruff et al 1981
Giant cell fibroblastoma	Shmookler & Enzinger 1982
Aggressive angiomyxoma	Steeper & Rosai 1983
Fibrolipomatous hamartoma of nerve	Silverman & Enzinger 1985
Fibroosseous pseudotumour of digits	Dupree &Enzinger 1986
Plexiform schwannoma	Fletcher & Davies 1986
Myofibroblastoma of breast	Wargotz et al 1987
Intranodal myofibroblastoma	Suster & Rosai 1989, Weiss et al 1989
So-called Borderline Malignancy	
Epithelioid haemangioendothelioma	Weiss & Enzinger 1982
Spindle-cell haemangioendothelioma	Weiss & Enzinger 1986
Plexiform fibrohistiocytic tumour	Enzinger & Zhang 1988
Malignant	
Primitive neuroectodermal tumour of thoracopulmonary region	Askin et al 1979
Angiomatoid malignant fibrous histiocytoma	Enzinger 1979
Calcifying synovial sarcoma	Varela-Duran & Enzinger 1982
Extrarenal rhabdoid tumour	Lynch et al 1983
Solid variant of alveolar rhabdomyosarcoma	Tsokos et al 1984

clinicopathological studies and trials of treatment, but has, by necessity, made it extremely difficult for many pathologists or clinicians to gain any worthwhile experience or expertise in this field. The development of regional or even national centres has alleviated this situation to some extent, most notably in the USA and Scandinavia, but in this respect the United Kingdom has been rather dilatory. Another very great help, at least from the pathologist's point of view, has been the publication of an excellent, definitive clinicopathological text on soft tissue tumours (Enzinger & Weiss 1983).

Despite this undoubted progress, the extent of our knowledge in this field is lagging way behind that of the more common carcinomas and lymphomas. With a few notable exceptions, the aetiology and pathogenesis of most tumour types remains almost totally unknown. In some ways, it is even more depressing to realise that the histogenetic origin of many soft tissue tumours also remains undecided. This is largely a reflection of the comparatively unspecialised nature of mesenchyme, neoplasms of which show very unpredictable differentiation, and of the striking diversity and multipotentiality of neural crest neoplasms, the peripherally located examples of which are traditionally regarded as connective tissue tumours. It is not surprising that an unidentified 'mesenchymal stem cell' is invoked as the progenitor in many cases, if one considers, for example, that most embryonal rhabdomyosarcomas arise at sites devoid of skeletal muscle and that extraskeletal osteosarcomas and chondrosarcomas develop, by definition, in tissue outside the osteoarticular system. At present, it is probably fair to say that a histogenetic theory of soft tissue neoplasia is untenable.

Even so, despite such a gloomy background, most of us are able to diagnose the bulk of soft tissue tumours, if only by pattern recognition which is, after all, the basis of diagnostic histopathology. By applying appropriate and strict criteria, most can be diagnosed on haematoxylin and eosin sections alone. Histochemistry, immunohistochemistry and electron microscopy may then be of use to confirm or prove the nature of the neoplasm. Unfortunately, such techniques are only infrequently of help if one has no clues at all on conventional sections. These methods have, however, been of great value in the study of tumour differentiation and hence have helped to refine recent classifications and, on occasion, have led to changes in nomenclature.

Examples of the influence of modern diagnostic techniques are legion. Prominent among these are the realisations that many lesions formerly classified as fribrosarcoma are more accurately designated as monophasic synovial sarcoma or malignant peripheral nerve sheath tumours; that, in similar fashion, the relatively common pleomorphic rhabdomyosarcoma of the past in fact only occasionally shows evidence of myogenous differentiation and, by many, is now regarded as pleomorphic MFH; that clear cell sarcoma of tendons and aponeuroses is in fact a malignant melanoma of soft tissues (Chung & Enzinger 1983); that synovial sarcoma bears very little relationship to true synovium and would be better relabelled by some as carcinosarcoma of soft tissues (Miettinen & Virtanen 1984); that many tumours previously categorised as Ewing's sarcoma or malignant small round cell tumours of the thoracopulmonary region (Askin tumours) represent primitive neuroectodermal tumours (neuroepitheliomas) (Dehner 1986, Linnoila et al 1986, Cavazanna et al 1987) and that so-called systemic angioendotheliomatosis is actually an angiocentric lymphoma (Sheibani et al 1986, Theaker et al 1986). Many of these advances are discussed in more detail in Chapter 14.

Other proposed alterations in nomenclature have had more to do with a better appreciation of the biological nature of a given tumour. For example, the term epithelioid haemangioma is preferred to angiolymphoid hyperplasia with eosinophilia, since it suggests the neoplastic (rather than reactive) nature of this lesion and describes the characteristic endothelial appearance. Similarly, the term atypical lipoma is gradually being introduced to describe well-differentiated liposarcomas arising in a limb, since, in a histologically pure form, they virtually never metastasise (Evans et al 1979, Kindblom et al 1982, Azumi et al 1987).

There is no doubt that further recategorisation of existing tumours is inevitable. Possible cases include dermatofibrosarcoma protuberans, which is almost certainly fibroblastic or perineural fibroblastic in origin rather than fibrohistiocytic (Escalona-Zapata et al 1981, Dupree et al 1985, Fletcher et al

1985, Fletcher et al 1988) and angiomatoid malignant fibrous histiocytoma, which bears very little clinical or histological resemblance to any of the other, more widely studied, forms of MFH.

Irrespective of these niceties, it should be remembered that the eventual beneficiary of these advances must be the patient. Currently the average 5 year survival of the more common sarcomas, such as the ubiquitous malignant fibrous histiocytoma, myxoid liposarcoma and leiomyosarcoma, is significantly better than that of the common carcinomas, like those of lung, breast or stomach. It is therefore not acceptable to write off the majority of cases as high-grade unclassifiable lesions, as has often happened in the past. Most impressively, the previously lethal rhabdomyosarcomas of childhood are proving curable by radical multimodal therapy, as has clearly been shown by the American Intergroup Rhabdomyosarcoma Study (Maurer et al 1977, Sutow et al 1982, Raney et al 1987).

The continued improvement in patient management is heavily dependent upon the efforts of pathologists to utilise standard diagnostic criteria and to make every effort to accurately classify a tumour where possible. Only then can clinical trials be of any value and only by these efforts can different sensitivities or response rates to varying forms of treatment be recognised in individual tumour types.

Despite our relative lack of insight into the true biology of soft tissue tumours, advances are being made at an impressive rate, particularly in the fields of cytogenetics and oncogene analysis. With the advent of ever more sophisticated techniques, this is an exciting period in which to be interested in these enigmatic neoplasms.

REFERENCES

Askin F B, Rosai J, Sibley R K, Dehner L P, McAllister H 1979 Malignant small cell tumour of the thoracopulmonary region in childhood. A distinctive clinicopathologic entity of uncertain histogenesis. Cancer 43: 2438–2451

Azumi N, Curtis J, Kempson R L, Hendrickson M R 1987 Atypical and malignant neoplasms showing lipomatous differentiation. A study of 111 cases. American Journal of Surgical Pathology 11: 161–183

Cavazzana A, Miser J S, Jefferson J, Triche T J 1987 Experimental evidence for a neural origin of Ewing's sarcoma. American Journal of Surgical Pathology 127: 507–518

Chung E B, Enzinger F M 1979 Fibroma of tendon sheath. Cancer 44: 1945–1954

Chung E B, Enzinger F M 1981 Infantile myofibromatosis. Cancer 48: 1807–1818

Chung E B, Enzinger F M 1983 Malignant melanoma of soft parts. A reassessment of clear cell sarcoma. American Journal of Surgical Pathology 7: 405–413.

Cooper P H, McAllister H A, Helwig E B 1979 Intravenous pyogenic granuloma. A study of 18 cases. American Journal of Surgical Pathology 3: 221–228

Dehner L P 1986 Peripheral and central primitive neuroectodermal tumours. A nosologic concept seeking a concensus. Archives of Pathology and Laboratory Medicine 110: 997–1005

Dupree W B, Enzinger F M 1986 Fibro-osseous pseudotumor of the digits. Cancer 58: 2103–2109

Dupree W B, Langloss J M, Weiss S W 1985 Pigmented dermatofibrosarcoma protuberans (Bednar tumour). A pathologic, ultrastructural and immunohistochemical study. American

Journal of Surgical Pathology 9: 630–639

Enjoji M, Hashimoto H 1984 Diagnosis of soft tissue sarcomas. Pathology Research and Practice 178: 215–226

Enzinger F M 1979 Angiomatoid malignant fibrous histiocytoma. A distinct fibrohistiocytic tumour of children and young adults simulating a vascular neoplasm. Cancer 44: 2147–2157

Enzinger F M, Weiss S W 1983 Soft tissue tumours. C V Mosby, St Louis

Enzinger F M, Zhang R 1988 Plexiform fibrohistiocytic tumour presenting in children and young adults. An analysis of 65 cases. American Journal of Surgical Pathology 12: 818–826

Escalona-Zapata J, Fernandez E A, Escuin F L 1981 The fibroblastic nature of dermatofibrosarcoma protuberans. A tissue culture and ultrastructural study. Virchows Archiv A (Pathological Anatomy) 391: 165–175

Evans H L, Soule E H, Winkelmann R K 1979 Atypical lipoma, atypical intramuscular lipoma and well differentiated retroperitoneal liposarcoma. A reappraisal of 30 cases formerly classified as well differentiated liposarcoma. Cancer 43: 574–584

Fletcher C D M, Davies S E 1986 Benign plexiform (multinodular) schwannoma: a rare tumour unassociated with neurofibromatosis. Histopathology 10: 971–980

Fletcher C D M, Martin-Bates E, 1987, Spindle cell lipoma: a clinicopathological study with some original observations. Histopathology 11: 803–817

Fletcher C D M, Evans B J, McCartney J C, Smith N, Wilson Jones E, McKee P H 1985 Dermatofibrosarcoma protuberans: a clinicopathological and immunohistochemical study with a review of the literature. Histopathology 9: 921–938

Fletcher C D M, Davies S E, McKee P H 1987 Cellular schwannoma: a distinct pseudosarcomatous entity. Histopathology 11: 21–35

Fletcher C D M, Theaker J M, Flanagan A, Krausz T 1988 Pigmented dermatofibrosarcoma protuberans (Bednar tumour): melanocytic colonisation or neuroectodermal differentiation? A clinicopathological and immunohistochemical study. Histopathology 13: 631–644

Gallager R L, Helwig E B 1980 Neurothekeoma — benign cutaneous tumor of neural origin. American Journal of Clinical Pathology 74: 759–764

Hajdu S I 1979 Pathology of soft tissue tumours. Lea and Febiger, Philadelphia

Hare H F, Cerny M J 1963 Soft tissue sarcoma. A review of 200 cases. Cancer 16: 1332–1337

Kindblom L G, Angervall L, Fassina A S 1982 Atypical lipoma. Acta Pathologica Microbiologica Scandinavica Section A 90: 27–36

Lauer D H, Enzinger F M 1980 Cranial fasciitis of childhood. Cancer 45: 401–406

Linnoila R I, Tsokos M, Triche T J, Marangos P J, Chandra R S 1986 Evidence for neural origin and PAS-positive variants of the malignant small cell tumour of thoracopulmonary region ('Askin tumour'). American Journal of Surgical Pathology 10: 124–133

Lynch H T, Shurin S B, Dahms B B, Izant R J, Lynch J, Danes B S 1983 Paravertebral malignant rhabdoid tumor in infancy. In vitro studies of a familial tumor. Cancer 52: 290–296

Maurer H M, Moon T, Donaldson M et al 1977 The Intergroup Rhabdomyosarcoma Study. A preliminary report. Cancer 40: 2015–2026

Miettinen M, Virtanen I 1984 Synovial sarcoma — a misnomer. American Journal of Pathology 117: 18–25

Patchefsky A S, Enzinger F M 1981 Intravascular fasciitis. A report of 17 cases. American Journal of Surgical Pathology 5: 29–36

Raney R B, Tefft M, Newton W A et al 1987 Improved prognosis with intensive treatment of children with cranial soft tissue sarcomas arising in nonorbital parameningeal sites. A report from the Intergroup Rhabdomyosarcoma Study. Cancer 59: 147–155

Russell W O, Cohen J, Enzinger F M et al 1977 A clinical and pathological staging system for soft tissue sarcomas. Cancer 40: 1562–1570

Shmookler B M, Enzinger F M 1981 Pleomorphic lipoma: a benign tumour simulating liposarcoma. A clinicopathologic analysis of 48 cases. Cancer 47: 126–133

Shmookler B M, Enzinger F M, 1982 Giant cell fibroblastoma: a peculiar childhood tumour. Laboratory Investigation 46: 76A (Abstract)

Sheibani K, Battifora H, Winberg C D et al 1986 Further evidence that 'malignant angioendotheliomatosis' is an angiotropic large-cell lymphoma. New England Journal of Medicine 314: 943–948

Silverman T A, Enzinger F M 1985 Fibrolipomatous hamartoma of nerve. A clinicopathologic analysis of 26 cases. American Journal of Surgical Pathology 9: 7–14

Steeper T A, Rosai J 1983 Aggressive angiomyxoma of the female pelvis and perineum. Report of nine cases of a distinctive type of gynecologic soft tissue neoplasm. American Journal of Surgical Pathology 7: 463–475

Suster S, Rosai J 1989 Intranodal haemorrhagic spindle-cell tumor with 'amianthoid' fibers. Report of six cases of a distinctive mesenchymal neoplasm of the inguinal region that simulates Kaposi's sarcoma. American Journal of Surgical Pathology 13: 347–357

Sutow W W, Lindberg R D, Gehan E A et al 1982 Three-year relapse free survival rates in childhood rhabdomyosarcoma of the head and neck. Report from the Intergroup Rhabdomyosarcoma Study. Cancer 49: 2217–2221

Theaker J M, Gatter K C, Esiri M M, Easterbrook F 1986 Neoplastic angioendotheliosis — further evidence supporting a lymphoid origin. Histopathology 10: 1261–1270

Tsokos M, Miser A, Pizzo P, Triche T 1984 Histologic and cytologic characteristics of poor prognosis childhood rhabdomyosarcoma. Laboratory Investigation 50: 61A (Abstract)

Varela-Duran J, Enzinger F M 1982 Calcifying synovial sarcoma. Cancer 50: 345–352

Wargotz E S, Weiss S W, Norris H J 1987 Myofibroblastoma of the breast. Sixteen cases of a distinctive benign mesenchymal tumour. American Journal of Surgical Pathology 11: 493–502

Weiss S W, Gnepp D R, Bratthauer G L 1989 Palisaded myofibroblastoma. A benign mesenchymal tumour of lymph node. American Journal of Surgical Pathology 13: 341–346

Weiss S W, Enzinger F M 1982 Epithelioid haemangioendothelioma. A vascular tumor often mistaken for a carcinoma. Cancer 50: 970–981

Weiss S W, Enzinger F M 1986 Spindle cell haemangioendothelioma. A low grade angiosarcoma resembling a cavernous haemangioma and Kaposi's sarcoma. American Journal of Surgical Pathology 10: 521–530

Woodruff J M, Godwin T A, Erlandson R A, Susin M, Martini N 1981 Cellular schwannoma. A variety of schwannoma sometimes mistaken for a malignant tumor. American Journal of Surgical Pathology 5: 733–744

2. Aetiology of soft tissue tumours

M. Enjoji   M. Tsuneyoshi

INTRODUCTION

Not a great deal is known of the aetiology of soft tissue tumours. In most clinical entities, the exact cause is either not clear or has remained unexplained.

Genetic factors are linked to certain types of sarcoma or benign soft tissue lesion, particularly lesions related to neurofibromatosis (von Recklinghausen's disease). This disease predisposes to the development of malignant schwannoma and other soft tissue sarcomas. Age, sex and racial factors are intrinsic to any tumour, as witness many of the fibroblastic tumours of infancy. Hormones may possibly be responsible for the development of some types of soft tissue lesion (e.g. abdominal desmoid), but this concept remains to be fully explored. Host-mediated immunity plays an important role in both experimentally induced animal tumours and in some tumours seen clinically.

Extrinsic factors may be physical, chemical or biological in nature. There are at least two major physical agents related to the development of soft tissue tumours. One is injury or trauma which is responsible for many benign soft tissue lesions such as keloids, fibromatoses or myositis ossificans, and also for sarcomas of various histological types. The other is ionising irradiation, prescribed to treat other tumours or non-neoplastic lesions.

Certain chemicals can cause sarcomas. One recent example has been the proposed association between phenoxyherbicides and the occurrence of soft tissue sarcomas. Asbestos has long been known to give rise to a particular type of sarcoma, i.e. malignant mesothelioma.

Among the biological factors, viruses are probably the major factors related to the cause of cancer. Several oncogenic viruses will induce a sarcoma in animals, but whether such is the case in humans remains an open question. Circumstantial evidence suggests that Kaposi's sarcoma is a viral-associated lesion which often occurs in immunodeficient patients.

Sarcomas can be produced in laboratory animals following subcutaneous injection of carcinogens such as aromatic hydrocarbons. While these experimentally induced tumours have not been carefully compared with specific human sarcomas, several investigators have reported the induction of specific types such as malignant fibrous histiocytoma.

This chapter is devoted to intrinsic and extrinsic factors in the development of benign and malignant soft tissue tumours in humans, including genetic, environmental and iatrogenic factors. The experimental induction of soft tissue sarcomas is also given attention.

INTRINSIC FACTORS

Heredity

Genetic factors are aetiologically important, at least in a minority of soft tissue tumours, yet the genetic background or determination in human cancer is not always easy to differentiate from various environmental factors. There are examples of families in which the same type of soft tissue tumour occurred in more than one individual and some soft tissue tumours occur in association with known genetic conditions. The familial aggregation of some combinations of soft tissue tumour and other neoplastic conditions (such as breast cancer) have also been reported.

A variety of soft tissue tumours may occur in families, including fibromatoses of various types, elastofibromas, keloids, xanthomas, multiple lipomas, angiolipomas, leiomyomas, multiple glomus tumours, paragangliomas, and neuroblastomas. Soft tissue lesions such as fibromatosis colli, myofibromatosis, juvenile hyaline fibromatosis, angiolipomatosis, and neuroblastoma have occurred in siblings.

Usui et al (1984) described the occurrence of soft tissue sarcomas (two malignant fibrous histiocytomas and one leiomyosarcoma) in three siblings with Werner's syndrome, an autosomal recessive disorder. This syndrome is characterised by juvenile cataracts, scleroderma-like skin changes, and a high frequency of malignant neoplasms. According to Epstein et al (1966), 13 of 125 patients had associated malignant tumours, often of connective tissue origin. Hrabko et al (1982) reported the finding, in a 57-year-old man with Werner' syndrome, of a fibrosarcoma of the mediastinum and multiple basal cell epitheliomas.

In addition to an inherited tendency toward the development of specific tumours, a state or condition that predisposes to the development of tumours may also be inherited. A long-established example is neurofibromatosis (von Recklinghausen's disease), a disorder inherited as an autosomal dominant trait. Attention has focussed on the occurrence of soft tissue sarcomas, such as malignant schwannoma, in association with neurofibromatosis. Von Recklinghausen's disease, which appears early in life with the onset of the café-au-lait spots, is later characterised by a large number of neurofibromas. Although these tumours are usually slowly growing lesions, malignant schwannomas (including malignant Triton tumours) develop in about 5% of cases as a result of malignant transformation of the neurofibromas (Enzinger & Weiss 1983). Moreover, von Recklinghausen's disease is sometimes associated with soft tissue tumours other than malignant schwannoma, such as ganglioneuroma, rhabdomyosarcoma, and liposarcoma. Gardner's syndrome is also a familial condition inherited as an autosomal dominant trait and is characterised by a combination of polyposis coli, dental abnormalities, epidermoid cysts, osteomas, fibromas and desmoid fibromatosis, especially of the intra-abdominal type.

Various familial aggregations involving soft tissue sarcomas together with a small number of other tumour types have been reported. Li & Fraumeni (1969) studied four families in which a pair of children had soft tissue sarcomas and their close relatives had early onset cancers, especially breast cancer in the mother. Birch et al (1984) found that, among the mothers of a series of 143 children with soft tissue sarcomas there were six cases of breast cancer, representing a three-fold excess risk of breast cancer. Soft tissue sarcomas may also be associated with adrenocortical carcinomas and brain tumours in the same family. Miller (1971) made a survey of death certificates and noted that in each of two families, one child died of rhabdomyosarcoma and another of adrenocortical carcinoma, defining such a combination as part of a familial cancer syndrome. A genetic influence also appears to underlie the tendency of soft tissue sarcomas to aggregate in siblings and to be associated with brain tumours, as reported by Chabalko et al (1974).

Recent interest has focussed on chromosome changes in certain malignant neoplasms. Although the biological significance of chromosomal translocations is not well understood for a particular malignancy, there is little doubt that such cytogenetic alternations may have diagnostic and therapeutic significance. There are chromosome abnormalities in the following soft tissue malignancies: neurogenic sarcoma, liposarcoma, synovial sarcoma, fibrosarcoma, malignant mesothelioma, leiomyosarcoma, rhabdomyosarcoma, haemangiopericytoma, Ewing's sarcoma and peripheral neuroepithelioma (Becher et al 1984). A particular translocation between chromosomes 11 and 22, t(11;22) (q24;q12), has been found in patients with Ewing's sarcoma as well as in those with a malignant neuroepithelioma (Whang-Peng et al 1984). Such findings support the hypothesis that these two entities share a common histogenesis or that the malignant transformation has a common basis (see Ch. 14).

Hormones

There is a striking difference in sex incidence of some specific soft tissue lesions. For instance, almost all cases of nasopharyngeal angiofibroma occur in adolescent males, whereas most cases of abdominal desmoid affect young women during or following pregnancy. Here, sex hormones may have a close relationship to the development or growth of the tumour. Some desmoid tumours fluctuate in size with menses and regress following the menopause (McDougall & McGarrity 1979), and grow during pregnancy, or in those using oral contraceptives (Waddell 1975). On the other hand, specific testosterone-binding receptors were detected in nasopharyngeal angiofibroma, thereby suggesting that this tumour is androgen-dependent (Lee et al 1980).

Lipomas also occur more frequently in women than in men, particularly in obese persons over age 45. Since 1966, the development of lipomatosis termed 'dewlap' has been reported. The lesion occurs in those on corticosteroids, usually in the mediastinum and episternal regions (Lucena et al 1966). Myelolipomas may also develop in association with endocrine disorders such as Cushing's disease or hermaphroditism.

Concerning malignant tumours, leiomyosarcomas more often occur in females and proliferation of cells of smooth muscle origin may be evoked by oestrogenic stimulation. However, there are no reliable data supporting endocrine relationships in soft tissue leiomyosarcoma. In addition, a few cases of hepatic angiosarcoma are associated with androgenic anabolic steroids and diethylstilboestrol.

Particular predisposing conditions

Some soft tissue tumours are accompanied by particular diseases. Dupuytren's disease, characterised by palmar and/or plantar fibromatosis, is more common in diabetics and in epileptics, as well as in those with chronic alcoholism. Dupuytren's disease was detected in 55% of patients with long-standing epilepsy, and in 25% of 60 alcoholic men (Pojer et al 1972). Epileptic patients were usually on anticonvulsant drugs such as phenobarbital, and the alcoholics often had associated liver disease. Abnormal liver enzymes were common in both epileptic and alcoholic groups in this particular study.

Chronic lymphoedema of the extremities is a particular condition implicated in the aetiology of lymphangiosarcoma (Stewart & Treves 1948). Most such patients have undergone radical mastectomy for carcinoma of the breast and had chronic lymphoedema for 4 to 14 years (Taswell et al 1962). Lymphangiosarcoma has also been noted in cases of traumatic, idiopathic and congenital lymphoedema. Although there had been no report that lymphangiosarcoma occurred in patients with filarial lymphoedema, a few cases have recently been reported (Muller et al 1987) and others have been seen from East Africa (C D M Fletcher − personal communication). Postoperative adjuvant radiotherapy may also be responsible for the development of postmastectomy lymphangiosarcoma, but the number of patients with a history of radiation therapy at the site of tumour development was not significant (Sordillo et al 1981).

Immunological factors

Host-mediated immunity plays an important role in the development of tumours. The best-known type of soft tissue sarcoma developing in immunodeficient persons is Kaposi's sarcoma. This multifocal cutaneous tumour is prevalent among patients with acquired immunodeficiency syndrome (AIDS), particularly homosexuals. Kaposi's sarcomas may also occur in immunosuppressed patients, including those who had been on the immunosuppressive drug prednisone (Hoshaw & Schwartz 1980), renal transplant recipients (Akhtar et al 1984), those with Hodgkin's disease or angioimmunoblastic lymphadenopathy (Varsano et al 1984).

EXTRINSIC FACTORS

Physical agents

Injury and trauma

Trauma is also an important factor in the pathogenesis of various benign and malignant soft tissue lesions. However, it is doubtful that a single injury can lead to the production of a soft tissue tumour. In lesions such as desmoid fibromatosis, a genetic defect or an endocrine factor coupled with trauma seems to be important in the pathogenesis. As formulated by Diamandopoulos and Meissner (1985), the essential criteria before a positive relationship between a tumour and a given trauma can be considered are as follows:

1. The part in which the tumour arose must be proved to have been normal before the injury
2. The tumour must develop within a reasonable time after the trauma
3. The tumour must be of a type that could originate from the cells traumatised
4. Trauma must have been adequate to produce tissue disruption and ecchymosis.

Antecedent injury or trauma, whether a single or repeated event, has been implicated in the development of the following benign conditions of the soft tissues: benign fibrous proliferations such as nodular fasciitis and proliferative myositis or fasciitis, fibromatoses including Dupuytren and desmoid types, some fibrous infantile lesions, lipoma, giant cell tumour of tendon sheath, intramuscular myxoma and the simple ganglion. Keloids develop in and near a scar induced often by furuncles, vaccinations, or cautery and, in women, frequently by the piercing of ear lobes. In our experience, this lesion often occurs in the scar of a BCG vaccination and presents in adolescents who received such treatment years before. Dermatofibrosarcoma protuberans has also been reported in vaccination sites (Morman et al 1979, Fletcher et al 1988).

The traumatic neuroma is a non-neoplastic proliferation in response to nerve transection, often occurring after surgery. The lesion may form a tumour-like nodule or be microscopic. Morton's neuroma, on the other hand, is occasioned by compression of the neural bundles by the adjacent metatarsal heads. Myositis ossificans, a non-progressive tumour-like condition, is the result of previous trauma in about a half of the cases.

Injury produced by friction is considered to be a causative agent in elastofibroma and in fibroma of the tendon sheath as well, although the exact cause of these lesions is unknown. In the case of elastofibroma dorsi, the tumours are considered to result from friction of the scapular apex against the ribbed thorax, as originally proposed by Järvi & Saxén (1961). Järvi & Länsimies (1975) later found subclinical elastofibroma-like changes in the subscapular thoracic fascia of 38 among 235 unselected autopsy cases examined.

As for soft tissue sarcomas, rare cases of fibrosarcoma occur at the site of a previous injury after a latent period of several years or even decades. In such cases, the sarcoma occurs often in scar tissue (cicatricial fibrosarcoma). Enzinger & Weiss (1983) reported personal experience of only four fibrosarcomas that clearly arose at the site of a former injury. In such cases, the causative factors included a chain saw injury, a sledge hammer injury, a healed shotgun wound, a draining sinus of chronic osteomyelitis (Morris & Lucas 1964), and a prosthetic vascular graft (Burns et al 1972). A further small group of fibrosarcomas are well recognised to arise in burn scars (Fleming & Rezek 1941, Enzinger & Weiss 1983). Examples of malignant fibrous histiocytomas, a more recently adopted entity, were noted at previous surgical sites (Inoshita & Youngberg 1984), and at fracture sites (Bader et al 1981), metal implants (Lee et al 1984), or a total hip replacement (Swann 1984). In certain cases, a haematoma developing after trauma preceded the onset of myxoid liposarcoma (Enzinger & Weiss 1983), and a case of osteogenic sarcoma arising from a calcified haematoma (Butler & Woolley 1936) was reported. There is reasonable evidence to suggest that a proportion of trauma-related cases are, in fact, induced by retained foreign material (Jennings et al 1988).

There are cases of rhabdomyosarcoma following severe trauma with a latent period of years (Cureton & Griffiths 1956–7). A peculiar case was that of a 4-year-old boy with embryonal rhabdomyosarcoma of the exstrophic bladder repaired shortly after birth, although no mention was made of a causal relationship between the surgery and the development of tumour (Semerdjian et al 1972). Trauma may also be responsible for some cases of synovial sarcoma. The question arises as to whether trauma contributes to the development of synovial sarcoma or is merely a coincidence. Extraosseous osteosarcomas may also be related to injury. Six (13%) of the 48 patients in the series of Sordillo et al (1983) related a history of trauma to the area where the extraosseous osteosarcoma had developed. Moreover, several cases of such extraosseous tumours developing in myositis ossificans have been reported (Shanoff et al 1967). Chase & Enzinger (1985) reported antecedent trauma to the area at which epithelioid sarcoma developed in 20% of their 241 patients, the mean time interval being 29 months from time of the trauma to presentation of the tumour. Fletcher (1987) has also recently described eight sarcomas, of varying histological type, which had apparently arisen in chronic tropical ulcers.

Solar radiation

Although solar radiation as a predisposing factor to soft tissue tumours has been given little attention, it is probably related to the occurrence of atypical fibroxanthoma, a rapidly growing, ulcerative lesion almost exclusively occurring in the sun-exposed skin of the elderly.

Ionizing radiation

Therapeutic radiation. The induction of malignant tumours by irradiation given for therapeutic purposes has been of great concern. Since a carcinoma of the hand developed in a physician in 1902, tumours have been induced experimentally or observed clinically in virtually every mammalian tissue that has been irradiated (Cade 1957). Individual cases of soft tissue sarcoma arising in previously irradiated tissue have frequently been reported, although the larger series of postradiation sarcomas have been concerned with lesions arising in bones (Kim et al 1978). A wide variety of histological types of tumour has been caused by external irradiation given for therapeutic purposes to treat other lesions, most often an independent primary tumour. Cahan et al (1948) suggested the following criteria for a sarcoma to be considered as radiation-induced:

1. The sarcoma should arise in the area subjected to the irradiation
2. A latent period in years must exist between the time of irradiation and development of the sarcoma
3. The sarcoma must be diagnosed as such histologically.

A number of cases of postradiation sarcomas were seen to conform to these criteria.

Among 116 radiation-induced soft tissue sarcomas reported in the literature up to 1986, fibrosarcomas (27 cases) and sarcomas not further classified (25 cases) appear to be the most common, followed by malignant fibrous histiocytoma (17 cases), extraskeletal osteosarcoma (16 cases), neurogenic sarcoma (12 cases) and angio- or lymphangiosarcoma (6 cases). However, it is likely that in the past the malignant fibrous histiocytoma, a formerly unrecognized entity, had been reported on many occasions as fibrosarcoma or under some other terms, such as pleomorphic sarcoma. Since the entity was established, malignant fibrous histiocytoma seems to be the most commonly observed postirradiation sarcoma (Davidson et al 1986) and this has been borne out by a recent large series from the Armed Forces Institute of Pathology (Laskin et al 1988). We have encountered 4 such cases (2%) out of a total of 201 malignant fibrous histiocytomas, following irradiation for breast carcinoma, uterine cervical carcinoma, haemangioma, and an unknown sacral lesion, respectively. In the literature, common preceding conditions were carcinoma of breast (31 cases), carcinoma of uterine cervix (14 cases), retinoblastoma (4 cases), testicular seminoma (4 cases), or even benign lesions. Although any site can give rise to a postradiation soft tissue tumour, the most common is the chest wall, including the axilla, as linked to breast carcinoma. The pelvis, head and neck are also frequently involved.

Regarding the methods of radiotherapy for the primary conditions, external, intracavitary and interstitial administrations have been used, modifying the dose given to meet particular needs. X-ray beams of a wide range of quality, as well as gamma-ray beams, or beta-ray beams from radioactive sources have been implicated. While the induction of a postirradiation tumour does not necessarily seem to be related to either the source or method of radiation, neoplasms are, to some degree, related to the site of absorption, the dose given, age of the patient and other unknown factors. The time interval between irradiation and diagnosis of sarcoma varies from 4 to 45 years, with an approximate average of 11 years. The dose given and the incidence of sarcomas appear to be related, though the precise dose is usually difficult to estimate. In virtually all reported cases, over 1000 roentgens have been given (Mindell et al 1977). About 2000 rad seems to be the lowest dose related to the development of tumour in adults; in some instances over 10 000 rad were given. In general the larger the dose, the higher the incidence of sarcoma (Kim et al 1978), and there appears to be an inverse relationship between the total dose and the latency period (Laskin et al 1988).

Thorotrast. Thorotrast, a 20% colloidal solution of radioactive thorium dioxide, was formerly used to visualise hollow organs, for arteriography, and for hepatolienography. Following injection of this substance, the material dispersed systemically and was typically deposited within the reticuloendothelial system, sometimes resulting in the development of a malignant neoplasm, most often in the liver. The latent period between the use of the substance and the clinical evidence of tumour ranged between 5 and 30 years. Falk et al (1979) reported that an epidemiological investigation of hepatic angiosarcoma in the United States, directed primarily during the years 1964–1974, identified 26 cases of thorotrast-induced hepatic angiosarcoma. In addition, several cases of human soft tissue sarcoma attributed to thorotrast, probably extravasated during the course of injection, have been reported (Hasson et al 1975). Since the first such report of a fibrosarcoma by Plenge and Krükenmeyer (1954), subsequent reports on soft tissue sarcomas such as neurogenic sarcoma, malignant mesothelioma and extraskeletal chondrosarcoma and osteosarcoma have followed. In 1961, we autopsied a 38-year-old woman with retroperitoneal leiomyosarcoma, in association with thorotrast storage in the liver, spleen, para-aortic lymph nodes and retroperitoneum.

Chemical agents

Although a wide variety of chemical compounds have been shown to produce a sarcoma when injected into deeper tissues of experimental animals, only a limited number of chemicals are known to give rise to a human soft tissue sarcoma.

Asbestos

Asbestos is the most notorious and best known among the chemical substances linked to human sarcomas, albeit related only to a particular type of sarcoma, i.e. malignant mesothelioma. The causal relationship between asbestos exposure and malignant mesothelioma was noted as late as 1960 when Wagner et al reported 47 cases of malignant mesothelioma from the asbestos region of South Africa. Exposure to asbestos occupationally involves not only workers in mining and heavy plant industries, but also those engaged in manufacturing a variety of asbestos-related products.

Phenoxyherbicides

Since 1977, Swedish studies suggested an association between exposure to phenoxyherbicides and soft tissue sarcoma (Hardell & Sandström 1979), malignant lymphoma and colonic carcinoma (Hardell 1981). These chemicals have been used in agriculture and forestry in Sweden since the end of the 1940s and similar studies were published from New Zealand (Smith et al 1984). The result of a case-control study in Sweden showed that exposure to phenoxyacetic acid or chlorophenols led to a 6-fold increase in the risk for soft tissue sarcomas (Eriksson et al 1981). However, further studies are needed to prove the relationship between exposure to these chemicals and the increased risk of sarcoma, particularly since doubt has recently been expressed about previous means of data collection (Lynge et al 1987).

Phenoxyherbicides include 2,4,5-trichlorophenoxyacetic acid (2,4,5-T) and chlorophenols, both of which contain polychlorinated dibenzodioxins and dibenzofurans. These are applied as herbicides, either by aerial or ground spraying. Not only agriculture and forestry workers, but also railroad workers were considered to show an increased incidence of tumour related to the exposure of phenoxyherbicides. Cases of soft tissue sarcoma have also been discovered among workers involved in the manufacture of 2,4,5-T and related compounds and among dioxin-exposed workers in the United States as well. Dioxins are contaminants occurring during the chemical manufacture of chlorinated phenoxyacetic acids and chlorophenols. The soft tissue sarcomas reported by Fingerhut et al (1984), as occurring in seven dioxin-exposed workers, were two each of maglinant fibrous histiocytoma, fibrosarcoma, liposarcoma and one of myxoid neurogenic sarcoma. A recent Scandinavian study (Hardell & Eriksson 1988) has shown that phenoxyacetic acids may be aetiologically more important than chlorophenols.

Iron compounds

Earlier experimental work revealed that repeated injections of iron compounds into rodents were associated with the development of sarcoma at the sites of injection. These compounds are given intramuscularly for the treatment of iron deficiency, particularly long-standing anaemia. Since the mid-1970s, there have been sporadic reports of this occurrence in humans, mostly from the United Kingdom, at injection sites in the buttocks or deltoid. However, Weinbren et al (1978), who reviewed eight published cases, reported that only four cases were acceptable as having arisen in the gluteal muscle injected with iron compounds. These soft tissue tumours varied histologically, including pleomorphic sarcoma, rhabdomyosarcoma, fibrosarcoma and reticulum cell sarcoma, although the experimentally-induced tumours were fairly uniform, being interpreted as either fibrosarcoma or histiocytic sarcoma (Weinbren et al 1978). Accordingly, these authors concluded that the findings do not support the view that such treatment carries a strong risk of tumour development.

Aluminium compounds

Aluminium compounds used in desensitising injections also induced sarcomas in laboratory studies. However, a retrospective survey by McIllmurray & Langman (1978) did not support the suggestion of a causal relationship between sarcoma formation and the injections.

Penicillin

Fibrosarcomas occurring at the site of injection of penicillin in sesame oil occurred in two young women, as reported by Goldenberg (1954) and there is also a report of extraosseous osteogenic sarcoma affecting the right thigh and buttock of a 29-year-old white male (Lee et al 1977). This patient had a nodule at the site of eventual tumour development for eight years following an intramuscular injection of penicillin.

Biological agents

Viruses

There is little evidence to suggest that micro-organisms other than viruses can cause human cancer.

In a recurring digital fibrous tumour now termed 'infantile digital fibromatosis', viral origin of the lesion was once favoured because of intracytoplasmic inclusion bodies present in the proliferating fibroblastic cells and because of the multiplicity of lesions, occasional recurrence and spontaneous regression of tumours (Reye 1965). Attempts to isolate viruses have been unsuccessful and the inclusions have been shown to be a tangled ball of actin filaments (Iwasaki et al 1980, 1983). A viral aetiology has also been considered for cases of juvenile xanthogranuloma, a lesion with an involutional nature, but there is, as yet, no convincing proof.

Kaposi's sarcoma is apparently virus-related, as based on a range of circumstantial evidence. These tumours appear to be multiple and multifocal lesions with no clear, single primary tumour and the clinical course varies enormously. There is a prevalence in Equatorial Africa and among homosexuals (Hutt 1984). Cytomegalovirus (CMV) antigens can be identified in the tumour cells of some cases (Walter et al 1984), but the proposed aetiological relationship between CMV and Kaposi's sarcoma is now thought to be improbable (Grody et al 1988, Van Den Berg et al 1989).

The precise role of immunodeficiency in the pathogenesis of AIDS-related and African Kaposi's sarcoma is not fully understood. There is no doubt, however, that many such patients have depressed cell-mediated immunity (Gottlieb & Ackerman 1982, Dorfman 1984) and that this is probably directly related to HIV infection, suggesting a possible defect in immune surveillance. It is also of interest that the sporadic, indolent form of Kaposi's sarcoma, seen predominantly in the elderly, is associated with a markedly increased incidence of other malignancies, particularly of the lymphoreticular system (Safai et al 1980, Ulbright & Santa Cruz 1981).

EXPERIMENTAL MODELS

Since the precise relevance of animal models to human soft tissue sarcomas is uncertain, this section really serves as a record of various experimental means of inducing sarcomas, which may be useful for controlled in vivo or in vitro studies, but which are of unknown significance.

Soft tissue sarcomas have long been induced in laboratory animals by giving subcutaneous injections of carcinogens such as polycyclic hydrocarbons. As to the histological types of experimental tumours, earlier reports included no specific typing, rather spindle cell sarcoma and pleomorphic sarcoma were the terms most often used. The term 'fibrosarcoma' was also frequently used, and probably included pleomorphic tumours resembling the malignant fibrous histiocytomas seen clinically.

Though not fully explored, soft tissue and bone malignant fibrous histiocytomas have been induced with a high incidence in rats, using 4-hydroxyaminoquinoline 1-oxide (4-HAQO) (Konishi et al 1982, Maruyama et al 1983). These lesions were induced at the site of injections by repeated weekly injections of 1 mg 4-HAQO/rat for 4 weeks. In other experiments, malignant fibrous histiocytomas were produced in mice with macrophages transformed by SV40 virus (Yumoto & Morimoto 1980) and in rats by intra-articular injection of 9,10-dimethyl 1-1,2-benzanthracene (Sakamoto 1986).

As for other specified soft tissue sarcomas, synovial sarcomas, together with fibrosarcomas, were produced in rats also by injecting 9,10-dimethyl 1-1, 2-benzanthracene (DMBA) into the joint cavity (Ghadially & Roy 1966). However, these tumours did not have the biphasic features of the tumour cells characteristic of synovial sarcoma. Rhabdomyosarcomas have been induced in rats by the injection of nickel sulphide (Corbeil 1968, Shibata et al 1989) and malignant nerve sheath tumours in rats may follow intrauterine exposure to ethylnitrosurea (Cardesa et al 1983).

Lacassagne and Vinzent (1929) seem to have been the first to induce fibrosarcoma as well as osteosarcoma in the legs of rabbits, by X-ray radiation.

Soft tissue sarcomas as well as osteosarcomas are also produced in animals by giving radioactive fission products. For example, inoculation of a colloidal suspension of radioactive cerium chloride induced bone and soft tissue tumours at the site of inoculation in 77% of the rats (Klein et al 1977). Here, the soft tissue tumours included fibrosarcomas, haemangiopericytomas, angiosarcomas and rhabdomyosarcomas. Thorotrast also produces sarcomas when injected subcutaneously into rats and mice (Selbie 1936).

SUMMARY

Genetic and extrinsic factors such as injury and trauma, radiation and some chemical agents play an important role in the development of at least some types of benign and malignant tumours of soft tissues. Whereas injury and trauma are linked to the development of a variety of benign fibrous proliferations, therapeutic radiation seems to be the most important identifiable cause of a significant number of sarcomas of varying histological type. Soft tissue tumours do not necessarily result from a single aetiological insult, but rather they may often be multifactorial. Genetic factors often work in combination with other causative agents in the development of tumours. Of great concern at present is Kaposi's sarcoma associated with AIDS, an entity possibly linked to both viruses and host immunosuppression.

REFERENCES

Akhtar M, Bunuan H, Ali M A et al 1984 Kaposi's sarcoma in renal transplant recipients. Ultrastructural and immunoperoxidase study of four cases. Cancer 53: 258–266

Bader H, Spohner F, Gerlitzky W et al 1981 Malignes fibroses Histiocytom nach suprakondylärer Oberschenkelfraktur. Deutsche Medizinische Wochenschrift 106: 336–339

Becher R, Wake N, Gibas Z et al 1984 Chromosome changes in soft tissue sarcomas. Journal of the National Cancer Institute 72: 823–831

Birch J M, Hartley A L, Marsden H B et al 1984 Excess risk of breast cancer in the mothers of children with soft tissue sarcomas. British Journal of Cancer 49: 325–331

Bloom D 1956 Heredity of keloids. Review of the literature and report of a family with multiple keloids in five generations. New York State Journal of Medicine 56: 511–519

Burns W A, Kanhouwa S, Tillman L et al 1972 Fibrosarcoma occurring at the site of a plastic vascular graft. Cancer 29: 66–72

Butler F E, Woolley I M 1936 Osteogenic sarcoma arising from a calcified hematoma. Radiology 26: 236–237

Cade S S 1957 Radiation-induced cancer in man. British Journal of Radiology 356: 393–402

Cahan W G, Woodard H Q, Higinbotham N L et al 1948 Sarcoma arising in irradiated bone. Report of eleven cases. Cancer 1: 3–29

Cardesa A, Llanes F, Merchan J, Alvarez T, Ludena M D, Mohr U 1983 Plexiform structures in malignant schwannomas after prenatal exposure to ethylnitrosurea. Experimental Pathology 24: 103–115

Chabalko J J, Creagan E T, Fraumeni J F 1974 Epidemiology of selected sarcomas in children. British Journal of National Cancer Institute 53: 675–679

Chase D R, Enzinger F M 1985 Epithelioid sarcoma. Diagnosis, prognostic indicators, and treatment. American Journal of Surgical Pathology 9: 241–263

Corbeil L B 1968 Antigenicity of rhabdomyosarcomas induced by nickel sulfide (Ni_3S_2) Cancer 21: 184–189

Cureton R J R, Griffiths J D 1956 Rhabdomyosarcoma of the hand following severe trauma. British Journal of Surgery 44: 509–513.

Davidson T, Westbury G, Harmer C L 1986 Radiation-induced soft tissue sarcoma. British Journal of Surgery 73: 308–309

Diamandopoulos G Th, Meissner W A 1985 Neoplasia. In: Kissane J M (ed) Anderson's pathology, 8th edn. C V Mosby, St. Louis, p 514–559

Dorfman R F 1984 Kaposi's sarcoma revisited. Human Pathology 15: 1013–1017

Enzinger F M, Weiss S W 1983 Soft tissue tumours. C V Mosby, St Louis

Epstein C J, Martin G M, Schultz A L et al 1966 Werner's syndrome. A review of its symptomatology, natural history, pathologic features, genetics and relationship to natural aging process. Medicine 45: 177–221

Eriksson M, Hardell L, Berg N O et al 1981 Soft tissue sarcomas and exposure to chemical substances. A case-reference study. British Journal of Industrial Medicine 38: 27–33

Falk H, Telles N C, Ishak K G et al 1979 Epidemiology of thorotrast-induced hepatic angiosarcoma in the United States. Environmental Research 18: 65–73

Fingerhut M A, Halperin W E, Honchar P A et al 1984 An evaluation of reports of dioxin exposure and soft tissue sarcoma pathology among chemical workers in the United States. Scandinavian Journal of Work Environment and Health 10: 299–303

Fleming R M, Rezek P R 1941 Sarcoma developing in an old burn scar. American Journal of Surgery 54: 457–465

Fletcher C D M 1987 Soft tissue sarcomas apparently arising in chronic tropical ulcers. Histopathology 11: 501–510

Fletcher C D M, Theaker J M, Flanagan A, Krausz T 1988 Pigmented dermatofibrosarcoma protuberans (Bednar tumour): melanocytic colonisation or neuroectodermal differentiation? A clinicopathological and immunohistochemical study. Histopathology 13: 631–643

Ghadially F N, Roy S 1966 Experimentally produced synovial sarcomas. Cancer 19: 1901–1908

Goldenberg I S 1954 Penicillin in sesame oil and fibrosarcoma. A report of two cases. Cancer 7: 905–909

Gottlieb G J, Ackerman A B 1982 Kaposi's sarcoma: an extensively disseminated form in young homosexual men. Human Pathology 13: 882–892

Grody W N, Lewin K J, Naeim F 1988 Detection of cytomegalovirus DNA in classic and epidemic Kaposi's sarcoma by in situ hybridization. Human Pathology 19: 524–528

Hardell L 1981 Relation of soft tissue sarcoma, malignant lymphoma and colon cancer to phenoxy acids, chlorophenols and other agents. Scandinavian Journal of Work Environment and Health 7: 119–130

Hardell L, Sandström A 1979 Case-control study: soft-tissue sarcomas and exposure to phenoxyacetic acid or chlorophenols. British Journal of Cancer 39: 711–717

Hasson J, Hartman K S, Milikow E, Mittelman J A 1975 Thorotrast-induced extraskeletal osteosarcoma of the cervical region. Report of a case. Cancer 36: 1827–1833

Hoshaw R A, Schwartz R A 1980 Kaposi's sarcoma after immunosuppressive therapy with prednisone. Archives of Dermatology 116: 1280–1282

Hrabko R P, Milgrom H, Schwartz R A 1982 Werner's syndrome with associated malignant neoplasms. Archives of Dermatology 118: 106–108

Hutt M S R 1984 Kaposi's sarcoma. British Medical Bulletin 40: 355–358

Inoshita T, Youngberg G A 1984 Malignant fibrous histiocytoma arising in previous surgical sites. Report of two cases. Cancer 53: 176–183

Iwasaki H, Kikuchi M, Mori R et al 1980 Infantile digital fibromatosis. Ultrastructural, histochemical and tissue culture observations. Cancer 46: 2238–2247

Iwasaki H, Kikuchi M, Ohtsuki I et al 1983 Infantile digital fibromatosis. Identification of actin filaments in cytoplasmic inclusions by heavy meromyosin binding. Cancer 52: 1653–1661

Järvi O, Saxén E 1961 Elastofibroma dorsi. Acta Pathologica et Microbiologica Scandinavica 51 (suppl 144): 83–84

Järvi O H, Länsimies P H 1975 Subclinical elastofibromas in the scapular region in an autopsy series. Acta Pathologica et Microbiologica Scandinavica, Section A 83: 87–108

Jennings T A, Peterson L, Axiotis C A, Friedlaender G E, Cooke R A, Rosai J 1988 Angiosarcoma associated with foreign body material. A report of three cases. Cancer 62: 2436–2444

Kim J H, Chu F C, Woodard H Q et al 1978 Radiation-induced soft-tissue and bone sarcoma. Radiology 129: 501–508

Klein B, Pals S, Masse R et al 1977 Studies of bone and soft-tissue tumours induced in rats with radioactive cerium chloride. International Journal of Cancer 20: 112–119

Konishi Y, Maruyama H, Mii Y et al 1982 Malignant fibrous histiocytomas induced by 4-(hydroxyamino) quinoline 1-oxide in rats. Journal of the National Cancer Institute 68: 859–865

Lacassagne A, Vinzent R 1929 Sarcomas provoques chez des Lapins par l'irradiation d'abces a Streptobacillus caviae. Société de Biologie 81: 249–251

Laskin W B, Silverman T A, Enzinger F M 1988 Postradiation soft tissue sarcomas. An analysis of 53 cases. Cancer 62: 2330–2340

Lee D A, Rao B R, Meyer J S et al 1980 Hormonal receptor determination in juvenile nasopharyngeal angiofibromas. Cancer 46: 547–551

Lee J H, Griffiths W J, Bottomley R H 1977 Extraosseous osteogenic sarcoma following an intramuscular injection. Cancer 40: 3097–3101

Lee Y-S, Pho R W H, Nather A 1984 Malignant fibrous histiocytoma at site of metal implant. Cancer 54: 2286–2289

Li F P, Fraumeni J F Jr 1969 Soft-tissue sarcomas, breast cancer, and other neoplasms. A familial syndrome? Annals of Internal Medicine 71: 747–752

Lucena G E, Bennett W M, Pierre R V 1966 'Dewlap', a corticosteroid-induced episternal fatty tumor. New England Journal of Medicine 275: 834–835

Lynge E, Storm H, Jensen O M 1987 The evaluation of trends in soft tissue sarcoma according to diagnostic criteria and consumption of phenoxy herbicides. Cancer 60: 1896–1901

McDougall A, McGarrity G 1979 Extra-abdominal desmoid tumours. Journal of Bone and Joint Surgery 61-B: 373–377

McIllmurray M B, Langman M J S 1978 Soft tissue sarcomas and intramuscle injections. An epidemiological survey. British Medical Journal 23: 864–865

Maruyama H, Mii Y, Emi Y et al 1983 Experimental studies on malignant fibrous histiocytoma. II. Ultrastructure of malignant fibrous histiocytomas induced by 4-(hydroxyamino)-quinoline-1-oxide in rats. Laboratory Investigation 48: 187–198

Miller R W 1971 Deaths from childhood leukemia and solid tumours among twins and other sibs in the United States, 1960–67. Journal of the National Cancer Institute 46: 203–209

Mindell E R, Shah N K, Webster J H 1977 Postradiation sarcoma of bone and soft tissues. Orthopedic Clinics of North America 8: 821–834

Morman M R, Ruey-Yen L, Petrozzi J W 1979 Dermatofibrosarcoma protuberans arising in a site of multiple immunizations. Archives of Dermatology 115: 1453

Morris J M, Lucas D B 1964 Fibrosarcoma within a sinus tract of chronic draining osteomyelitis. Case report and review of literature. Journal of Bone and Joint Surgery 46-A: 538–857

Muller R, Hajdu S I, Brennan M F 1987 Lymphangiosarcoma associated with chronic filarial lymphedema. Cancer 59: 179–183

Plenge K, Krückenmeyer K 1954 Über ein Sarkom am Ort der Thorotrastinjektion. Zentralblatt für Allgemeine Pathologie und Pathologische Anatomie 92: 255–260

Pojer J, Radivojevic M, Williams T F 1972 Dupuytren's disease: its association with abnormal liver function in alcoholism and epilepsy. Archives of Internal Medicine 129: 561–566

Reye R D K 1965 Recurring digital fibrous tumours of childhood. Archives of Pathology 80: 228–231

Safai B, Mike V, Giraldo G, Beth E, Good R A 1980 Association of Kaposi's sarcoma with second primary malignancies. Possible etiopathologic implications. Cancer 45: 1472–1479

Sakamoto K 1986 Malignant fibrous histiocytoma induced by intra-articular injection of 9, 10-dimethyl 1-1, 2-benzanthracene in the rat. Pathologic and enzyme histochemical studies. Cancer 57: 2313–2322

Selbie F R 1936 Experimental production of sarcoma with thorotrast. Lancet 2: 847–848

Semerdjian H S, Texter J H, Yawn D H 1972 Rhabdomyosarcoma occurring in repaired exstrophied bladder. A case report. Journal of Urology 108: 354–356

Shanoff L B, Spira M, Hardy S B 1967 Myositis ossificans: evolution to osteogenic sarcoma. Report of a histologically verified case. American Journal of Surgery 113: 537–541

Shibata M, Izumi K, Sano N, Akagi A, Otsuka H 1989 Induction of soft tissue tumours in F344 rats by subcutaneous, intramuscular, intra-articular and retroperitoneal injection of nickel sulphide (NiS$_2$). Journal of Pathology 157: 263–274

Smith A H, Pearce N E, Fisher D O et al 1984 Soft tissue sarcoma and exposure to phenoxyherbicides and chlorophenols in New Zealand. Journal of the National Cancer Institute 73: 1111–1117

Sordillo P P, Chapman R, Hajdu S I et al 1981 Lymphangiosarcoma. Cancer 48: 1674–1679

Sordillo P P, Hajdu S I, Magill G B et al 1983 Extraosseous osteogenic sarcoma. A review of 48 patients. Cancer 51: 727–734

Stewart F W, Treves N 1948 Lymphangiosarcoma in postmastectomy lymphedema. A report of six cases in elephantiasis chirurgica. Cancer 1: 64–81

Swann M 1984 Malignant soft tissue tumour at the site of a total hip replacement. Journal of Bone and Joint Surgery 66-B: 629–631

Taswell H F, Soule E H, Coventry M B 1962 Lymphangiosarcoma arising in chronic lymphedematous extremities. Report of thirteen cases and review of literature. Journal of Bone and Joint Surgery 44-A: 277–294

Ulbright T M, Santa Cruz D J 1981 Kaposi's sarcoma: relationship with hematologic, lymphoid and thymic neoplasia. Cancer 57: 963–873

Usui M, Ishii S, Yamawaki S et al 1984 The occurrence of soft tissue sarcomas in three siblings with Werner's syndrome. Cancer 54: 2580–2586

van den Berg F, Schipper M, Jiwa M, Rook R, van de Rijke F, Tigges B 1989 Implausibility of an aetiological association between cytomegalovirus and Kaposi's sarcoma shown by four techniques. Journal of Clinical Pathology 42: 128–131

Varsano S, Manor Y, Steiner Z et al 1984 Kaposi's sarcoma and angioimmunoblastic lymphadenopathy. Cancer 54: 1582–1585

Waddell W R 1975 Treatment of intra-abdominal and abdominal wall desmoid tumours with drugs that affect the metabolism of cyclic 3', 5'-adenosine monophosphate. Annals of Surgery 181: 299–302

Wagner J C, Sleggs C A, Marchand P 1960 Diffuse pleural mesothelioma and asbestos exposure in the North Western Cape Province. British Journal of Industrial Medicine 17: 260–271

Walter P R, Philippe E, Nguemby-Mbina C, Chamlian A 1984 Kaposi's sarcoma: presence of Herpes-type virus particles in a tumor specimen. Human Pathology 15: 1145–1146

Weinbren K, Salm R, Greenberg G 1978 Intramuscular injections of iron compounds and oncogenesis in man. British Medical Journal i: 683–685

Whang-Peng J, Triche T J, Knutsen T et al 1984 Chromosome translocation in peripheral neuropithelioma. New England Journal of Medicine 311: 584–585

Yumoto T, Morimoto K 1980 Experimental approach to fibrous histiocytoma. Acta Pathologica Japonica 30: 767–778

3. Epidemiology of soft tissue tumours

A. C. Templeton

INCIDENCE AND PREVALENCE

The science of epidemiology is based upon the construction of a ratio between the frequency of a given event and the population in which it occurs. Most often these ratios are expressed as prevalence or incidence (Feinstein & Esdaile 1987). Incidence is the frequency with which an event occurs in a given population in a given unit of time. For reporting cancer, the event is the first diagnosis of a tumour, expressed in terms of 100 000 people at risk in the period of 1 year. Thus, the overall incidence of cancer in the USA is 400 per 100 000 per year or 0.4% annually. The prevalence is the proportion of the population found to be suffering from a given disease at a given moment of time. With cancer it is usual to quote incidence figures because these are easier to obtain and more accurate. Such figures are used in the assessment of environmental risks and the number of patients expected to require initial treatment in a given area. Prevalence is much more difficult to estimate. Calculation requires surveillance of the apparently well population as well as the sick and requires a very much more precise definition of disease than is needed for calculation of the incidence (vide infra). Such figures would be very valuable in determining the feasibility of screening programmes or in calculating how many personnel would be required to care for patients with cancer. Absence of reliable prevalence data helps to explain why planning for construction of facilities and some screening progammes is so difficult.

At first sight, it would appear that incidence and prevalence are but slightly different ways of presenting the same information. There are considerable differences however. Let us consider a disease such as Kaposi's sarcoma which has a wide range of clinical pattern varying from a slowly progressive disease lasting many years, which does not prevent the subject from working or caring for himself, to a rapidly lethal disease killing the subject within six weeks of first symptoms. In between these extremes some people suffer from a slowly progressive, but locally destructive infiltrating tumour. Incidence figures, unless they are collected very assiduously, tend to exaggerate the number of patients with rapid lethal disease. Prevalence data by contrast will exaggerate the more chronic pattern. Both figures require the following pieces of precise information if they are to be useful.

1. Diagnostic criteria

It may appear self-evident that one needs to know precisely whether the disease in question is present or not and that this question is susceptible to a precise answer. In terms of generating incidence figures it is indeed rather easy. The question becomes, 'Are you sufficiently certain of the diagnosis to decide upon treatment.' If the answer is yes, then mark down a case, if no, then wait a while for the question to become clearer. In prevalence data, one is not allowed such a luxury. At what point along the progression from initiation to promotion to progression through dysplasia to invasion to metastasis is a cancer present? After diagnosis and initial treatment is a patient still suffering from the disease? Thus, is a woman who has recently undergone hysterectomy for leiomyosarcoma still suffering from the disease? The surgeon usually says no, because there is no macroscopic evidence of persistence and no justification for surgical intervention at this juncture. The psychiatrist says yes, because the emotional response is life-long. The pathologist says probably, because the natural history indicates that most such patients will declare pulmonary metastases in time. The chemotherapy consultant who is placed on the horns of this dilemma will answer the question with a firm maybe!

In addition, in the specific context of soft tissue neoplasms, there is a much more fundamental problem — that of obtaining reproducible diagnostic criteria at the histological level. This is a particular problem in determining the relative incidences of different types of sarcoma, in which interobserver variation in classification is a major problem. A typical example would be pleomorphic malignant fibrous histiocytoma, a term for which some pathologists have diagnostic criteria while others use it as a wastebin for the undiagnosable (Fletcher 1987, Dehner 1988). Clearly, histological precision can have a great influence on epidemiological statistics.

2. Availability of diagnostic facilities

One obviously needs to know the proportion of cases diagnosed and would intuitively guess that the more accessible the facilities, the higher the proportion of cases diagnosed. This is indeed correct, but the impact of quality and availability of diagnosis is more subtle. Thus, a poor medical service would conclude that Kaposi's sarcoma was an unusual, invasive neoplasm of the limbs. This is because those with the rapidly fatal generalised forms of the disease would not reach hospital and those with minimal constitutional effect would not bother to make the journey. Young people are more likely to be seen than the elderly and those with superficial diseases more than those with deep lesions. Thus, the efficiency of reporting retinoblastoma in Africa is many times higher than the efficiency of reporting hepatocellular carcinoma (Templeton & Bianchi 1972). It is usually believed that inadequate health services will always give rise to under-reporting, so correction merely requires an estimate of its extent. Unfortunately, over-reporting can also occur due to harvesting. If a new facility or a new staff member arrives in a poorly served area, the first year's diagnoses are usually relatively few. When word gets around the community that treatment is available, there is often a large number of diagnoses made in the second year. This figure is often extrapolated upwards and wildly exaggerated estimates of the true incidence results. In fact, the second year figure is itself an overestimate and is often closer to the prevalence rather than the incidence rate. By the time the third year rolls around, the backlog of the cases has largely been dealt with and new cases appear much less frequently. It is not until the fourth or fifth year after a given service has been introduced that true incidence is reflected in the number of cases treated annually. The more prolonged the disease process, the greater the errors. Thus, the incidence of Kaposi's sarcoma, desmoid tumour and subcutaneous leiomyoma, among others, are liable to substantial miscalculation.

3. Population statistics

Obviously, information on age, numbers of people and their sex is required and is usually recorded. Less frequently available but also useful are occupation, address and previous residence, social habits, gynaecological history and race among many other factors. The age distribution of the population at risk requires to be known and taken into account. Thus, European populations tend to be rather older than any other and still show the effects of the carnage of the World Wars and the 1919 influenza epidemic. African populations tend to show a Christmas-tree-like distribution to the age pyramid, a result of significant mortality in each successive age group. The US population shows the effects of massive immigration and the 'baby boom and bust cycles' of the recent past, and is now rapidly ageing. The mathematical constructs for correcting for age distribution are many and various, but none of them completely compensate, which makes world comparisons hazardous. Population statistics are least reliable at the extremes of life so that many statistics are quoted for the so-called truncated population usually aged 20–60 or so. These figures are often accurate, but ignore the very population in which many tumours are most common.

4. Death rates

Information as to the fact and date of death is required and is recorded in most cases. This enables one to calculate the absolute survival rate. The cause and manner of death is often not available. Whether a person dies of, with, or after cancer is obviously important in assessing the effectiveness of different treatments, for example, but is information that is often not available. Statisticians therefore use survival tables for the populations as a whole and in effect ascribe any excess mortality to the presence of the tumour (the relative survival).

5. Medical migration

Medical migration for the purposes of diagnosis and treatment, both into and out of the designated survey area, adds further confounding variables. This is greatest when a part of a single country is considered, but international migration effects the apparent incidence and prevalence of both high-risk, rapidly fatal diseases of young people and the more prolonged diseases of any age. Thus a survey of rheumatoid arthritis in an area including a spa town might come to rather startling conclusions as to the incidence and prevalence of this group of diseases.

It is easiest to obtain both incidence and prevalence figures in areas that are homogeneous, isolated, possessed of a good, available, cheap medical service which serves a racially homogeneous population of about 2–4 million. These conditions are met in New Zealand, but virtually everywhere else one or other factors makes for problems. The Scandinavian countries are probably the next best in terms of available figures because of their highly developed social system. Great Britain and the State of Connecticut are a step or two behind! All other countries have considerable inaccuracies embedded in the reporting procedure and require caution in interpretation. This is especially true in registries in the third world where very significant inaccuracies occur. There is considerable under-reporting of cases, most especially of those tumours that occur in older people in deep-seated locations and produce non-specific symptoms.

In the particular instance of soft-tissue tumours there are difficulties at every step. The total number of cases that occur in a given time is small; therefore, one must survey a large population for a long period of time to accumulate statistically analysable figures. Diagnostic criteria for inclusion within the group as a whole are soft and susceptible to intra- and interobserver error. Benign connective tissue lesions are in aggregate much more common than malignant lesions. Thus, only small changes in diagnostic differentiation between, say leiomyomata and leiomyosarcoma will have substantial statistical impact. Benign versus malignant fibrous histiocytoma and granulation tissue versus Kaposi's sarcoma are other examples that readily come to mind. In one survey from Finland the authors rejected 33% of cases originally recorded in the cancer registry (Rantakokko & Ekfors 1979).

Registration convention also varies somewhat. All registries file sarcomas of the limbs under a single rubric. There are, however, variations that are sometimes difficult to detect when scanning registry compilations. For example, tumours of the peripheral nervous system, ranging from neurilemmoma, neurofibrosarcoma, tumours of the autonomic ganglia including phaeochromocytoma and peripheral round cell tumours, are sometimes classified as soft-tissue tumours and sometimes together with tumours of the nervous or even endocrine system. Happily many of these lesions are rare so that this registration variation does not have great effect upon published totals. Of more importance is the difficulty of identifying soft-tissue tumours of defined organs, such as stomach or uterus or even retroperitoneal masses, which sometimes appear under the anatomical site and sometimes under the soft-tissue rubric. There is also variation due to problems in histological interpretation. Mesothelioma is an important example. The epithelial variant frequently being classified as a metastatic carcinoma, the fibrous variant as a soft tissue tumour and the mixed tumour as a lesion of the pleura or peritoneum. Regrettably, the epidemiology of mesothelioma has been obscured by superb examples of circular reasoning. Thus, when confronted with somewhat equivocal data the diagnosis of mesothelioma is made when the history of asbestos exposure is obtained and avoided when it is not (Wright et al 1984)!

When individual histopathological entities are concerned, the problem becomes magnified. There are many tumours described. For example the WHO-sanctioned International Histological Classification, notes 25 separate types of soft tissue sarcoma. Even if distinctions between these entities were sharp and readily made, this 'proliferation of proliferations' would constitute an epidemiologist's nightmare. But of course there is little clear agreement on such diagnoses. The relentless advance of malignant fibrous histiocytoma, which has virtually swallowed pleomorphic rhabdomyosarcoma and bids fair to putting fibrosarcoma out of business, is a case in point (Fletcher 1987, Dehner 1988). It is a small wonder therefore that the bemused epidemiologist is usually reduced to bundling all these tumours together, making a few calculations and then forgetting about the whole tissue.

When this is done the results are understandably not terribly useful. The successive volumes of *Cancer incidence in Five Continents* (Waterhouse et al 1982) report a total incidence of soft tissue sarcoma that varies from 2 to 4 cases per 100 000 per year (truncated population) in most countries. A much higher rate is reported from Hawaii, particularly among Hawaiian males. However in the publication of SEER data, the same Hawaiian registry reports no increase in incidence over other areas of the United States (National Cancer Institute 1981). Presumably some reclassification of doubtful data occurred in the meantime. By contrast, the incidence rate among Maori New Zealanders, who are racially related to Hawaiians, is probably low, though calculations from the New Zealand registry are based upon very small numbers. An incidence figure of 6.3 cases per 100 000 is reported among males in Bulawayo, a result of the high incidence of Kaposi's sarcoma in that city. Low incidence levels of soft-tissue sarcoma are reported from Miyagi and Osaka prefectures in Japan, but other prefectures show a similar level to the rest of the world. Singapore Chinese rates also seem to be low. No distinct pattern emerges from this data except that the incidence is higher in males than females at all ages and that there is a small peak of incidence in early childhood and then, among adults, a relatively slow arithmetic rise with age. This contrasts with the exponential increase that occurs with most epithelial tumours. There is no consistent strong geographical effect except for the well-known distribution of Kaposi's sarcoma discussed below. The apparently greater proportion of all malignancies accounted for by soft tissue sarcomas in Malawi (Fletcher — unpublished data) reflects not only the high incidence of Kaposi's sarcoma, but also the relative youth of the population and the dearth of the more common carcinomas seen in 'developed' countries. In the US, blacks show an excess of smooth muscle tumours of the uterus and peripheral nerve tumours but other soft-tissue neoplasms show no racial predilection (Polednak 1986). Among children the rate in US whites is about twice that in blacks (Young & Miller 1975). Analysis of SEER data shows no significant variation with race or geography within the USA (National Cancer Institute 1981). Rates in Puerto Rico are lower than in other areas but the rate in the Spanish population of New Mexico is rather higher than in whites in that state. Analysis of data from the Connecticut registry shows a steady rise in the incidence of soft-tissue tumours which doubled during the period 1935–1968.

CARCINOGENS

One of the implicit aims of epidemiology is to correlate the incidence of a particular disease with a potential carcinogen, be it genetic or environmental. Genetic studies have shown the association of soft-tissue tumours with a variety of syndromes. Thus, von Recklinghausen's disease (Sorensen et al 1986) is associated with gliomas and neurofibrosarcoma. Gardner's syndrome shows an association between soft tissue tumours and polyposis coli. Some families show many soft-tisse hamartomas (Bowdens syndrome) and retino-blastoma is associated with a risk of osteosarcoma. These examples provide some insight into the carcinogenic process, but most are rare and do not have great impact on the epidemiology of soft tissue tumours in general.

Epidemiology hopes to detect the influence of environmental factors in a number of ways. First and most obvious, one hopes to find an altered incidence of a particular tumour in a particular group of people. This is much easier to discern if the lesion in question is rare and readily diagnosable. The association of polyvinyl chloride precursors or thorotrast with angiosarcoma of the liver is a case in point. These relationships came to light, not only because of geographical and temporal proximity, but also because the disease is rare, the histology was distinctive and the site provocative. Unfortunately, these very important features are not discernible in the cancer registry data of most soft-tissue tumours. Date of registration is known but seldom published. Location of tumour and precise site of origin are seldom noted in registry returns because the numbers of soft-tissue neoplasms are small and the complexity of registering all this information would be too great. To take as a theoretical example, exposure to a carcinogen that is preferentially stored in adipose tissue and gives rise to tumours there. Exactly which histological form such a tumour might take is conjectural; logically one might expect liposarcomas, but more likely a mixture of histological types would occur. Thus it might be useful to know the exact site of liposarcomas, whether they occur in adipose parts of the body, or whether the patient was fat or thin. One would need to survey the registry data to note an association of sarcomas occurring in the fat-bearing areas of overweight people in order to reveal the effects of such a carcinogen. Another characteristic feature of the action of powerful carcinogens is to induce multiple tumours, particularly in people younger than the conventional age for liposarcoma. Multiplicity is fairly easy to discern in epithelial tumours, but in soft tissue sarcomas there is a problem in separating multiple primary tumours from metastasis (Enzinger & Weiss 1983). In most cases, multiple sites of involvement by soft tissue tumours are assumed to be a result of metastasis, thereby obfuscating potentially valuable data. If data of this degree of sophistication are not available, it is likely that the effect of a new carcinogen would be missed. The complexity of obtaining, registering and retrieving such data are daunting in the extreme.

With these remarks as a preface, it is truly remarkable that anything of consequence has emerged from the epidemiology of soft tissue tumours. The remainder of this chapter will be devoted to specific instances in which epidemiological data has hinted at, or discerned precisely, the action of a carcinogen. In descending order of certainty the following will be discussed: angiosarcoma and its association with thorotrast and polyvinyl chloride precursors, mesothelioma with asbestos, soft-tissue tumours with herbicides and insecticides and Kaposi's sarcoma with a variety of potential agents.

Angiosarcoma and thorotrast

Radioisotopes of thorium have a very desirable property of being very opaque to X-rays and were therefore used as a contrast medium, particularly for cerebral angiography. The disadvantage of the very long half-life is that large doses of irradiation are received by organs storing the material. Of a given dose of thorium administered intravenously, 60% is stored in the liver and 30% in the spleen with the balance predominantly being located within the bone marrow. The widespread use of thorium dioxide (thorotrast) as a radiological contrast medium was followed by the development of angiosarcoma of the liver 20–50 years later. Subsequently, this agent has been implicated in the development of many different tumours, hepatocellular carcinoma and osteosarcoma among them. The epidemiology of these tumours follows administration faithfully after an induction period of up to 50 years. There are many surveys in different countries of the risk of induction of tumours. A recently published series from Germany will serve as representative (Kauch et al 1986). Of their series of 1964 patients receiving thorotrast, 347 developed liver cancers. Most of these patients also had cirrhosis, 35 showed myeloproliferative disorders and 20 developed aplastic anaemia. There was a close correlation between the incidence of tumour and the dose to which the organ was exposed.

Angiosarcoma and PVC

The association of polyvinyl chloride and the same tumour came to light following the astute observation of a family practitioner who noted the development of a neoplasm with which he had been previously unfamiliar, in two of his patients (Block 1974, Creech & Johnson 1974).

Polyvinyl chloride is widely used in the manufacture of clothes and accessories, furniture and automobiles. The injurious agent is the monomer, which is seen in large concentrations only in the manufacturing process or after combustion. Other proposed uses for the monomer were as a hair spray propellant, mouth wash and in cigarettes. The polymer is relatively harmless, though some monomer persists which has caused some concern since polyvinyl components are used as food containers. In experimental, and in rare human, conditions vinyl chloride monomer has been shown to produce a variety of vascular proliferations within the liver, including peliosis hepatis, benign angiomas, epitheloid haemangiomas and angiosarcomas possibly in sequence. A common feature of all these lesions is the marked overproduction of vimentin in tumour cells. The surrounding liver may or may not show fibrosis. The exposure time to polyvinyl chloride monomer in patients showing one or other of these lesions has varied from 4 to 30 years. The prompt adaption of manufacturing methods and protection of workers has resulted in a dramatic reduction of exposure and of ascribable tumours (Forman 1985). It is certain that, had either of these agents produced a common tumour, such as bronchial carcinoma, or even a less distinctive soft tissue at another site, the association would probably not have been made.

Vascular neoplasms of the liver are also seen in women taking various contraceptive steroids. In this instance, the most frequent histological pattern seen is the epithelioid haemangioendothelioma (Dean et al 1985).

Mesothelioma and asbestos

The epidemiology of this association is a splendid story of the international detective work spanning the entire globe and deserves the many plaudits it has received (Wagner 1986). However, the strength of the association, the relative risk of different fibre types and the proper societal response thereunto has yet to be settled. The incidence of this disease has risen in most industrialised countries in recent years. For example, in Great Britain 150 cases were reported to the mesothelioma registry in 1968 compared with 600 in 1984 (Jones & Thomas 1986). At least in part, this increase is due to increased awareness of the entity, both on the part of clinicians and pathologists, but there has fairly certainly been a real increase too. It is to be hoped that the rate will start to fall as the workers, exposed to high concentrations of fibre in the 1940s, age and die. The incidence of peritoneal mesothelioma has also risen in Great Britain, but less sharply (Gardner et al 1985). It too shows an association with asbestos exposure. The relative risk of different occupations seems to be in the order of two- or three-fold in Sweden (Malker et al 1985).

The diagnosis of mesothelioma is a difficult one and, as already stated, is liable to circular reasoning that has probably overstated the strength of the association (Kannerstein et al 1979). Perhaps now that stains for specific keratins are available and the place of electron microscopy in diagnosis established a more accurate definition of the entity will be available. Many of the epidemiological studies should be repeated and hopefully cleaned up. The definition of significant asbestos exposure also requires reanalysis. Virtually every resident of a modern city has some asbestos material in the lung, so that denominator for many epidemiological calculations requires to be reconsidered. More recently, the potential carcinogenicity of other man-made mineral fibres has come under question and a number of surveys have shown an increased incidence of lung cancer among production workers in such industries as fibreglass insulation manufacture. The precise risk, or whether any risk exists at all, is hotly argued.

Soft tissue sarcomas and phenoxyherbicides

Phenoxyherbicides are a class of compounds used to kill broad-leafed plants. They may be divided into three major groups known as T, D and M groups. T-type herbicides are used in forestry, D and M mainly as weed-control agents in cereal crops.

A series of papers published in 1977 and 1981 from Sweden showed a strong association between phenoxyherbicide exposure and the development of soft-tissue lesions; an attributable risk of six-fold was discerned (Hardell 1977, Hardell & Sandstrom 1979, Ericksson et al 1981). This data gave rise to international concern most particularly in association with the use of Agent Orange in Vietnam and the exposure of large numbers of US veterans to this material. Agent Orange is a 1:1 mixture of T and D material. More recent studies, however, have tended either to deny or substantially diminish the attributable risk of such exposure. Thus studies on farmers in New Zealand (Smith et al 1984) and USA (Hoar et al 1986), manufacturers of phenoxy-herbicides in Denmark (Lynge 1985) and veterans of Vietnam in the United States (Greewald et al 1984) have shown little or no association of soft-tissue lesions with phenoxyherbicide exposure. Problems in data collection methods may be responsible for some of these differences (Lynge et al 1987) and the validity of this association remains sub judice.

Much concern has been expressed over the hazards of exposure to a related compound, tetrachlorodibenzo-p-dioxin, (Sterling 1984). Perhaps the best data is that from the survey of the population exposed to dioxin following the 1976 explosion in Sevesco. This shows that even before the accident, the eventually polluted area showed an increase in soft-tissue tumours (Puntoni et al 1986). The authors suggest that this material does indeed cause soft tissue sarcomas and that it had been doing so for some years prior to the factory explosion that achieved such notoriety.

The epidemiology of Kaposi's sarcoma

From the epidemiologist's viewpoint, Kaposi's sarcoma may be divided into two groups, the endemic and epidemic (acquired immunodeficiency syndrome — AIDS — associated) forms. Endemic Kaposi's sarcoma was originally described as occurring predominantly in elderly Jewish males from Southern Europe. The pattern of disease usually seen in this group was the development of acral nodules causing a slowly progressive non-life-threatening disease. Immigrant studies showed a disease incidence of about 500 times higher in such people in America as compared with immigrants of other religions from other areas (Rothman 1962). This suggested a strong genetic effect, an impression that was confirmed by scattered reports of familial disease and by segregation of disease with certain HLA tissue types.

In the 1930s it became apparent that Kaposi's sarcoma was extremely common in Africa. There is an extensive literature on this subject, recently reviewed by Gigase (1984). Over the next three decades, information on tumour incidence from different parts of Africa showed that the highest incidence was in North Eastern Zaire, where the disease accounted for about 15% of malignant tumours in males. In the region of the tropical rain forest from Ghana to Uganda the incidence of this lesion is high and rates fall rapidly once beyond this region, whether travelling through the Savanna belt to the desert in the north, eastward through the dry highland country of East Africa, or southward beyond the Zambesi. It has often been suggested that the geographical distribution Kaposi's sarcoma is similar to that of Burkitt's tumour. In fact, though the broad distribution of these two tumours is rather similar in detail, they are very different. In Uganda, for example, Kaposi's sarcoma is very common in the high country bordering on Zaire. Here, Burkitt's tumour is virtually absent; whereas, both are seen with great frequency in the relatively low-lying West Nile district. It is difficult therefore to argue that both tumours must be produced by similar agents. These features point strongly towards an environmental factor, since Africans of widely different ethnic origins all developed this disease at high incidence when in Africa, whereas their descendents in the Americas had a much lower incidence. The nature of these environmental factors is uncertain. Cytomegalovirus titres among patients with Kaposi's sarcoma in America were noted to be higher than among controls (Giraldo et al 1980). In Africa, patients also showed high titres, but these levels are similar to those in control Africans without disease. Europeans and Asians resident in high incidence areas do not develop this tumour in any greater frequency than would be expected from their ethnic heritage (Chopra & Templeton 1971). Thus, European Jews show the highest incidence and northern Europeans and Indians show only a rare case. These epidemiological features suggest a possible genetic predisposition, but these results could also be explained on environmental grounds, in that black, white and brown residents of Africa have very different lifestyles. These apparently genetically conditioned effects persist among renal transplant recipients. Thus, Saudis (Qunibi et al 1988) and Jews resident in North America (Harwood et al 1979) or Australia (Sheil 1977), undergoing renal transplantation for a variety of reasons, show an incidence of Kaposi's sarcoma hundreds of times higher than Anglo Saxons. The precise nature of the genetic factor is uncertain. There is no constant relationship with any particular HLA type. Thus, in Saudi Arabia HLA A2 was found in excess (Qunibi et al 1988) but there was no association with HLA DR5 which has been reported in both endemic (Pollack et al 1983) and epidemic disease (Friedman-Kien et al 1982) in other parts of the world.

This worldwide distribution and incidence of Kaposi's sarcoma seems to have been fairly stable over a period of at least 50 years from before 1930 to 1970, though experience from the earlier period is only anecdotal. Within the overall disease incidence, three patterns or types of disease were discerned. These are nodular, locally aggressive and generalized (Taylor et al 1971). In central Africa up to the period of the mid 1970s these patterns accounted for roughly 75%, 20% and 5% of cases respectively. The nodular pattern occurs almost exclusively in elderly males and follows the slowly progressive course noted in European subjects. Locally aggressive disease showed an appearance much closer to that of other soft tissue sarcomas in that the lesions invade local structures, ulcerate, fungate and metastasize. Most of these patients had some signs of nodular disease elsewhere in the skin. Many patients gave a history of having had nodular disease for many years prior to the development of the locally infiltrative lesion. It is assumed that the aggressive lesion results from altered behaviour of a pre-existing nodular lesion. This is the only pattern of disease which can be truly said to metastasize with involvement of neighbouring nodes being particularly frequent. The generalised pattern of disease has attracted great interest, though until recently this accounted for only about 5% of cases. Patients with generalised disease present with the virtually simultaneous onset of numerous proliferations of Kaposi's sarcoma in many areas of the body. About half of this latter group of cases occurred in adults and about half in children. In children, these nodules occur almost exclusively in lymph nodes, producing a clinical appearance strongly suggestive of malignant lymphoma. In considerable contrast to the sex ratio in other patterns of disease, girls are affected almost as often as boys. Among adults, generalized disease presents with nodules occurring under epithelial surfaces, within parenchymal organs and in lymph nodes. The sex ratio among adults with generalized disease showed a male preponderance of about 2 to 1. This figure contrasts with the 10 to 1 ratio seen in endemic nodular or locally aggressive disease both in African and European subjects. Pregnant women seemed to be particularly likely to show this pattern of disease. There have been many speculations as to the cause of this anomalous sex ratio. The known effect of oestrogens on vascular reactivity, as in the hot flush of the menopause, the incidence of vascular tumours in people taking oral contraceptive pills and the increased risk of thrombosis in pregnancy and in pill users, give hints of a strong relationship between oestrogens and endothelial cells; however, no explanation has been forthcoming. Oestrogen administration has been used without effect in therapy for Kaposi's sarcoma. Prior to 1975, endemic disease among Europeans showed a nodular pattern disease in virtually all subjects. Very few showed locally aggressive lesions though Kaposi himself was aware of this possible form of the disease. About 4% of patients showed the generalized disorder, most of whom were children (Dutz & Stout 1960).

Another striking feature of Kaposi's sarcoma is its relationship to abnormal immune function. In Africa, there is an association with leprosy. In Europe, an association with malignant lymphoma has long been known. It is this feature that may explain its relationship to renal transplantation and with AIDS.

Patients with nodular disease maintain a capacity to respond to cutaneous challenges with dinitrochlorobenzene (DNCB). The development of an aggressive tumour is associated with loss of such reaction (Master et al 1970). Whether the tumour suppresses the immune reaction or immune suppression allows tumour progression is uncertain. Points in favour of the former include the reactivation of DNCB response following tumour excision and the presence of nodular rather than aggressive disease in some patients with lepromatous leprosy.

In most of the world, before 1975 Kaposi's sarcoma was conspicuous by its absence. There were two or three cases reported from India and Sri Lanka and none from China, Southeast Asia or South America. The incidence of Kaposi's sarcoma in the Caribbean Islands has recently become of great interest, but unfortunately reliable figures are hard to come by. There are anecdotal verbal reports of cases noted in Haiti and the Dominican Republic, but no records exist of cases in Jamaica and Cuba. Haitians in the US were among the first groups of patients known to be affected by AIDS and a large proportion of these men developed Kaposi's sarcoma (MMWR 1982). It was widely assumed at that time that the AIDS epidemic in the USA had started following infection acquired by homosexual males while vacationing in Haiti. It has now been realised that the incidence of AIDS in Haiti is rather lower than in the USA (Lange & Jaffe 1987) and it seems just as likely that AIDS was carried to Haiti from New York as in the opposite direction. The incidence of Kaposi's sarcoma in Haiti, though not accurately known, is certainly low and seems to be largely, if not exclusively, confined to the population at risk for AIDS. There also seems little doubt that the rise in incidence occurred in 1979 (Mitacek et al 1986). In North Africa, the disease was and is extremely rare. In South Africa, it was common among blacks and occurred in whites as would be appropriate for their European ancestry. The incidence in Northern Europe and Russia is extremely low and virtually all cases reported from these regions have occurred in Jewish men who trace their ancestry back to Southern Europe. This high risk survived the journey to wherever these people migrated. Thus, Rothman (1962) calculated that the incidence of Kaposi's sarcoma among Jews in the USA was about 500 times higher than among Gentiles. A recent study in Sardinia confirms the genetic effect on disease incidence (Scappaticci et al 1986).

Upon this apparently stable endemic pattern, dramatic changes have occurred in the incidence and type of disease. In the 1950s it was noted that Kaposi's sarcoma was developing with undue frequency in renal transplant recipients. As noted above, the incidence of Kaposi's sarcoma among Jews or Arabs undergoing renal transplantation is much higher than among non-Semites. This suggests that the procedure revealed a genetic susceptibility to the disease, but is insufficient to induce tumours in most of our species. These lesions would usually regress if immunosuppressive agents were withdrawn. These observations strengthened the already close association of Kaposi's sarcoma with perturbations of the immune system. Subsequently, Kaposi's sarcoma was also noted to occur in patients who were receiving steroid therapy for a wide variety of disorders.

In the early 1980s a rash of cases were noted to occur in association with AIDS. AIDS associated (epidemic) Kaposi's sarcoma shows a histological appearance which is in every way identical to that seen in the endemic disease. However, the clinical pattern is very different. The individual cutaneous lesions follow a similar evolution as is seen in endemic disease, but are more commonly located on the face, trunk and palate, whereas in endemic disease nodules develop almost exclusively on the limbs. Involvement of internal organs is much more common in epidemic disease, with nodules and/or plaques in the gastrointestinal tract and along the bronchi being particularly common. Most patients developing Kaposi's sarcoma with AIDS have already had several episodes of infectious disease and have a profound immune perturbation. In this group the survival is in the order of 6 months. It seems that Kaposi's sarcoma predicts this poor outlook rather than causing it, since the lesions themselves are seldom the cause of significant symptoms. The exception to this rule is involvement of the lungs where the plaque-like spread along bronchi results in marked respiratory difficulty and closely mimics the effect of cardiac failure, both in terms of symptoms and X-ray appearance (Nash & Fligiel 1984). There is a small group of HIV antibody-positive patients who develop Kaposi's sarcoma before the development of infections and sometimes before an alteration of helper/suppressor ratio. These patients may have a prolonged survival and follow a protracted course. Such patients have been successfully managed for several years with no systemic treatment beyond local radiation therapy to cosmetically obvious tumours.

The proportion of patients with AIDS who develop Kaposi's varies. It seems to be much more common in homosexuals with the disease than in drug addicts or haemophiliacs. At least some of the variations are due to familiarity with both AIDS and Kaposi's sarcoma on the part of the physician. In the first years of the epidemic, there was often reluctance to diagnose AIDS without histological demonstration of Kaposi's sarcoma, which policy probably exaggerated the association. More recently there has been a tendency to diagnose any haemorrhagic blemish in a homosexual man as Kaposi's sarcoma. In fact, many vascular connective tissue lesions are more common in such hosts and this has lead to an artifically high diagnostic rate. During the patch phase of the disease, it is often difficult to be certain of the diagnosis even with an adequate biopsy. The initial reports of AIDS from both Europe and North America reported an incidence of Kaposi's sarcoma in about 35% of cases. Most of these early series were composed of predominantly young white homosexual subjects. And it seems that this subgroup showed the highest risk of developing Kaposi's sarcoma. In more recent reports, the frequency of the disease has been much smaller. For example, the proportion of AIDS patients in San Francisco diagnosed as having Kaposi's sarcoma has fallen from 70% to about 35% in 5 years (Drew et al 1986). It may be of significance that the frequency and level of cytomegalovirus titres have fallen in parallel. The frequency of Kaposi's sarcoma in AIDS patients is smallest in Hispanic drug addicts. For example, a recent review from Puerto Rico showed only 5 of 70 patients with AIDS had Kaposi's sarcoma (De Vinatea et al 1988).

It is uncertain as to why this variation should occur, but hypotheses include:

1. There may be differences in genetic susceptibility of the patient involved
2. Drug addicts with AIDS have a different range of infections which may influence the liability to develop Kaposi's sarcoma
3. The duration of the disease may be different in the different subtypes of patients susceptible to AIDS
4. Sophistication in the use of hospitals and standards of medical care are different in the two groups
5. Histological criteria are very varied, especially in regard to the so-called inflammatory variant of Kaposi's sarcoma. For example, in a series from Florida, the authors diagnosed Kaposi's sarcoma in virtually all cases and claim that lymph nodes are involved in virtually every case (Moskowitz et al 1985).

In Africa, there has been a marked increase in the incidence of generalised Kaposi's sarcoma and almost all of these patients have HIV antibodies against Type 1 virus or overt AIDS. In Uganda, for example, this pattern was seen in 33 of 194 cases of Kaposi's sarcoma registered in the Kampala cancer registry between 1980 and 1984 (Serwadda et al 1986). This proportion contrasts with a figure of 3% seen a decade earlier in the same area. The same phenomenon has been noted in North Tanzania, although not always in HIV-positive patients (Craighead et al 1988). Patients with locally aggressive or nodular pattern of Kaposi's sarcoma do not have HIV antibodies (Bayley et al 1985). It would be very interesting to know what proportion of Africans with AIDS develop Kaposi's sarcoma. Unfortunately, the incidence of AIDS in Africa is not known with any precision. One might predict that Kaposi's sarcoma would occur in Africans with AIDS less commonly than elsewhere, since AIDS in Africa would be expected to have a much more rapidly lethal course than in Northern Europe, for example. Patients with immune deficiency and chronic infections are liable to die from recrudescence of pre-existing malaria or parasitic infection. Conversely, whether the high incidence of Kaposi's sarcoma in equatorial Africa is due to an environmental or genetic effect, one might expect Kaposi's sarcoma to develop even more rapidly there than in other parts of the world. Regrettably, there is not yet sufficient data even to address this question. There are suggestions that human immunodeficiency virus or something closely related was present in parts of Uganda in 1972 (Saxinger et al 1985). HIV antibody is present in about 10% of the Ugandan population (Serwadda et al 1985) and the majority of these people are symptom free. Slim disease occurs fairly commonly in the subpopulation but does not appear to be inevitable. The majority of people with Slim disease do not have Kaposi's sarcoma. There are insufficient numbers of patients in Africa who have successfully undergone renal transplantation to know whether this group of people is more or less likely to develop Kaposi's sarcoma than Caucasian residents in temperate climates. The collection and analysis of statistics in both these groups could be very valuable. There is so far no information available on differences, if any, between the relative risks of developing Kaposi's sarcoma in AIDS due to type I or type II HIV virus.

REFERENCES

Bayley A C, Downing R G, Cheingsong-Popov R et al 1985 HTLV III Serology distinguishes atypical and endemic Kaposi's sarcoma in Africa. Lancet 1: 359–364
Bhana D, Templeton A C, Master S P 1970 Kaposi's sarcoma of lymph nodes. British Journal of Cancer 24: 464–470
Block J B 1974 Vinyl chloride and angiosarcoma. Journal of the Kentucky Medical Association 72: 483–485
Cerimele D, Contu L, Scapaticci S, Cottoni F 1984 Kaposi's sarcoma in Sardinia: An epidemiologic and genetic investigation. Annals of the New York Academy of Sciences 437: 216–227
Chopra S, and Templeton A C 1971 Cancer in East African Indians. International Journal of Cancer 8: 176–183
Craighead J, Moore A, Grossman H et al 1988 Pathogenetic role of HIV infection in Kaposi's sarcoma of equatorial East Africa. Archives of Pathology and Laboratory Medicine 112: 259–265
Creech J L, Johnson M N 1974 Angiosarcoma of the liver in the manufacture of vinyl chloride. Journal of Occupational Medicine 16: 150–151
Dean, P J, O'Hara C J, Haggitt R C 1985 Malignant epitheloid hemangioendothelioma of the liver in young women. American Journal of Surgical Pathology 9: 695–704

Dehner L P 1988 Malignant fibrous histiocytoma. Non-specific morphologic pattern, specific pathologic entity or both? Archives of Pathology and Laboratory Medicine 112: 236–237

De Vinatea M, Malher G, Lasala C, Climent C, Lopez E, Angritti P 1988 Journal of Laboratory Investigation 24A (suppl)

Drew W L, Mills J, Hauer L, Gottlieb A, Miner R 1986 Journal of Laboratory Investigation 55 (suppl): 8

Dutz W, Stout A P 1960 Kaposi's sarcoma in infants and children. Cancer 13: 684–694

Enzinger F M, Weiss S W 1983 Liposarcoma. In: Soft tissue tumours. C. V. Mosby, St. Louis, p 242–280

Eriksson M, Hardell L, Berg N, Moller T, Axelson O 1981 Soft-tissue sarcomas and exposure to chemical substances. British Journal of Industrial Medicine 38: 27–33

Feinstein A R, Esdaile J M 1987 Incidence prevalence and evidence. American Journal of Medicine 82: 113–119

Fletcher C D M 1987 Malignant fibrous histiocytoma? Histopathology 11: 433–438

Forman D 1985 Exposure to vinyl chloride and angiosarcoma of the liver. British Journal of Industrial Medicine 42: 750–753

Friedman-Kien A E, Laubenstein L J, Rubinstein P et al 1982 Disseminated Kaposi's sarcoma in homosexual men. Annals of Internal Medicine 96: 693–700

Gardner M J, Jones R D, Pippard E C, Saiton N 1985 Mesothelioma of the peritoneum during 1967–82 in England and Wales. British Journal of Cancer 51: 121–126

Gigase P L 1984 Epidemiologie du sarcome de Kaposi en Afrique. Bulletin de la Societe de Pathologie Exotique et de ses Filiales 77: 546–559

Giraldo G, Beth E, Huang E S 1980 Kaposi's sarcoma and its relationship to cytomegalovirus. International Journal of Cancer 26: 23–29

Greenwald P, Kovasznay B, Collins D N, Therriault G 1984 Sarcomas of soft-tissue after Vietnam service. Journal of the National Cancer Institute 73:1107–1109

Hardell L 1977 Maligna mesenkymala tumöres och exposition för fenoxisyror – en klinisk observation. Lakastidningen 74: 2753–2754

Hardell L, Ericksson M 1981 Soft tissue sarcomas, phenoxyherbicides and chlorinated phenols. Lancet 2: 250–252

Hardell L, Sandstrom A 1979 Case control studies. Soft tissue sarcomas and exposure to phenoxyacetic acids or chlorophenols. British Journal of Cancer 39: 711–717

Harwood A R, Osaba D, Hofstader S L et al 1979 Kaposi's sarcoma in recipients of renal transplants. American Journal of Medicine 67: 759–765

Hoar S K, Blair A, Holmes F F et al 1986 Agricultural herbicide use and risk of lymphoma and soft tissue sarcoma. Journal of the American Medical Association 1986; 256: 1141–1147

Jones B, Thomas P 1986 Incidence of mesothelioma in Britain. Lancet i: 1275

Kannerstein M, Churg J, McCaughen W T E 1979 Function of mesothelioma panels. Annals of the New York Academy of Sciences 330: 433–438

Kauch G, von Wesch H, Luhrs H, Lieberman D 1986 Radiation induced primary liver tumours in thorotrast patients. In: Bannasch P, Zerban H (eds) Pathogenesis of primary liver tumours induced by chemicals. Recent results in cancer research, vol 100. Springer, Berlin, p 16–22

Lange W R, Jaffe J M 1987 AIDS in Haiti. New England Journal of Medicine 316: 1409–1410

Lynge E 1985 A follow-up study of cancer incidence among workers in manufacture of phenoxyherbicides in Denmark. British Journal of Cancer 52: 259–270

Lynge E, Storm H H, Jensen O M 1987 The evaluation of trends in soft tissue sarcoma according to diagnostic criteria and consumption of phenoxy herbicides. Cancer 60: 1896–1901

Malker H S, McLaughlin J K, Malker R K et al 1985 Occupational risks for pleural mesothelioma in Sweden 1961–79. Journal of the National Cancer Institute 74: 61–66

Master S P, Taylor J F, Kyalwazi S, Ziegler J L 1970 Immunological studies on Kaposi's sarcoma in Uganda. British Medical Journal 1: 600–602

Mitacek E J, St Vallieres D, Polednak A P 1986 Cancer in Haiti 1979–84. Distribution of various forms of cancer according to geographical area and sex. International Journal of Cancer 88: 9–16

MMWR 1982 Opportunistic infections and Kaposi's sarcoma among Haitians in the United States. Morbidity and Mortality Weekly Reports 31: 353–361

Moskowitz E B, Hensley G T, Gould E W, Weiss S D 1985 Frequency and anatomic distribution of lymphadenopathic Kaposi's sarcoma in the acquired immunodeficiency syndrome. Human Pathology 6: 447–456

Nash G, Fligiel S 1984, Kaposi's sarcoma presenting as pulmonary disease in the acquired immunodeficiency syndrome. Diagnosis by lung biopsy. Human Pathology 15: 999–1001

National Cancer Institute 1981 SEER incidence and mortality data 1973–77. National Cancer Institute Monograph 57

Polednak P 1986 Incidence of soft tissue cancers in black and whites in New York state. International Journal of Cancer 38: 21–30

Pollack M S, Safai B, Myskowski P L, Gold J W, Pandey J, Dupont B 1983 Frequencies of HLA and GM immunogenetic markers in Kaposi's sarcoma. Tissue antigens 21: 1–8

Puntoni R, Merio F, Fini A, Meazza L, Santi L 1986 Soft tissue sarcomas in Sevesco. Lancet ii: 525

Qunibi W Y, Akhtar M, Sheth K et al 1988 Kaposi's sarcoma: The most common tumour after renal transplantation in Saudi Arabia. American Journal of Medicine 84: 225–232

Rantakokko V, Ekfors T O 1979 Sarcomas of the soft tissues in the extremities and limb girdles. Acta Clinica Scandinavia 145: 385

Rothman S 1962 Remarks on sex, age and racial distribution of Kaposi's sarcoma and on possible pathogenetic factor. Acta Unio Internationalis Contra Cancrum 18: 322

Saxinger W C, Levine P M, Dean A G 1985 Evidence of exposure to HTLV III in Uganda before 1973. Science 2278: 1036–1038

Scappaticci S, Cerimele D, Cottoni F, Pasquali F, Fraccaro M 1986 Chromosomal aberrations in lymphocyte and fibroblast cultures of patients with the sporadic type of Kaposi's sarcoma. Human Genetics 72: 311–317

Serwadda D, Sewankambo N K, Carswell J W 1985 Slim disease, a new disease in Uganda and its association with HTLV III infection. Lancet ii: 849

Serwadda D, Carswell W, Ayuko W O, Wamukota W, Madda P, Downing R G 1986 Further experience with Kaposi's sarcoma in Uganda. British Journal of Cancer 53: 497–500

Sheil A F 1977 Cancer in renal allograft recipients in Australia and New Zealand. Transplant Proceedings 9: 1133–1136

Smith A M, Pearce N E, Fisher D O, Gilesh J, Teague C A, Howard J K 1984 Soft tissue sarcoma and exposure to phenoxyherbicides and chlorophenols. Journal of the National Cancer Institute. 73: 1111–1117

Sorensen S A, Mulvihill J J, Nielsen A 1986 Long-term follow-up of von Recklinghausen neurofibromatosis. New England Journal of Medicine 314: 1010–1015

Sterling T D 1984 Health effects of dioxin. Science 223: 120

Taylor J F, Templeton A C, Vogel C L, Ziegler J L, Kyalwazi S K 1971 Kaposi's sarcoma in Uganda, a clinicopathologic study. International Journal of Cancer 8: 122–135

Templeton A C, Bianchi A 1972 Bias in an African cancer registry. International Journal of Cancer 10: 186–193

Wagner J C 1986 Mesothelioma and mineral fibers. Cancer 57: 1905–1911

Waterhouse J A M, Muir C S, Shanmugaratnam K, Powell J 1982 Cancer incidence in five continents. Publication 42, IARC, Lyons

Young J L, Miller R W 1975 Incidence of malignant tumours in US children. Journal of Pediatrics 86: 254–260

Wright W E, Sherwin R P, Dickson E A, Bernstein L, Field T B, Henderson B E 1984 Malignant mesothelioma incidence asbestos exposure and reclassification of histopathology. British Journal of Industrial Medicine 41: 39–45

4. Current classification of soft tissue tumours

E. B. Chung

Soft tissue tumours constitute a group of proliferative lesions of mesenchymal tissue which vary greatly with respect to site of origin, histological structure and biological behaviour. The greatest contribution to the modern classification of these tumours is presented in the soft tissue fascicle of the *Atlas of Tumour Pathology*, originally by Stout in 1953 and reissued with Lattes in 1967. While many attempts have been made to create a practical but comprehensive system of classification, that of the World Health Organization (Enzinger & Shiraki) has provided the most useful, particularly in terms of understanding those characteristics determining effective management and predicting prognosis.

Advances in the study of various soft tissue tumours have necessitated re-evaluation of their classification (Enzinger & Weiss 1983). This chapter is presented with the intention of providing an up-to-date system of classification (Table 4.1).

TUMOURS AND TUMOURLIKE LESIONS OF FIBROUS TISSUE

On the basis of biological behaviour and age-incidence, these lesions are categorised into four groups:

1. Benign fibroblastic proliferations
2. Fibromatoses
3. Fibrous tumours of infancy and childhood
4. Malignant-fibrosarcomas.

Benign fibroblastic proliferations

These are for the most part reactive rather than neoplastic in origin. Some are often mistaken for sarcomas, and therefore have been designated as 'pseudosarcomatous proliferative lesions of soft tissue' (Dahl & Angervall 1977).

1. Nodular fasciitis

This lesion was originally designated 'subcutaneous pseudosarcomatous fibromatosis' (Konwaler et al 1955). Parosteal fasciitis (Hutter et al 1962),

Table 4.1   Classification of soft tissue tumours

Tissue type/cell	Benign tumours and tumour-like lesions	Tumours of intermediate malignancy	Malignant tumours
Fibrous tissue	*Fibroblastic proliferation* 1. Nodular fasciitis 2. Proliferative fasciitis 3. Proliferative myositis 4. Fibroma of tendon sheath 5. Elastofibroma 6. Nasopharyngeal angiofibroma 7. Keloid		1. Adult fibrosarcom 2. Congenital and infantile fibrosarcoma

	Fibromatoses
	1. Superficial (fascial)
	  a. Palmer fibromatosis
	  b. Planter fibromatosis
	  c. Penile fibromatosis
	  d. Knuckle pads
	2. Deep (musculoaponeurotic)
	  a. Abdominal and intra-abdominal fibromatoses
	  b. Extra-abdominal fibromatosis		

	Fibrous tumours of infancy and childhood 1. Fibrous hamartoma of infancy 2. Infantile digital fibromatosis 3. Infantile myofibromatosis: Solitary and multicentric types 4. Juvenile hyalin fibromatosis 5. Gingival fibromatosis 6. Fibromatosis colli 7. Infantile (desmoid-type) fibromatosis 8. Calcifying aponeurotic fibroma 9. Giant cell fibroblastoma		
Fibrohistiocytes	1. Xanthoma 2. Juvenile xanthogranuloma 3. Reticulohistiocytoma 4. Fibrous histiocytoma	1. Dermatofibrosarcoma protuberans 2. Bednar tumor 3. Plexiform fibrohistiocytic tumour	1. Atypical fibroxanthoma 2. Myxoid malignan fibrous histiocytoma (MFH) 3. Inflammatory M▶ 4. Pleomorphic MF 5. Giant cell MFH 6. Angiomatoid MF

Table 4.1 Classification of soft tissue tumours (*Continued*)

Tissue type/cell	Benign tumours and tumour-like lesions	Tumours of intermediate malignancy	Malignant tumours
Adipose tissue	1. Lipoma 2. Angiolipoma 3. Spindle cell and pleomorphic lipoma 4. Lipoblastoma and lipoblastomatosis 5. Angiomyolipoma 6. Myelolipoma 7. Intramuscular lipoma 8. Diffuse lipomatosis 9. Hibernoma		1. Well-differentiated liposarcoma 2. Myxoid liposarcoma 3. Round cell liposarcoma 4. Pleomorphic liposarcoma 5. Dedifferentiated liposarcoma
Muscle	*Smooth muscle tumours* 1. Leiomyoma 2. Angiomyoma 3. Epithelioid leiomyoma		1. Leiomyosarcoma 2. Epithelioid leiomyosarcoma
	Striated muscle tumours 1. Adult rhabdomyoma 2. Fetal rhabdomyoma 3. Genital rhabdomyoma		1. Embryonal rhabdomyosarcoma 2. Alveolar rhabdomyosarcoma 3. Pleomorphic rhabdomyosarcoma 4. Mixed rhabdomyosarcoma 5. Rhabdomyosarcoma with ganglion cells
Blood vessels	*Localized superficial haemangiomas* 1. Capillary haemangioma 2. Cavernous haemangioma 3. Arteriovenous haemangioma 4. Venous haemangioma 5. Epithelioid haemangioma 6. Granulation tissue-type haemangioma	1. Epithelioid haemangioendo-thelioma 2. Spindle cell haemangioendo-thelioma 3. Malignant endovascular papillary angioendothelioma	1. Angiosarcoma 2. Kaposi's sarcoma 3. Malignant glomus tumour 4. Malignant haemangioperi-cytoma
	Deep Haemangiomas 1. Intramuscular haemangioma 2. Synovial haemangioma 3. Intraneural haemangioma		
	Glomus tumour		
	Haemangiopericytoma		
	Reactive vascular proliferations mimicking angiosarcoma 1. Papillary endothelial hyperplasia 2. Nodal angiomatosis		

Table 4.1   Classification of soft tissue tumours (*Continued*)

Tissue type/cell	Benign tumours and tumour-like lesions	Tumours of intermediate malignancy	Malignant tumours
Lymph vessels	1. Lymphangioma 2. Lymphangiomatosis 3. Lymphangiomyoma and lymphangiomyomatosis		1. Lymphangio-sarcoma
Synovial tissue	1. Localised giant cell tumour of tendon sheath 2. Diffuse giant cell tumour of tendon sheath		1. Malignant giant c tumour of tend sheath 2. Synovial sarcoma

Peripheral nerve	1. Traumatic neuroma
	2. Morton's neuroma
	3. Neuromuscular hamartoma
	4. Nerve sheath ganglion
	5. Neurilemmoma
	6. Solitary circumscribed neuroma
	7. Solitary neurofibroma
	8. Neurofibromatosis
	  a. Localized neurofibroma
	  b. Plexiform neurofibroma
	  c. Diffuse neurofibroma
	9. Granular cell tumour
	10. Myxoid tumour of nerve sheath
	11. Extracranial meningioma
	12. Pigmented neuroectodermal tumour of infancy
			1. Malignant schwannoma
			  a. Malignant schwannoma with rhabdomyoblas differentiation
			  b. Malignant schwannoma with grandular differentiation
			  c. Malignant epithelioid schwannoma
			2. Malignant granul. cell tumour
			3. Malignant melanoma of soft parts
			4. Malignant pigmented neuroectodermal tumour of infanc
			5. Peripheral neuropithelioma
			6. Olfactory neuroblastoma
			7. Soft tissue ependymoma

Autonomic nerve	1. Ganglineuroma 2. Melanocytic schwannoma		1. Neuroblastoma 2. Ganglioneuro-blastoma 3. Malignant melanocytic schwannoma
Cartilage-forming tissue	Extraskeletal chondroma		1. Extraskeletal wel differentiated chondrosarcoma 2. Extraskeletal myxoid chondrosarcoma 3. Extraskeletal mesenchymal-chondrosarcoma

Table 4.1   Classification of soft tissue tumours (*Continued*)

Tissue type/cell	Benign tumours and tumour-like lesions	Tumours of intermediate malignancy	Malignant tumours
Bone-forming tissue	1. Panniculitis ossificans 2. Myositis ossificans 3. Fibrodysplasia (myositis) ossificans progressiva 4. Extraskeletal osteoma		1 Extraskeletal osteosaroma
Uncertain histogenesis	1. Congenital (gingival) granular cell tumour 2. Tumoural calcinosis 3. Myxoma 4. Amyloid tumour 5. Parachordoma		1. Alveolar soft part sarcoma 2. Epithelioid sarcoma 3. Extraskeletal Ewing's sarcoma 4. Extrarenal rhabdoid tumour 5. Malignant mesenchymoma

Unclassified soft tissue tumours and tumourlike lesions

cranial fasciitis (Lauer & Enzinger 1979) and **intravascular fasciitis** (Patchefsky & Enzinger 1981) have now been recognised as variants.

2. Proliferative fasciitis

This lesion of adult life is similar to nodular fasciitis with respect to location, rapidity of growth, and self-limited nature, however it is distinguished by the presence of large basophilic cells resembling ganglion cells (Chung & Enzinger 1975).

3. Proliferative myositis

Often misinterpreted as sarcoma, this is the muscular counterpart of proliferative fasciitis (Enzinger & Dulcey 1967).

4. Fibroma of tendon sheath

This fibrous nodule is firmly attached to the tendon sheath and most frequently found in the hands and feet (Chung & Enzinger 1979, Pulitzer et al 1989).

5. Elastofibroma

This is a poorly circumscribed tumour-like degenerative lesion involving almost exclusively the subscapular region of elderly individuals (Järvi & Saxén 1961).

6. Nasopharyngeal angiofibroma

This is a relatively uncommon benign tumour that occurs almost exclusively in teenage males. Some believe that the lesion represents a variant of the angioma (Sternberg 1954).

7. Keloid

This overgrowth of scar tissue occurs primarily in the corium and is characterised by the presence of thick glassy collagen bundles (Blackburn & Cosma 1966).

Fibromatoses

These non-metastasising fibrous tumours tend to invade locally and recur after surgical excision (Stout 1954, Allen 1977).

1. Superficial (fascial) fibromatoses

Palmar fibromatosis. This aponeurotic nodular proliferation often leads to contracture of the fingers (Dupuytren's contracture).

Plantar fibromatosis (Ledderhose's disease). This rarely causes contracture of the toes.

Penile fibromatosis (Peyronie's disease). This lesion affects the fascial structures and fibrous septa of the corpora cavernosa and the corpus spongiosum. Some have suggested that this subtype may have an inflammatory or vasculitic aetiology.

Knuckle pads. Knuckle pads may be associated with both palmar and plantar fibromatosis (Lagier & Meinecke 1975). The lesion is marked by flat or dome-shaped fibrous thickening over the extensor surfaces of the proximal interphalangeal or metacarpophalangeal joints.

2. Deep (musculoaponeurotic) fibromatoses

Unlike superficial fibromatoses, these lesions tend to be locally aggressive in behaviour and principally involve the deep musculature of the trunk and the extremities.

Abdominal and intra-abdominal fibromatoses. Abdominal fibromatosis is a locally aggressive, infiltrative fibroblastic tumour, arising from musculoaponeurotic structures of the abdominal wall. Intra-abdominal fibromatosis, essentially a variant of abdominal fibromatosis, may be subclassified into 'pelvic fibromatosis' or 'mesenteric fibromatosis', and is often associated with Gardner's syndrome.

Extra-abdominal fibromatosis. This chiefly affects the muscles of the shoulder, pelvic girdles and thighs of adolescents and young adults. Because of its innocuous microscopic appearance, its potential to infiltrate neighbouring tissues, and its high recurrence rate, this tumour poses a difficult problem in recognition and management.

Fibrous tumours of infancy and childhood

Fibromatoses occurring in adults are usually well-defined and clearly recognisable lesions; however, those affecting infants and children show more variability and differ in their histological appearance. Since Stout's original series on juvenile fibromatosis (1954) many fibromatous tumours have been recognised and categorised as distinct entities (Chung 1985).

1. Fibrous hamartoma of infancy

This unique tumour was originally reported by Reye in 1956 as a 'subdermal fibromatous tumour of infancy'; however, because of its organoid growth pattern of superfluous tissue, Enzinger in 1965 (1965a) suggested this now widely accepted designation.

2. Infantile digital fibromatosis

This tumour of the fingers and toes (Shapiro 1969) is characterised by a high local recurrence rate (Rosenberg et al 1978) and the presence of distinctive intracytoplasmic inclusion bodies within proliferating fibroblasts (Reye 1965).

3. Infantile myofibromatosis: solitary and multicentric types

Congenital generalized fibromatosis was first described by Stout in 1954. Additional cases have since been reported under different names reflecting the various histological appearances and histogenetic hypotheses (Beatty 1962). The term 'myofibromatosis' is preferred because of the tumour's microscopic resemblance to smooth muscle tissue and the need for a clearer distinction from the more locally aggressive infantile fibromatosis of the desmoid type.

These lesions clinically present as two major types, solitary and multicentric. In larger lesions, there is usually a distinct zoning phenomenon with a central hemangiopericytoma-like area and peripheral short fascicles of myofibroblasts (Chung & Enzinger 1981).

4. Juvenile hyalin fibromatosis

Exhibiting an autosomal recessive pattern of inheritance (Kitano et al 1972), this disease is characterised by the presence of multiple cutaneous tumours throughout the body particularly in the scalp, clinically resembling turban tumours (Drescher et al 1967). The lesions are composed of streaks of spindle cells embedded in abundant homogeneous eosinophilic ground substance (Remberger et al 1985).

5. Gingival fibromatosis

This condition is marked clinically by a slowly-growing, ill-defined swelling of the gums and manifests as an autosomal dominant disease that often affects several members of the family. These lesions are commonly observed during the eruption of deciduous teeth (Farrer-Brown et al 1972).

6. Fibromatosis colli

This lesion usually appears during the first weeks of life, often associated with muscular torticollis or wryneck. Congenital muscular torticollis represents fibromatosis limited to the sternocleidomastoid muscle (Coventry et al 1960).

7. Infantile (desmoid-type) fibromatosis

This exhibits considerable histomorphological variation, ranging from immature mesenchymal lesions to mature lesions which closely resemble adult musculoaponeurotic fibromatosis. Its more cellular variant has been known as 'agressive infantile fibromatosis', implying difficulty in distinguishing it from infantile fibrosarcoma (Chung & Enzinger 1976).

8. Calcifying aponeurotic fibroma

This distinctive tumour, first described as juvenile aponeurotic fibroma (Keasbey 1953), shows a predilection for the palms and soles. Some consider it to be a cartilage analogue of fibromatosis (Lichtenstein & Goldman 1964).

9. Giant cell fibroblastoma

This new entity, described in 1982 by Shmookler and Enzinger occurs most often in children younger than 10 years of age with a slight predilection for the back and thigh. Tumours are characterised histologically by a mixture of fibroblasts and floret giant cells in a myxoid or collagenised fibrous tissue and the presence of clefts and cystic or sinusoidal spaces (Dymock et al 1987, Fletcher 1988)

Malignant tumours of fibrous tissue

Before the era of electron microscopy and immunohistochemistry, fibrosarcomas were greatly overdiagnosed.

1. 'Adult' fibrosarcomas

Comprising less than 12% of all sarcomas (Pritchard et al 1974), fibrosarcoma consists of interlacing fascicles of spindle cells surrounded by abundant reticulin fibers, often forming a herringbone pattern. There have been well-documented cases of fibrosarcoma arising in scar tissue — cicatricial fibrosarcoma (Fleming & Rezek 1941, Stout 1948) and radiation-induced fibrosarcoma (Schwartz & Rothstein 1968, Gane et al 1970).

2. Congenital and infantile fibrosarcoma

Compared with adult fibrosarcoma, congenital (Balsaver et al 1967), infantile or juvenile fibrosarcoma (Stout 1962b) is similar in its histological picture; however, its clinical course is much more favourable. Despite rapid growth and a high degree of cellularity, most are cured by wide local excision (Chung & Enzinger 1976).

FIBROHISTIOCYTIC TUMOURS

The designation of 'fibrohistiocytic lesions' is more descriptive than conceptual. Both benign and malignant fibrohistiocytic tumours are marked by the presence of cells resembling normal histiocytes and fibroblasts.

Benign fibrohistiocytic tumours

1. Xanthoma

This reactive histiocytic proliferation often occurs in response to alterations in serum lipids.

2. Juvenile xanthogranuloma

Originally termed 'naevo-xantho-endothelioma' (McDonagh 1912) this lesion is distinct from ordinary xanthomas; however, the cells are neither naevoid nor endothelial (Helwig & Hackney 1954). Up to 15% arise in adolescence or early adulthood (Sonoda et al 1985).

3. Reticulohistiocytoma

This lesion may occur either as a localised cutaneous form (reticulohistiocytoma or reticulohistiocytic granuloma), or as a part of a systemic disease (multicentric reticulohistiocytosis or lipoid dermatoarthritis) (Albert et al 1960). Both forms occur almost exclusively in adults and are regarded as exaggerated reactive processes to an unknown stimulus (Purvis & Helwig 1954, Barrow & Holubar 1969).

4. Fibrous histiocytoma

This benign unencapsulated tumour is composed of a variable admixture of fibroblastic and histocytic cells often arranged in the dermis in a storiform or cartwheel pattern and accompanied by foamy macrophages and siderophages.

Cutaneous fibrous histiocytoma. This lesion is alternatively known as dermatofibroma, nodular subepidermal fibrosis, histiocytoma or sclerosing hemangioma (Gross & Wolbach 1943, Rentiers & Montgomery 1949, Niemi 1970).

Deeply situated fibrous histiocytoma. This subtype tends to be larger and better circumscribed than the cutaneous form (Fletcher 1990).

Fibrohistiocytic tumours of intermediate malignancy

1. Dermatofibrosarcoma protuberans (DFSP)

Bearing a histological similarity to fibrous histiocytoma, often with a distinct storiform pattern, this lesion has a greater propensity for local recurrence and gives rise to mestastases rarely (Fletcher et al 1985).

2. Bednář tumour

Originally described as 'storiform neurofibroma' (Bednář 1957), these cutaneous tumours resemble DFSP in both biological behaviour and appearance. They are distinguished by the presence of melanin-bearing dendritic cells — pigmented dermatofibrosarcoma protuberans (Dupree et al 1985, Fletcher et al 1988).

3. Plexiform fibrohistiocytic tumour

This recently described entity affects mainly young patients, is centred on the dermal/subcutaneous junction and frequently recurs. Rarely, it may metastasise to lymph nodes (Enzinger & Zhang 1988).

Malignant fibrohistiocytic tumours

Malignant fibrous histiocytoma (MFH), also known as maglinant fibrous xanthoma (O'Brien & Stout 1964, Enzinger 1979a,b) or fibroxanthosarcoma (Merkow et al 1971, Kempson & Kyriakos 1972), is most common in patients in the fifth to seventh decades of life, typically occurring in the extremities and the retroperitoneum.

1. Atypical fibroxanthoma (Malignant fibrous histiocytoma: superficial type)

First described in 1963 by Helwig, this tumour is histologically indistinguishable from the pleomorphic type of MFH and is best regarded as a superficial form of MFH (Enzinger 1979a). Metastasis is exceedingly rare.

2. Malignant fibrous histiocytoma: myxoid type

Also known as myxofibrosarcoma (Angervall et al 1977), more than half of this tumour appears myxoid (Weiss & Enzinger 1977). Subcutaneous origin is common.

3. Malignant fibrous histiocytoma: inflammatory type

This group has also been called malignant fibrous xanthoma and xanthosarcoma (Kahn 1973), and shows a predilection for the retroperitoneum.

4. Malignant fibrous histiocytoma: pleomorphic type

This relatively common form of MFH has a highly variable morphological pattern and in the past has been diagnosed as pleomorphic forms of fibrosarcoma, liposarcoma or rhabdomyosarcoma (Weiss & Enzinger 1978).

5. Malignant fibrous histiocytoma: giant cell type

This is also known as malignant giant cell tumour of soft parts (Guccion & Enzinger 1972).

6. Malignant fibrous histiocytoma: angiomatoid type

A more recently described entity occurring in a significantly younger age group (Enzinger 1979b), this condition is characterised by solid nodular masses of fibroblast- and histocyte-like cells that surround blood-filled spaces accompanied at the periphery by a marked lymphoplasmacytic infiltrate. It carries a much better prognosis than the other subtypes.

TUMOURS AND TUMOURLIKE LESIONS OF ADIPOSE TISSUE

Benign tumours of adipose tissue

1. Lipoma

Often presenting as a single subcutaneous, painless mass, this lesion is composed of mature adipose tissue with no cellular atypia, but may contain an appreciable amount of fibrous tissue (fibrolipoma) or diplay extensive myxoid change (myxolipoma).

Approximately 6–7% of all patients with lipomas have multiple tumours (Adair et al 1932). Not uncommonly, multiple lipomas are arranged in a symmetrical distribution. Some cases demonstrate a familial involvement with an autosomal dominant inheritance pattern (Stephens & Isaacson 1959).

2. Angiolipoma

Angiolipoma occurs chiefly as a subcutaneous nodule on the forearm of young adults. Multiple angiolipomas are more common than solitary ones (Howard & Helwig 1960).

3. Spindle cell and pleomorphic lipoma

Spindle cell lipoma typically occurs in the regions of the shoulder and posterior neck of elderly men (Enzinger & Harvey 1975). It is composed of an admixture of mature lipocytes and uniform spindle cells set in a mucinous and fibrous background.

The clinical setting and gross appearance of the **pleomorphic lipoma** are similar to those of spindle cell lipoma; however, it is distinguished by the presence of bizarre giant cells having a floret arrangement of nuclei and stromal fibrosis. Superficially, it resembles of sclerosing or pleomorphic liposarcoma (Shmookler & Enzinger 1981).

4. Lipoblastoma and lipoblastomatosis

Lipoblastomatosis is usually noted during the first three years of life, primarily affecting the extremities (Vellios et al 1958). Two subtypes are: lipoblastoma which is encapsulated and confined to the subcutis and lipoblastomatosis which tends to be infiltrative and deeply situated (Chung & Enzinger 1973).

5. Angiomyolipoma

This benign tumour occurs in the kidney or rarely as a separate tumour in close proximity to the kidney.

6. Myelolipoma

This tumour-like lesion occurs most commonly in the adrenal glands but may also be found in the retroperitoneal and pelvic regions. It is usually unassociated with any haematopoietic disorder (Enzinger et al 1969).

7. Intramuscular lipoma

Also referred to as infiltrating lipomas, these tumours chiefly affect adults in the muscles of the lower extremities, especially those of the thigh, and trunk (Enzinger 1977, Fletcher & Martin-Bates 1988).

8. Diffuse lipomatosis

This is a rare diffuse overgrowth of mature adipose tissue involving a large portion of an extremity or the trunk. It chiefly affects children.

9. Hibernoma

This is an uncommon benign tumour which chiefly affects adults and predominates in the interscapular region followed by the axilla, mediastinum, and neck (Levine 1972, Allen 1981). This histological similarity of the tumour to the brown fat of hibernating animals is supported by ultrastructural findings (Seemayer et al 1975).

Malignant tumours of adipose tissue

Liposarcoma is one of the most common soft tissue sarcomas and primarily occurs in adults. It is most frequently found in the extremities, particularly the thigh, and the retroperitoneum (Enzinger & Winslow 1962).

1. Well-differentiated liposarcoma

These tumours, particularly the lipoma-like and sclerosing types which display characteristic tumour cells with large hyperchromatic nuclei but equivocal lipoblasts, are nearly always non-metastasising neoplasms, suggesting the term 'atypical lipoma' (Evans et al 1979, Azumi et al 1987). However, they may recur and cause a compression effect by their large size.

The inflammatory type is marked by a prominent lymphoplasmacytic infiltrate with a background of lipogenic tumour with only occasional lipoblasts or atypical cells with hyperchromatic nuclei.

2. Myxoid liposarcoma

By far the most common type of liposarcoma (Enzinger & Winslow 1962, Evans 1979, Allen 1981), this is composed of widely separated round to fusiform or stellate mesenchymal cells and lipoblasts set in a myxoid stroma accompanied by a delicate plexiform capillary network.

3. Round cell liposarcoma

This represents a poorly differentiated form of myxoid liposarcoma (Evans 1979), but deserves separate recognition because of its prominent tendency to metastasise.

4. Pleomorphic liposarcoma

The most anaplastic type of liposarcoma (Enzinger & Winslow 1962, Allen 1981), this may be difficult to distinguish from MFH in the absence of characteristic lipoblasts.

5. Dedifferentiated liposarcoma

Also called mixed liposarcoma (Allen 1981), this lesion exhibits mixed histological patterns showing either the well-differentiated liposarcoma or sometimes the myxoid liposarcoma with poorly differentiated areas that may resemble MFH or be composed of undifferentiated mesenchymal cells (Evans 1979).

TUMOURS OF MUSCLE TISSUE

Smooth muscle tumours – benign tumours of smooth muscle

These tumours occur more frequently in the female genital and gastrointestinal tracts and less commonly in the skin and subcutis (Stout & Lattes 1967). They are typified by the presence of longitudinal myofibrils. Leiomyomatosis peritonealis disseminata and intravenous leiomyomatosis are usually not considered to be soft tissue tumours.

1. Leiomyoma

The cutaneous leiomyomas are subcategorised into two types: leiomyomas of pilar arrector origin and genital leiomyomas (Stout 1937).

Leiomyomas of deep soft tissue are uncommon. Most are located in the extremities, within the abdominal cavity or retroperitoneum and are prone to undergo regressive changes. Rarely these tumours display areas of nuclear atypia, unassociated with mitotic activity, which are usually attributable to degenerative changes and such cases are referred to as pleomorphic leiomyomas.

2. Angioleiomyoma

Also called vascular leiomyoma (Stout 1937), this solitary tumour arises from the wall of blood vessels typically located in the subcutis of the lower extremities (Hachisuga et al 1984).

3. Epithelioid leiomyoma

Alternatively known as bizarre leiomyoma and leiomyoblastoma (Stout 1962a, Appelman & Helwig 1976), this lesion is characterised by round or polygonal cells with acidophilic cytoplasm and a perinuclear clear zone. Their smooth muscle nature has been confirmed by electron microscopy (Salazar & Totten 1970). These tumours show a striking predilection to occur in the abdominal cavity, gastrointestinal tract and sometimes the uterus.

Malignant tumours of smooth muscle

1. Leiomyosarcoma

These are more prevalent in the gastrointestinal and female genital tracts. In soft tissue, they are found most commonly in the retroperitoneum, and less often in the omentum and mesentery (Russell et al 1977) and in the skin and subcutaneous tissue of the proximal extremities (Dahl & Angervall 1974).

2. Epithelioid leiomyosarcoma

Although similar to their benign counterparts, these neoplastic cells are less mature and exhibit a greater degree of pleomorphism and mitotic activity. Non-visceral, soft tissue origin is rare.

Striated muscle tumours — benign tumours of striated muscle

Rhabdomyomas are usually classified clinically as well as histomorphologically.

1. Adult rhabdomyoma

These occur principally in adults with a mean age of 56 years (Corio & Lewis 1979) and are virtually confined to the head and neck region, particularly in the tongue and larynx (Moran & Enterline 1964).

2. Fetal rhabdomyoma

First reported by Dehner et al 1972, this relatively rare tumour occurs chiefly in children before the age of 3 years, most commonly in the subcutaneous tissues of the head and neck, especially the posterior auricular area (Dehner et al 1972).

3. Genital rhabdomyoma

Although this bears some resemblance to both adult and fetal rhabdomyomas (particularly to the latter), it usually presents as a polypoid mass in the vagina or vulva of women in their 30s and 40s (di Sant' Agnese & Knowles 1980) and tends to have a myxoid quality (Gee & Finckh 1977).

Malignant tumours of striated muscle

The most common childhood soft tissue sarcomas are rhabdomyosarcomas (Gonzalez-Crussi & Black-Schaffer 1979). These tumours are divided into three major categories: embryonal, alveolar and pleomorphic. The embryonal and alveolar types are also collectively known as juvenile rhabdomyosarcoma as opposed to adult rhabdomyosarcoma, the pleomorphic type (Stout & Lattes 1967).

1. Embryonal rhabdomyosarcoma

This is the most common type of rhabdomyosarcoma (Gonzalez-Crussi & Black-Schaffer 1979). It occurs predominantly in younger children, commonly in the head and neck region, retroperitoneum, bile ducts and urogenital tract (Masson & Soule 1965). When growing beneath a mucous membrane the tumour often assumes the shape of large polypoid masses resembling a bunch of grapes, hence the name **sarcoma botryoides**.

2. Alveolar rhabdomyosarcoma

This predominates in older children and young adults (Enterline & Horn 1958, Enzinger & Shiraki 1969), occurring more frequently in the extremities and is associated with a worse prognosis than the embryonal type (Enzinger & Shiraki 1969).

3. Pleomorphic rhabdomyosarcoma

This is the least common of the three basic types of rhabdomyosarcoma. It almost always occurs in adults primarily in the large muscles of the extremities especially the thigh (Enzinger 1965b).

4. Mixed rhabdomyosarcoma

Occasionally, there is an overlapping among the aforementioned types of rhabdomyosarcoma, i.e. embryonal rhabdomyosarcoma with areas of alveolar or pleomorphic features, sometimes referred to as mixed rhabdomyosarcoma.

5. Rhabdomyosarcoma with ganglion cells (malignant ectomesenchymoma)

This is a rare tumour that occurs mostly in the retroperitoneum, scrotum, perineum and face of infants and small children (Kawamoto et al 1987). The lesion consists of a mixture of rhabdomyosarcomatous features, ganglion cells and neuroma-like areas which are believed to be derived from the migratory neural crest (ectomesenchyme), hence the designation **ectomesenchymoma** (Karcioglu et al 1977).

TUMOURS AND TUMOURLIKE LESIONS OF BLOOD VESSELS

Benign tumours of blood vessels

Haemangiomas are broadly divided into two groups:

A. Localized haemangiomas are far more common and usually these are superficially located with a predilection for the head and neck region (Martin & MacCollum 1961) however, they may also involve deep structures, such as skeletal muscle.

B. Diffuse haemangiomas, commonly known as angiomatosis, involve large segments of the body such as an entire extremity and deserve specific recognition.

A. Localized haemangioma

1. Capillary haemangioma

Capillary haemangiomas represent the most common of all types.

Juvenile haemangioma is an immature form of capillary haemangioma which occurs in the first year of life. It is variously known as hypertrophic angioma, cellular haemangioma of infancy, infantile or juvenile haemangio-endothelioma, benign haemangioendothelioma of infancy and strawberry naeves.

2. Cavernous haemangioma

These are composed of large dilated blood-filled vessels lined by a flattened endothelium.

3. Arteriovenous haemangioma

These are divided into two subtypes: deep and superficial. The deep form usually occurs in young persons and is generally regarded as an arteriovenous malformation (Ward & Horton 1940). The superficial form occurs exclusively in adults as a small asymptomatic cutaneous nodule (Girard et al 1974).

4. Venous haemangioma

These are typically present during adult life and occur most commonly in deep locations, particularly in the retroperitoneum and the mesentery.

5. Epithelioid haemangioma

Also known as Kimura's disease (Kawada et al 1965), angiolymphoid hyperplasia with eosinophilia (Wells & Whimster 1969), pseudopyogenic granuloma (Kandil 1970) and histiocytoid haemangioma (Rosai et al 1979), these lesions characteristically occur in young adults in the head and neck region, particularly in the vicinity of ear. Despite the prominent inflammatory response, these lesions are regarded as neoplastic processes (Weiss & Enzinger 1982).

6. Granulation tissue-type haemangioma

This histological picture of an uncomplicated early lesion of granuloma pyogenicum, or eruptive haemangioma (Marsch 1981) is essentially that of an ordinary lobulated capillary haemangioma, except for its distinctive polypoid appearance. The gingiva is a common site and pregnancy is often a precipitating factor (granuloma gravidarum). The intravenous form of pyogenic granuloma, in contrast to the mucocutaneous form, shows virtually no inflammatory changes (Cooper et al 1979).

Deep haemangioma: 1. Intramuscular haemangioma

Among the vascular tumours of deep soft tissue, the intramuscular haeman-gioma is the most common form, most frequently occurring in young adults in the lower extremity, particularly the muscles of the thigh. Intermingled with the proliferating blood vessels there is often overgrowth of adipose tissue giving an impression of angiolipoma (Allen & Enzinger 1972).

2. Synovial haemangioma

This type of intra-articular cavernous haemangioma grows either as a discrete polypoid lesion or as a diffuse process, usually in the knee joint (Cobey 1943).

3. Intraneural haemangioma

Most of these extremely rare tumours are basically cavernous haemangiomas (Losli 1952).

B. Diffuse haemangioma

Popularly known as angiomatosis, this is characterised by an irregular vascular pattern in which vessels of varying size are often accompanied by a large amount of mature fat. Angiomatosis prevails in children during the early growth period.

Telangiectasia is a relatively common vascular lesion (Johnson 1976). The vascular ectasias, including systemic angiomatosis of congenital origin, are all excluded from this classification.

Glomus tumour

Also known as **glomangioma**, this is predominantly a tumour of adult life. It is derived from the neuromyoarterial glomus (Stout 1935b) and found most commonly in the distal portion of the extremities. Occasional cases contain smooth muscle (glomangiomyoma).

Haemangiopericytoma

This uncommon neoplasm was first described by Stout and Murray in 1942 as a less organoid type of glomus tumour. It is often deep seated and most commonly found in the lower extremity, retroperitoneum, head and neck region and trunk (Enzinger & Smith 1976).

Congenital or infantile haemangiopericytoma merits distinction as a specific entity because of its exclusive occurrence during infancy and its benign clinical behaviour, despite the presence of mitotic activity and necrosis which are often the diagnostic features that indicate malignancy in adult haemangiopericytoma (Enzinger & Smith 1976). It is located almost exclusively in the subcutaneous tissue as a multilobular mass.

REACTIVE VASCULAR PROLIFERATIONS MIMICKING ANGIOSARCOMA

1. Papillary endothelial hyperplasia

Also called vegetant intravascular haemangioendothelioma (Masson 1970), this lesion is thought to be a peculiar variant of an organising thrombus (Clearkin & Enzinger 1976).

2. Nodal angiomatosis

Reactive vascular proliferation is occasionally encountered in the subcapsular region of draining lymph nodes where there is obstruction of afferent lymphatics, particularly in axillary lymph nodes at the time of mastectomy for breast carcinoma (Fayemis & Toker 1975). This lesion may sometimes mimic nodal involvement by Kaposi's sarcoma in its early development.

Vascular tumours of borderline or intermediate malignancy

The term haemangioendothelioma is currently used to indicate borderline or intermediate malignancy (Weiss & Enzinger 1982), although it is often regarded as a synonym for angiosarcoma by some (Taxy & Gray 1979).

1. Epithelioid haemangioendothelioma

This tumour of adult life occurs in either superficial or deep soft tissue, most commonly in the extremities. The solid growth pattern and the epithelioid appearance of the tumour cells frequently lead to confusion with metastatic carcinoma (Weiss & Enzinger 1982, Weiss et al 1986).

2. Spindle cell haemangioendothelioma

This low grade angiosarcoma is characterised by combined features of both a cavernous haemangioma and Kaposi's sarcoma (Weiss & Enzinger 1986). Typically, it develops in the dermis and subcutaneous tissue of the distal extremities in a multifocal pattern and only rarely metastasises.

3. Malignant endovascular papillary angioendothelioma

This rare but distinctive tumour occurs primarily in the skin and subcutis of infants and young children (Dabska 1969, Manivel et al 1986). It is characterised by intravascular tuftlike or glomeruloid papillations, often with central hyaline cores.

Malignant vascular tumours

Although rare, these have been described in most organs and systems and are known generically as angiosarcoma (Rosai et al 1976). By inference, angiosarcomas arising in the clinical setting of lymphoedema have been designated lymphangiosarcoma, yet, may reveal both haemangiomatous and lymphangiomatous differentiation.

1. Angiosarcoma

This is characterised by the formation of irregular anastomosing vascular channels lined by one or more layers of atypical endothelial cells often of immature appearance. They occur most commonly in the skin and soft tissue, especially in the scalp or face of elderly and less so in the breast. Cutaneous angiosarcomas of this type are not associated with lymphoedema (Holden et al 1987).

Postmastectomy lymphangiosarcoma is a well-defined clinicopathological entity (Stewart & Treves 1948), arising in most cases after lymphoedema of around 20 years duration (Woodward et al 1972). Histologically, these lesions are essentially identical to those of cutaneous angiosarcoma unassociated with lymphoedema. It is now realised that any type of lymphoedema (including congenital and filarial) may develop this complication.

Angiosarcoma of the breast, a rare tumour, occurs exclusively in women usually during the third or fourth decade. It is the most malignant of all breast tumours (McDivitt et al 1966).

2. Kaposi's sarcoma

Kaposi's sarcoma occurs predominantly in elderly males, young African blacks and homosexual men (Dorfman 1984). The mature phase of Kaposi's sarcoma is characterised by the presence of spindle cell areas containing vascular slits with erythrocytes and deposits of hemosiderin. Ultrastructural studies have provided the best evidence in support of the vascular origin of this lesion (Mottaz & Zelickson 1966).

3. Malignant glomus tumour

Also called glomangiosarcomas, these exceedingly rare lesions have arisen in a pre-existing glomus tumour and consist of short spindle cells having features resembling the immature form of fibrosarcoma or leiomyosarcoma. None has metastasised (Kuhn & Rosai 1969, Lumley & Stansfeld 1972).

4. Malignant haemangiopericytoma

Haemangiopericytomas that metastasise often exhibit increased cellularity, brisk mitoses, foci of haemorrhage and necrosis (Enzinger & Smith 1976).

TUMOURS OF LYMPH VESSELS

Benign tumours of lymph vessels

Most of the benign tumours of lymph vessels represent hamartomas or malformations rather than true neoplasms.

1. Lymphangioma

Although traditionally divided into three types: capillary, cavernous and cystic, these all comprise a single group of lesions (Bill & Summer 1965). Capillary lymphangiomas are exceedingly rare and are difficult to distinguish from capillary haemangiomas. **Cystic lymphangiomas or hygromas** occur in the regions of neck and axilla. **Cavernous lymphangiomas** are found most commonly in the mouth, tongue and cheek.

More than half are present at birth (Bill & Summer 1965). Those which appear during adult life are localised lymphangioma circumscriptum or superficial cutaneous lymphangiomas, some of which apparently represent acquired lymphangiectasias (Fisher & Orkin 1970).

2. Lymphangiomatosis

An extremely rare disease in which lymphangiomas involve soft tissue and other organs in a diffuse or multifocal manner, this is essentially the lymphatic counterpart of angiomatosis. Like angiomatosis, this disease occurs principally in children.

3. Lymphangiomyoma and Lymphangiomyomatosis

Lymphangiomyoma is the currently accepted term for a benign tumour originally named lymphangiopericytoma (Cornog & Enterline 1966, Wolff 1973). When it involves large segments of the lymphatic chain, the term lymphangiomyomatosis is the preferred designation. These lesions are characterised by a tumour-like proliferation of smooth muscle in the lymphatics of the mediastinum, retroperitoneum and the lung, in close association with the thoracic duct and its tributaries (Wolff 1973). It occurs exclusively in females.

Malignant tumours of lymph vessels

Lymphangiosarcoma

These tumours have been observed exclusively in conjunction with chronic long-standing lymph stasis, usually secondary to radical mastectomy (post-mastectomy lymphangiosarcoma) or chronic lymphoedema of the lower extremities (Herrman 1965). They are composed of areas resembling haemangiosarcoma and groups of endothelium-lined empty spaces suggesting lymphatics. Thus the collective term angiosarcoma is used for this type of tumour instead of lymphangiosarcoma.

TUMOURS AND TUMOUR-LIKE LESIONS OF SYNOVIAL TISSUE

Benign tumours and tumour-like lesions of synovial tissue

Giant cell tumour of tendon sheath (GCTTS) is the most common tumour of synovial tissue.

1. Localized giant cell tumour of tendon sheath

Often referred to as nodular tenosynovitis, this primarily affects the fingers arising from the synovium of tendon sheath or region of the interphalangeal joint. As a rule, those on the feet are larger and more irregular in shape than those on the hands (Jones et al 1969).

2. Diffuse giant cell tumour of tendon sheath

This form occurs in areas adjacent to large weight-bearing joints, such as the knee and ankle, and in most cases it represents an extra-articular extension of pigmented villonodular synovitis.

Malignant tumours of synovial tissue

1. Malignant giant cell tumour of tendon sheath

This designation should be reserved for lesions in which benign GCTTS coexists with, or recurs as, an obvious malignant tumour (Carstens & Howell 1979).

2. Synovial sarcoma

Although most prevalent in the extremities about the large joints, this neoplasm is also encountered in areas without apparent relationship to synovial structures, as in the parapharyngeal region, abdominal wall and trunk. It occurs most commonly in young adults and is classified histologically into a biphasic type with distinct epithelial and spindle elements, a predominantly monophasic fibrous or epithelial type and a poorly differentiated type. Actual origin from synovium is now regarded as exceedingly unlikely.

TUMOURS AND TUMOUR-LIKE LESIONS OF PERIPHERAL NERVES

Benign tumours and tumour-like lesions of peripheral nerves

1. Traumatic neuroma

Also known as **amputation neuroma**, this non-neoplastic proliferation of nerve fibres, Schwann cells and scar tissue occurs in response to injury such as surgical or blunt trauma.

2. Morton's neuroma

This represents a reactive overgrowth of perineurial connective tissue that disrupts the nerves (Ariel 1983). It arises from one of the interdigital plantar nerves to form an extremely painful mass near the head of the metastarsal bones. It occurs most frequently in women (Harkin & Reed 1969).

3. Neuromuscular hamartoma

This extremely rare tumour-like lesion is composed of mature nerve and differentiated skeletal muscle fibres and occurs during infancy, intimately associated with a major nerve (Markel & Enzinger 1982).

4. Nerve sheath ganglion

Ganglion cysts rarely occur in intraneural locations. They represent a degenerative process and are usually located within the peroneal nerve (Cobb & Moiel 1974).

5. Neurilemoma

This well-demarcated or encapsulated tumour arises from the sheaths of Schwann (schwannoma) and is distinguished by a pattern of alternating Antoni A and B areas with or without Verocay bodies. Occasionally, the tumours composed exclusively of Antoni A areas displaying hypercellularity are referred to as cellular neurilemmomas that may be easily confused with sarcomas (Woodruff et al 1981, Fletcher et al 1987). Rarely, the cutaneous schwannoma may manifest as a plexiform growth simulating a plexiform neurofibroma. Plexiform neurilemmomas are, however, only rarely associated with von Recklinghausen's disease (Fletcher & Davies 1986, Iwashita & Enjoji

1987). In large tumours, there are often areas of degenerative change which include perivascular hyalinisation, clusters of foamy macrophages, gaping vessels with thrombi and bizarre nuclear atypia without any mitoses. Large neurilemmomas of long duration showing pronounced degenerative changes are known as ancient schwannoma. Neurilemmomas pursue a benign clinical course and rarely recur. For all practical purposes, they virtually never undergo malignant transformation (Abell et al 1970).

6. Solitary circumscribed neuroma

This entity, first described as 'palisaded, encapsulated neuroma' (Reed et al 1972), arises predominantly on the face or adjacent to a mucocutaneous junction and is not associated with either neurofribromatosis or the multiple endocrine neoplasia syndromes (Fletcher 1989).

7. Solitary neurofibroma

These occur in young persons and most of the lesions are superficially located. They may be highly myxoid (myxoid neurofibroma), and may contain a few structures reminiscent of tactile corpuscles that may sometimes predominate (Pacinian neurofibromas). In rare instances, a large portion of the lesion is composed of nests and cords of rounded Schwann cells embedded in a sclerotic stroma (epithelioid neurofibroma). Some tumours exhibit foci of melanocytic differentiation (pigmented neurofibroma). In occasional cases there are groups of cells with granular eosinophilic cytoplasm similar to a granular cell tumour (granular cell neurofibroma).

8. Neurofibromatosis

Commonly known as von Recklinghausen's disease, this autosomal dominant disease has several histological variants.

Localized neurofibroma. This is the most common type. It is typically located in the dermis and subcutis and histologically resemble solitary neurofibroma.

Plexiform neurofibroma. Virtually pathognomic of von Recklinghausen's disease (Harkin & Reed 1969), these lesions are usually deeply situated and involve major nerve trunks. When the lesion involves an entire region such as an extremity and is accompanied by redundant and hyperpigmented skin the condition is known as elephantiasis neuromatosa.

Diffuse neurofibroma. This uncommon but distinctive form occurs principally in the head and neck region of children and young adults. Characteristically, this form contains Wagner-Meissner corpuscles.

9. Granular cell tumour

Granular cell tumours are now accepted as growths of nerve sheath origin, and some prefer the term granular cell schwannma (Fisher & Wechler 1962).

The tumour may arise at virtually any site. Some of the cutaneous and submucosal lesions are associated with marked pseudoepitheliomatous hyperplasia of the overlying squamous epithelium.

10. Myxoid tumour of nerve sheath

Originally known as a myxoma of nerve sheath (Harkin & Reed 1969), it was renamed as neurothekeoma to emphasise its nerve sheath origin (Gallager & Helwig 1980). Usually these are tumours of childhood and early adult life and are most commonly found in the dermis and subcutis of the head, neck and shoulder regions.

11. Extracranial meningioma

These rare tumours arise from the ectopic arachnoid lining cells and are histologically indistinguishable from ordinary intracranial meningiomas. They occur in the skin or soft tissue of the scalp and along the vertebral axis.

12. Pigmented neuroectodermal tumour of infancy

Also known as retinal anlage tumour, melanotic progonoma, melanotic or melanocytic neuroectodermal tumour, this pigmented tumour occurs during the first year of life and usually involves the head and neck region especially the maxilla and sometimes the epididymis, mediastinum and other sites (Dehner et al 1979). It is now believed to be of neural crest origin; however, embryological evidence contradicts the theory of retinal anlage tumour (Borello & Gorlin 1966, Young & Gonzalez-Crussi 1985).

Malignant tumours of peripheral nerves

1. Malignant schwannoma

Also called neurofibrosarcoma, neurogenic sarcoma and neurosarcoma, this arises within a peripheral nerve or from a pre-existing neurofibroma and often resembles a fibrosarcoma. This is typically a disease of adult life and develops in 3–13% of patients with von Recklinghausen's disease (Guccion & Enzinger 1979). There are several histological variants.

Malignant schwannoma with rhabdomyoblastic differentiation. Conventionally known as malignant Triton tumour (Woodruff et al 1973), the hallmark of this tumour is scattered rhabdomyoblasts otherwise indistinguishable from an ordinary malignant schwannoma. Most tumours occur in patients with von Recklinghausen's disease.

Malignant schwannoma with glandular differentiation. Usually referred to as glandular malignant schwannoma, this is characterised histologically by the presence of glands embedded in a background of oridinary malignant schwannoma. They may also contain other heterotopic elements, such as bone and cartilage (Woodruff 1976).

Malignant epithelioid schwannoma. These closely resemble a carcinoma or melanoma (Stout 1935a, DiCarlo et al 1986), but originate in major nerves. They may be found in von Recklinghausen's disease.

The superficial form of malignant epithelioid schwannoma, also known as a neurotropic melanoma (Reed & Leonard 1979), appears to combine features of both malignant melanoma and malignant schwannoma. These tumours occur most commonly on the exposed areas of the head and neck. These lesions are located in the dermis and subcutis and they are made up of short fascicles of spindle to oval cells set in a desmoplastic stroma.

2. Malignant granular cell tumour

This extremely rare tumour is histologically similar to the benign form but can be distinguished on the basis of cellular pleomorphism and mitotic activity. Typically, it recurs before metastasising.

3. Malignant melanoma of soft parts

Since 1965 when Enzinger (Enzinger 1965d) described clear cell sarcoma of tendons and aponeuroses, this tumour has been widely recognised as a distinct entity and has steadily gained acceptance as a tumour of neural crest origin. It affects mainly young adults and occurs almost exclusively in the extremities, particularly in the region of the foot and ankle. In more than two-thirds of the cases, intracellular melanin is demonstrated and S-100 protein is positive (Chung & Enzinger 1983). The presence of melanin may easily be overlooked. Some have considered it as a variant of synovial sarcoma (Hajdu et al 1977), although this would now seem inappropriate.

4. Malignant pigmented neuroectodermal tumour of infancy

Although traditionally considered benign, rare metastases have developed. The metastatic lesions may be devoid of melanin pigment and appear similar to neuroblastoma (Dehner et al 1979).

5. Peripheral neuroepithelioma (adult neuroblastoma)

By definition these tumours do not arise from the sympathetic nervous system and therefore occur mostly outside the vertebral axis of the body, usually in the extremities. Urinary catecholamine metabolites are generally not elevated (Allan et al 1986).

6. Olfactory neuroblastoma

Also called olfactory neuroepithelioma or aesthesioneuroblastoma (Elkon et al 1979), these arise from the nasal cavity and rarely metastasise.

7. Soft tissue ependymoma

Primary soft tissue ependymomas are rare and are thought to arise from the misplaced neural tube. They are typically located in the subcutaneous tissues over the sacrococcygeal area without any underlying spinal lesion. Their appearance, both histological and electron microscopic, is similar to myxo-papillary ependymoma of the filum terminale and cauda equina (Helwig & Stern 1984).

TUMOURS OF AUTONOMIC NERVES

Benign tumours of autonomic nerves

1. Ganglioneuroma

This biologically benign tumour is most often located in the posterior medastinum and retroperitoneum, and composed of relatively mature ganglion cells set in a background of neurofibromatous or neuromatous stroma.

2. Melanocytic schwannoma

This is a rare but distinctive neoplasm of adult life and usually arises from the sympathetic nervous system. It occurs most commonly in the posterior mediastinum followed by the retroperitoneum. Tumours with a low mitotic count apparently pursue a benign clinical course (McGavran et al 1978).

Malignant tumours of autonomic nerves

1. Neuroblastoma

This is one of the most common malignant neoplasms of childhood, most being detected between birth and age four. It originates from primitive neuroblasts within the adrenal medulla or the sympathetic ganglia and is characterised by the presence of Homer-Wright rosettes.

2. Ganglioneuroblastoma

These are intermediate between neuroblastomas and ganglioneuromas in their histological appearance and behaviour. They characteristically occur along the thoracolumbar sympathetic chain.

3. Malignant melanocytic schwannoma

This is a very rare tumour that is essentially similar to its benign counterpart in its distribution. The clinical behaviour of the tumours varies depending on the level of mitotic activity and the feasibility of local wide excision (Mennemeyer et al 1979).

TUMOURS AND TUMOURLIKE LESIONS OF CARTILAGE FORMING TISSUE

Benign cartilaginous tumours of soft tissue

Extraskeletal chondroma

Chondroma of soft parts occurs predominantly in the third and fourth decades of life. These tumours chiefly affect the hands and feet; the fingers are by far the most common site. These lesions are firmly attached to tendon or aponeurosis and are composed of mature hyaline cartilage that often undergoes calcification (Chung & Enzinger 1978).

Malignant cartilaginous tumours of soft tissue

1. Extraskeletal well-differentiated chondrosarcoma

This very rare tumour is usually found in the extremities, deeply seated in muscle. The histological appearance is comparable to chondrosarcomas in bone.

2. Extraskeletal myxoid chondrosarcoma

Also known as **chordoid sarcoma** (Weiss 1976), this tumour occurs primarily in the deep tissues of the extremities (Enzinger & Shiraki 1972). The prognosis is usually good.

3. Extraskeletal mesenchymal chondrosarcoma

This is a tumour of young adults, principally found in the head and neck region, followed by the lower extremities. Unlike myxoid chondrosarcoma, it is a highly malignant neoplasm that pursues a rapid clinical course and metastasises in a high percentage of cases (Guccion et al 1973).

TUMOURS AND TUMOURLIKE LESIONS OF BONE-FORMING TISSUE

Benign osseous tumours and tumourlike lesions of soft tissue

1. Panniculitis ossificans

This benign ossifying process, also referred to as fibro-osseous pseudotumour (Dupree & Enzinger 1986), usually affects young persons and presents as a solitary well circumscribed mass in the subcutaneous tissue of the fingers and the hands.

2. Myositis ossificans

This is by far the most common benign bone-forming lesion of soft tissue. About 50% of cases follow mechanical trauma. In general, the lesion is well circumscribed and characterised histologically by the presence of a distinct zonal pattern reflecting different phases of cellular maturation (Johnson 1948).

3. Fibrodysplasia (myositis) ossificans progressiva

This is a rare hereditary disease that primarily affects children. These lesions are found most commonly in the neck, shoulder and back along the paravertebral region and are almost always associated with symmetrical malformation of the digits. Histologically the early lesion may mimic infantile (desmoid-type) fibromatosis, gradually followed by collagenisation and, later, irregular ossification (Cramer et al 1981).

4. Extraskeletal osteoma

This uncommon benign bone-forming tumour usually occurs in the scalp and extremities of newborn infants or may arise in later life in various locations. Primary cutaneous ossification can occur in Albright's hereditary osteodystrophy and as osteoma cutis (Brook & Valman 1971).

Malignant osseous tumours of soft tissue

Extraskeletal osteosarcoma

This uncommon tumour more often affects older individuals than the histologically identical osteosarcoma of bone. It occurs most commonly in the lower extremities, with a predilection for the thigh, followed by the upper extremities and retroperitoneum (Chung & Enzinger 1987).

TUMOURS AND TUMOUR-LIKE LESIONS OF UNCERTAIN HISTOGENESIS

Benign tumours and tumour-like lesions of uncertain histogenesis

1. Congenital (gingival) granular cell tumour

This tumour is virtually indistinguishable histologically from the conventional granular cell tumour of nerve sheath origin. The lesion occurs exclusively in infants and is characterised clinically by a pedunculated epulis-like growth at birth. Occasional tumours have been shown to regress spontaneously. Some consider it to be a peculiar reactive or degenerative process, modulated in part by hormonal factors. Others suggests that granular cells arise from epithelium related to the dental lamina (Lack et al 1981).

2. Tumoural calcinosis

This distinct entity is characterised by a large periarticular deposition of calcium, resembling a neoplasm, most commonly in the regions of the large joints. Although some suggest it is due to an inborn error of metabolism (Lafferty et al 1965), there are no demonstrable abnormalities in calcium metabolism, and the pathogenesis of tumoural calcinosis remains obscure.

3. Myxoma

These are benign tumours of unknown histogenesis that occur in a variety of locations, such as the heart, jaw bones, skin, aponeurotic tissue and skeletal muscle (Stout & Lattes 1967). These lesions are characterised by the presence of abundant myxoid material, a small number of inconspicous stellate or spindle-shaped cells and a paucity of blood vessels. Well-known myxoid lesions include: cutaneous focal mucinosis, cutaneous myxoid cyst, juxtaarticular myxoma and meniscal cyst, localized myxedema, and ganglion (cyst). The skeletal muscle lesion poses considerable problems in diagnosis.

Intramuscular myxoma is a tumour of adult life and most frequently affect the large muscles of the thigh, shoulder and buttocks (Enzinger 1965c). The great majority are solitary. Nearly all multiple myxomas are associated with fibrous dysplasia of bone, usually the monostotic type (Wirth et al 1971).

A locally aggressive myxoid tumour affecting the soft tissue of the female pelvis and perineum has been reported under the designation of angiomyxoma (Steeper & Rosai 1983).

4. Amyloid tumour

Amyloid tumours in soft tissue, unassociated with plasmacytoma or secondary amyloidosis, are extremely rare. They occur in the region of the groin, abdominal wall, breast, neck and orbit. Tumours of small size have also been observed in the eyelids and the skin. In general, serum proteins are normal in these patients, and the histogenesis remains uncertain.

5. Parachordoma

This rare tumour of uncertain histogenesis affects both children and adults and occurs most commonly in the extremities or peripheral parts of the body. It usually involves the soft tissues adjacent to tendon, synovium or osseous structures and consist of nests of pale staining or vacuolated rounded cells resembling those of the chorda dorsalis or notochord in an embryo (Dabska 1977).

Malignant tumours of uncertain histogenesis

1. Alveolar soft part sarcoma

Originally named in 1952 by Christopherson et al, this tumour has also been designated as malignant organoid granular cell myoblastoma and malignant non-chromaffin paraganglioma, although there is no evidence to support it to be of paraganglionic, schwannian or myogenic origin (Auerbach & Brooks 1987).

This distinct clinicopathological entity is characterised by small organoid aggregates of polygonal, coarsely granular cells separated by thin-walled cleft-like vascular spaces. The neoplastic cells often contain needle-like crystalline material that ultrastructurally represents unique, rhomboid, rod shaped membrane-bound crystals (Shipkey et al 1964).

2. Epithelioid sarcoma

First described by Enzinger in 1970, this tumour most commonly involves the dermis, subcutis or deeper soft tissue of the distal extremities, particularly the fingers, hands and forearms of young adults. It is often misinterpreted histopathologically as a necrobiotic granuloma and sometimes confused with squamous cell carcinoma and malignant melanoma. The histogenesis of epithelioid sarcoma remains uncertain. Primitive mesenchymal cells, histiocytes, fibroblasts and synovial cells have all been implicated (Chase & Enzinger 1985).

3. Extraskeletal Ewing's sarcoma

These are morphologically indistinguishable from Ewing's sarcoma of bone (Angervall & Enzinger 1975). They primarily affect young adults and most commonly involve the soft tissues of the lower extremity and the paravertebral region.

They present clinically as a rapidly growing deep-seated mass. Catecholamines are within normal limits and the histogenesis of Ewing's sarcoma remains unknown; however, recent studies indicate the strong possibility of neuroectodermal origin (Yunis 1986, Cavazzana et al 1987).

4. Extrarenal rhabdoid tumour

Originally described in the kidney (Haas et al 1981), this rare tumour may present at a wide variety of sites and is commonest in childhood (Sotelo-Avila et al 1986). It is characterised by intracytoplasmic hyaline inclusions, corresponding to paranuclear whorls of intermediate filaments, and is immunohistochemically heterogeneous.

Malignant mesenchymoma

This is a heterogenous group of neoplasms, which are composed of two or more unrelated malignant elements (Stout & Lattes 1967). Some are characterised by the coexistence of rhabdomyosarcomatous and liposarcomatous elements, while others consist of a specific type of sarcoma together with focal malignant cartilaginous or osseous tissue. Although the malignant Triton tumour and malignant ectomesenchymoma meet the same criteria, they deserve separate recognition.

These occur most commonly in the extremities and the retroperitoneum and are generally thought to arise from uncommitted primitive mesenchymal cells that have differentiated into multiple cell lines.

UNCLASSIFIED SOFT TISSUE TUMOURS AND TUMOURLIKE LESIONS

This category includes any primary tumour of soft tissue that cannot be placed in one of the aforementioned categories. It is estimated that approximately 10% of all sarcomas cannot be classified because of the quality of the available material and irrespective of the experience and knowledge of examining pathologists (Enzinger & Weiss 1983).

REFERENCES

Adair F E, Pack G T, Farrior J H 1932 Lipomas. American Journal of Cancer 16: 1104–1120
Albert J, Bruce W, Allen A C, Blank H 1960 Lipoid dermato-arthritis. Reticulohistocytoma of the skin and joints. American Journal of Medicine 28: 661–667
Allan S G, Cornbleet M A, Carmichael J, Arnott S J, Smyth J J 1986 Adult neuroblastoma. Report of three cases and review of the literature. Cancer 57: 2419–2421
Allen P W 1977 The fibromatoses: A clinicopathologic classification based on 140 cases. American Journal of Surgical Pathology 1: 255–270
Allen P W 1981 Tumors and proliferations of adipose tissue: a clinicopathologic approach. Masson Publishing, New York
Allen P W, Enzinger F M 1972 Hemangioma of skeletal muscle. An analysis of 89 cases. Cancer 29: 8–29
Angervall L, Enzinger F M 1975 Extraskeletal neoplasm resembling Ewing's sarcoma. Cancer 36: 240–251
Angervall L, Kindblom L-G, Merck C 1977 Myxofibrosarcoma: a study of 30 cases. Acta Pathologica et Microbiologica Scandinavica Section A 85: 127–140
Appelman H D, Helwig E B 1976 Gastric epithelioid leiomyoma and leiomyosarcoma (leiomyoblastoma). Cancer 38: 708–728
Ariel I M 1983 Tumours of the peripheral nervous system. Ca-A Cancer Journal for Clinicians 33: 282–299
Auerbach H E, Brooks J J 1987 Alveolar soft part sarcoma: A clinicopathologic and immunohistochemical study. Cancer 60: 66–73
Azumi N, Curtis J, Kempson R L, Henderickson M R 1987 Atypical and malignant neoplasms showing lipomatous differentiation. A study of 111 cases. American Journal of Surgical Pathology 11: 161–183

Balsaver A M, Butler J J, Martin R G 1967 Congenital fibrosarcoma. Cancer 20: 1607–1616

Barrow M V, Holubar K 1969 Multiple reticulohistiocytosis. A review of 33 patients. Medicine 48: 287–305

Beatty E C Jr 1962 Congenital generalized fibromatosis in infancy. American Journal of Diseases of Children 103: 620–624

Bednář B 1957 Storiform neurofibroma of the skin, pigmented and nonpigmented. Cancer 10: 368–376

Bill A H Jr, Sumner D S 1965 A unified concept of lymphangioma and cystic hygroma. Surgery Gynecology and Obstetrics 120: 79–86

Blackburn W R, Cosman R 1966 Histologic basis of keloid and hypertrophic scar differentiation. Clinicopathologic correlation. Archives of Pathology 82: 65–71

Borello E D, Gorlin R J 1966 Melanotic neuroectodermal tumour of infancy — A neoplasm of neural crest origin. Report of a case associated with high urinary excretion of vanilmandelic acid. Cancer 19: 196–206

Brook C G D, Valman H B 1971 Osteoma cutis and Albright's hereditary osteodystrophy. British Journal of Dermatology 85: 471–475

Carstens P H B, Howell R S 1979 Malignant giant cell tumour of tendon sheath. Virchows Archiv A Pathological Anatomy and Histopathology 382: 237–243

Cavazzana A O, Jefferson J, Triche T J 1987 Experimental evidence for a neural origin of Ewing's sarcoma of bone. American Journal of Pathology 127: 507–518

Chase D R, Enzinger F M 1985 Epithelioid sarcoma. Diagnosis, prognostic indicators, and treatment. American Journal of Surgical Pathology 9: 241–263

Christopherson W M, Foote F W Jr, Stewart F W 1952 Alveolar soft-part sarcomas: Structurally characteristic tumors of uncertain histogenesis. Cancer 5: 100–111

Chung E B 1985 Pitfalls in diagnosing benign soft tissue tumours in infancy and childhood. Pathology Annual 20 (Part II): 323–386

Chung E B, Enzinger F M 1973 Benign lipoblastomatosis. An analysis of 35 cases. Cancer 32: 482–492

Chung E B, Enzinger F M 1975 Proliferative fasciitis. Cancer 36: 1450–1458

Chung E B, Enzinger F M 1976 Infantile fibrosarcoma. Cancer 38: 729–739

Chung E B, Enzinger F M 1978 Chondroma of soft parts. Cancer 41: 1414–1424

Chung E B, Enzinger F M 1979 Fibroma of tendon sheath. Cancer 44: 1945–1954

Chung E B, Enzinger F M 1981 Infantile myofibromatosis. Cancer 48: 1807–1818

Chung E B, Enzinger F M 1983 Malignant melanoma of soft parts. A reassessment of clear cell sarcoma. American Journal of Surgical Pathology 7: 405–413

Chung E B, Enzinger F M 1987 Extraskeletal osteosarcoma. Cancer 60: 1132–1142

Clearkin K P, Enzinger F M 1976 Intravascular papillary endothelial hyperplasia. Archives of Pathology and Laboratory Medicine 100: 441–444

Cobb C A III, Moiel R H 1974 Ganglion of the peroneal nerve. Report of two cases. Journal of Neurosurgery 41: 255–259

Cobey M C 1943 Hemangioma of joints. Archives of Surgery 46: 465–468

Cooper P H, McAllister H A, Helwig E B 1979 Intravenous pyogenic granuloma: A study of 18 cases. American Journal of Surgical Pathology 3: 221–228

Corio R L, Lewis D M 1979 Intraoral rhabdomyomas. Oral Surgery 48: 525–531

Cornog J L Jr, Enterline H T 1966 Lymphangiomyoma, a benign lesion of chyliferous lymphatics synonymous with lymphangiopericytoma. Cancer 19: 1909–1930

Coventry M B, Harris L E, Bianco A J Jr, Bulbulian A H 1960 Congenital muscular toticollis (wryneck). Postgraduate Medicine 28: 383–392

Cramer S F, Ruehl A, Mandel M A 1981 Fibrodysplasia ossificans progressiva: a distinctive bone-forming lesion of the soft tissue. Cancer 48: 1016–1021

Dabska M 1969 Malignant endovascular papillary angioendothelioma of the skin in childhood. Clinicopathologic study of 6 cases. Cancer 24: 503–510

Dabska M 1977 Parachordoma: A new clinicopathologic entity. Cancer 40: 1586–1592

Dahl I, Angervall L 1974 Cutaneous and subcutaneous leiomyosarcoma — a clinicopathologic study of 47 patients. Pathologia Europaea 9: 307–315

Dahl I, Angervall L 1977 Pseudosarcomatous proliferative lesions of soft tissue with or without bone formation. Acta Pathologica et Microbiologica Scandinavica Section A 85: 577–589

Dehner L P, Enzinger F M, Font R L 1972 Fetal rhabdomyoma. An analysis of nine cases. Cancer 30: 160–166

Dehner L P, Sibley R K, Sauk J J Jr et al 1979 Malignant melanotic neuroectodermal tumor of infancy: A clinical, pathologic, ultrastructural and tissue culture study. Cancer 43: 1389–1410

DiCarlo E F, Woodruff J M, Bansal M, Erlandson R A 1986 The purely epithelioid malignant peripheral nerve sheath tumour. American Journal of Surgical Pathology 10: 478–490

Di Sant' Agnese P A, Knowles D M II 1980 Extracardiac rhabdomyoma: a clinicopathologic study and review of the literature. Cancer 46: 780–789

Dorfman R F 1984 Kaposi's sarcoma revisited. Human Pathology 15: 1013–1017

Drescher E, Woyke S, Markiewicz C, Tegi S 1967 Juvenile fibromatosis in siblings (fibromatosis hyalinica multiplex juvenilis). Journal of Pediatric Surgery 2: 427–430

Dupree W B, Enzinger F M 1986 Fibro-osseous pseudotumor of the digits. Cancer 58: 2103–2109

Dupree W B, Langloss J M, Weiss S W 1985 Pigmented dermatofibrosarcoma protuberans (Bednar tumor). A pathologic, ultrastructural and immunohistochemical study. American Journal of Surgical Pathology 9: 630–639

Dymock R B, Allen P W, Stirling J W, Gilbert E F, Thornbery J M 1987 Giant cell fibroblastoma. A distinctive, recurrent tumor of childhood. American Journal of Surgical Pathology 11: 263–271

Elkon D, Hightower S I, Lim M L, Cantrell R W, Constable W C 1979 Esthesioneuroblastoma. Cancer 44: 1087–1094

Enterline H T, Horn R C Jr 1958 Alveolar rhabdomyosarcoma. A distinctive tumor type. American Journal of Clinical Pathology 29: 356–366

Enzinger F M, Winslow D J 1962 Liposarcoma. A study of 103 cases. Virchows Archiv Pathological Anatomy and Histopathology 335: 367–388

Enzinger F M 1965a Fibrous hamartoma of infancy. Cancer 18: 241–248

Enzinger F M 1965b Recent trends in soft tissue pathology. In: Tumours of bone and soft tissues. Year Book Medical Publishers, Chicago, p 315–332

Enzinger F M 1965c Intramuscular myxoma. A review and follow-up study of 34 cases. American Journal of Clinical Pathology 43: 104–113

Enzinger F M 1965d Clear-cell sarcoma of tendons and aponeuroses. An analysis of 21 cases. Cancer 18: 1163–1174

Enzinger F M 1970 Epithelioid sarcoma. A sarcoma simulating a granuloma or a carcinoma. Cancer 26: 1029–1041

Enzinger F M 1977 Benign lipomatous tumors simulating a sarcoma. In: Management of primary bone and soft tissue tumors. Year Book Medical Publishers, Chicago, p 11–24

Enzinger F M 1979a Atypical fibroxanthoma and malignant fibrous histiocytoma. American Journal of Dermatopathology 1: 185

Enzinger F M 1979b Angiomatoid malignant fibrous histiocytoma: A distinct fibrohistiocytic tumor of children and young adults simulating a vascular neoplasm. Cancer 44: 2147–2157

Enzinger F M, Dulcey F 1967 Proliferative myositis. Report of 33 cases. Cancer 20: 2213–2223

Enzinger F M, Shiraki M 1969 Alveolar rhabdomyosarcoma. An analysis of 110 cases. Cancer 24: 18–31

Enzinger F M, Shiraki M 1972 Extraskeletal myxoid chondrosarcoma: An analysis of 34 cases. Human Pathology 3: 421–435

Enzinger F M, Harvey D A 1975 Spindle cell lipoma. Cancer 36: 1852–1859

Enzinger F M, Smith B H 1976 Hemangiopericytoma: an analysis of 106 cases. Human Pathology 7: 61–82

Enzinger F M, Weiss S W 1983 Soft tissue tumours. C V Mosby, St. Louis, p 1–8

Enzinger F M, Zhang R 1988 Plexiform fibrohistiocytic tumor presenting in children and young adults. An analysis of 65 cases. American Journal of Surgical Pathology 12: 818–826

Evans H L 1979 Liposarcoma: A study of 55 cases with a reassessment of its classification. American Journal of Surgical Pathology 3: 507–523

Evans H L, Soule E H, Winkelmann R K 1979 Atypical lipoma, atypical intrasmuscular lipoma and well-differentiated retroperitoneal liposarcoma. A reappraisal of 30 cases formerly classified as well differentiated liposarcoma. Cancer 43: 574–584

Farrer-Brown G, Lucas R B, Winstock D 1972 Familial gingival fibromatosis: an unusual pathology. Journal of Oral Pathology 1: 76–83

Fayemi A O, Toker C 1975 Nodal angiomatosis. Archives of Pathology 99: 170 172

Fisher E R, Wechsler H 1962 Granular cell myoblastoma – a misnomer. Electron microscopic and histochemical evidence concerning its Schwann cell derivation and nature (granular cell schwannoma). Cancer 15: 936–954

Fisher I, Orkin M 1970 Acquired lymphangioma (lymphangiectasis). Report of a case. Archives of Dermatology 101: 230–234

Fleming R M, Rezek P R 1941 Sarcoma developing in an old burn scar. American Journal of Surgery 54: 457–465

Fletcher C D M 1988 Giant cell fibroblastoma of soft tissue. A clinicopathological and immunohistochemical study. Histopathology 13: 499–508

Fletcher C D M 1989 Solitary circumscribed neuroma of the skin (so-called palisaded, encapsulated neuroma). A clinicopathologic and immunohistochemical study. American Journal of Surgical Pathology 13: 574–580

Fletcher C D M 1990 Benign fibrous histiocytoma of deep soft tissue. A clinicopathologic analysis of 21 cases. American Journal of Surgical Pathology – in press.

Fletcher C D M, Davies S E 1986. Benign plexiform (multinodular) schwannoma: a rare tumour unassociated with neurofibromatosis. Histopathology 10: 971–980

Fletcher C D M, Martin-Bates E 1988 Intramuscular and intermuscular lipoma: neglected diagnoses. Histopathology 12: 275–287

Fletcher C D M, Evans B J, McCartney J C, Smith N, Wilson Jones E, McKee P H 1985 Dermatofibrosarcoma protuberans: a clinicopathological and immunohistochemical study with a review of the literature. Histopathology 9: 921–938

Fletcher C D M, Davies S E, McKee P H 1987 Cellular schwannoma: a distinct pseudosarcomatous entity. Histopathology 11:21–35

Fletcher C D M, Theaker J M, Flanagan A, Krausz T 1988 Pigmented dermatofibrosarcoma protuberans (Bednar tumour): melanocytic colonisation or neuroectodermal differentiation? A clinicopathological and immunohistochemical study. Histopathology 13: 631–643

Gallager R L, Helwig E B 1980 Neurothekeoma – a benign cutaneous tumor of neural origin. American Journal of Clinical Pathology 74: 759–764

Gane N F C, Lindup R, Strickland P, Bennett M H 1970 Radiation-induced fibrosarcoma. British Journal of Cancer 24: 705–711

Gee D C, Finckh E S 1977 Benign vaginal rhabdomyoma. Pathology 9: 263–267

Girard C, Graham J H, Johnson W C 1974 Arteriovenous hemangioma (arteriovenous shunt). A clinicopathological and histochemical study. Journal of Cutaneous Pathology 1: 73–87

Gonzalez-Crussi F, Campbell R J 1970 Juvenile xanthogranuloma. Ultrastructural study. Archives of Pathology 89: 65–72

Gonzalez-Crussi F, Black-Schaffer S 1979 Rhabdomyosarcoma of infancy and childhood. Problems of morphologic classification. American Journal of Surgical Pathology 3: 157–171

Gross R E, Wolbach S B 1943 Sclerosing hemangiomas: Their relationship to dermatofibroma, histiocytoma, xanthoma and to certain pigmented lesions of the skin. American Journal of Pathology 19: 533–551

Guccion J G, Enzinger F M 1972 Malignant giant cell tumor of soft parts. An analysis of 32 cases. Cancer 29: 1518–1529

Guccion J G, Enzinger F M 1979 Malignant schwannoma associated with von Recklinghausen's neurofibromatosis. Virchows Archiv A Pathological Anatomy and Histopathology 383: 43–57

Guccion J G, Font R L, Enzinger F M, Zimmerman L E 1973 Extraskeletal mesenchymal chondrosarcoma. Archives of Pathology 95: 336–340

Hachisuga T, Hashimoto H, Enjoji M 1984 Angioleiomyoma. A clinicopathologic reappraisal of 562 cases. Cancer 54: 126–130

Hajdu S I, Shiu M H, Fortner J G 1977 Tendosynovial sarcoma: A clinicopathological study of 136 cases. Cancer 39: 1201–1217

Harkin J C, Reed R J 1969 Tumors of the peripheral nervous system. In: Atlas of tumour pathology. Armed Forces Institute of Pathology, 2nd series, fascicle 3

Hass J E, Palmer N F, Weinberg A G, Beckwith J B 1981 Ultrastructure of the malignant rhabdoid tumor of the kidney. A distinctive renal tumor of children. Human Pathology 12: 646–657

Helwig E B 1963 Atypical fibroxanthoma. Texas State Journal of Medicine 59: 664–667

Helwig E B, Hackney V C 1954 Juvenile xanthogranuloma (nevoxanthoendothelioma). American Journal of Pathology 30: 625–626

Helwig E B, Stern J B 1984 Subcutaneous sacrococcygeal myxopapillary ependymoma. A clinicopathologic study of 32 cases. American Journal of Clinical Pathology 81: 156–161

Herrmann J B 1965 Lymphangiosarcoma of the chronically edematous extremity. Surgery Gynecology and Obstetrics 121: 1107–1115

Holden C A, Spittle M F, Jones E W 1987 Angiosarcoma of the face and scalp, prognosis and treatment. Cancer 59: 1046–1057

Howard W R, Helwig E B 1960 Angiolipoma. Archives of Dermatology 82: 924–931

Hutter R V P, Stewart F W, Foote F W Jr 1962, Fasciitis — A report of 70 cases with follow-up proving the benignity of the lesion. Cancer 15: 992–1003

Iwashita T, Enjoji M 1987 Plexiform neurilemoma: a clinicopathological and immunohistochemical analysis of 23 tumours from 20 patients. Virchows Archiv A Pathological Anatomy and Histology 411: 305–309

Järvi O, Saxén E 1961 Elastofibroma dorsi. Acta Pathologica et Microbiologica Scandinavica Section A 51 (suppl 144): 83–84

Johnson L C 1948 Histogenesis of myositis ossificans. American Journal of Pathology 24: 681–682

Johnson W C 1976 Pathology of cutaneous vascular tumors. International Journal of Dermatology 15: 239–270

Jones F E, Soule E H, Coventry M B 1969 Fibrous xanthoma of synovium (giant-cell tumour of tendon sheath, pigmented nodular synovitis). A study of 118 cases. Journal of Bone and Joint Surgery 51A: 76–86

Kahn L B 1973 Retroperitoneal xanthogranuloma and xanthosarcoma (malignant fibrous xanthoma). Cancer 31: 411–422

Kandil E 1970 Dermal angiolymphoid hyperplasia with eosinophilia versus pseudopyogenic granuloma. British Journal of Dermatology 83: 405–408

Karcioglu Z, Someren A, Mathes S J 1977 Ectomesenchymoma: a malignant tumor of migratory neural crest (ectomesenchyme) remnants showing ganglionic, schwannian, melanocytic and rhabdomyoblastic differentiation. Cancer 39: 2486–2496

Kawada A, Takahashi H, Anzai T 1965 Eosinophilic lymphofolliculosis of the skin (Kimura's disease). Japanese Journal of Dermatology 76: 61–72

Kawamoto E H, Weidner N, Agostini R M Jr, Jaffe R 1987 Malignant ectomesenchymoma of soft tissue: Report of two cases and review of the literature. Cancer 59: 1791–1802

Keasbey L E 1953 Juvenile aponeurotic fibroma (calcifying fibroma). A distinctive tumor arising in the palms and soles of young children. Cancer 6: 338–346

Kempson R L, Kyriakos M 1972 Fibroxanthosarcoma of the soft tissues. A type of malignant fibrous histiocytoma. Cancer 29: 961–976

Kern W H 1960 Proliferative myositis. A pseudosarcomatous reaction to injury. Archives of Pathology 69: 209–216

Kitano Y, Horiki M, Aoki T, Sagami S 1972 Two cases of juvenile hyalin fibromatosis. Some histological, electron microscopic, and tissue culture observations. Archives of Dermatology 106: 877–883

Konwaler B E, Keasbey L, Kaplan L 1955 Subcutaneous pseudosarcomatous fibromatosis (fasciitis). Report of 8 cases. American Journal of Clinical Pathology 25: 241–252

Kuhn C III, Rosai J 1969 Tumors arising from pericytes. Ultrastructure and organ culture of a case. Archives of Pathology 88: 653–663

Lack E E, Crawford B E, Worsham G F, Vawter G F, Callihan M D 1981 Gingival granular cell tumors of the newborn (congenital 'epulis'). A clinical and pathologic study of 21 patients. American Journal of Surgical Pathology 5: 37–46

Lafferty F W, Reynolds E S, Pearson O H 1965 Tumoral calcinosis: A metabolic disease of obscure etiology. American Journal of Medicine 38: 105–118

Lagier R, Meinecke R 1975 Pathology of 'knuckle pads'. Study of four cases. Virchows Archiv Pathological Anatomy and Histopathology 365: 185–191

Lauer D H, Enzinger F M 1980 Cranial fasciitis of childhood. Cancer 45: 401–406

Levine G D 1972 Hibernoma: an electron microscopic study. Human Pathology 3: 351–359

Lichtenstein L, Goldman R L 1964 The cartilage analogue of fibromatosis: A reinterpretation of the condition called 'juvenile aponeurotic fibroma' Cancer 17: 810–816

Losli E J 1952 Intrinsic hemangiomas of the peripheral nerves. A report of two cases and a review of the literature. Archives of Pathology 53: 226–232

Lumley J S P Stansfeld A G 1972 Infiltrating glomus tumor of lower limb. British Medical Journal i: 484–485

McDivitt R W, Stewart F W, Berg J W 1966 Tumors of the breast. In: Atlas of tumor pathology. Armed Forces Institute of Pathology, 2nd series, fascicle 2

McDonagh J E R 1912 A contribution to our knowledge of the naevo-xantho-endotheliomata. British Journal of Dermatology 24: 85–99

McGavran W L III, Sypert G W, Ballinger W E 1978 Melanocytic schwannoma. Neurosurgery 2: 47–51

Manivel J C, Wick M R, Swanson P E, Patterson K, Dehner L P 1986 Endovascular papillary angioendothelioma of childhood: A vascular lesion possibly characterised by 'high' endothelial cell differentiation. Human Pathology 17: 1240–1244

Markel S R, Enzinger F M 1982 Neuromuscular hamartoma – a benign 'triton tumor' composed of mature neural and striated muscle elements. Cancer 49: 140–144

Marsch W C 1981 The ultrastructure of eruptive haemangioma ('pyogenic granuloma'). Journal of Cutaneous Pathology 8: 144–145

Martin L W, MacCollum D W 1961 Hemangiomas in infants and children. American Journal of Surgery 101: 571–580

Masson P 1970 Vegetant intravascular hemangioendothelioma. In: Human tumours, histology, diagnosis and technique, 2nd edn. Wayne State University Press, Detroit p 306–308

Masson J K, Soule E H 1965 Embryonal rhabdomyosarcoma of the head and neck. Report on eighty-eight cases. American Journal of Surgery 110: 585–591

Mennemeyer R P, Hammar S P, Tytus J S, Hallman K O, Raisis J E, Bockus D 1979 Melanotic schwannoma. Clinical and ultrastructural studies of three cases with evidence of intracellular melanin synthesis. American Journal of Surgical Pathology 3: 3–10

Merkow L P, Frich J C Jr, Slifkin M, Kyreages C G, Pardo M 1971 Ultrastructure of a fibroxanthosarcoma (malignant fibroxanthoma). Cancer 28: 372–383

Moran J J, Enterline H T 1964 Benign rhabdomyoma of the pharynx. A case report, review of the literature, and comparison with cardiac rhabdomyoma. American Journal of Clinical Pathology 42: 174–181

Mottaz J H, Zelickson A S 1966 Electron microscope observations of Kaposi's sarcoma. Acta Dermato-Venereologica 46: 195–200

Neimi K M 1970 The benign fibrohistiocytic tumours of the skin. Acta Dermato-Venereologica 50 Suppl 63: 1–66

O'Brien J E, Stout A P 1964 Malignant fibrous xanthomas. Cancer 17: 1445–1455

Okike N, Bernatz P E, Woolner L B 1978 Localized mesothelioma of the pleura: Benign and malignant variants. Journal of Thoracic and Cardiovascular Surgery 75: 363–372

Patchefsky A S, Enzinger F M 1981 Intravascular fasciitis: a report of 17 cases. American Journal of Surgical Pathology 5: 29–36

Pritchard D J, Soule E H, Taylor W F, Ivins J C 1974 Fibrosarcoma — a clinicopathologica and statistical study of 199 tumours of the soft tissues of the extremities and trunk. Cancer 33: 888–897

Pulitzer D R, Martin P C, Reed R J 1989 Fibroma of tendon sheath. A clinicopathologic study of 32 cases. American Journal of Surgical Pathology 13: 472–479

Purvis W E, Helwig E B 1954 Reticulohistiocytic granuloma (reticulohistiocytoma) of the skin. American Journal of Clinical Pathology 24: 1005–1015

Reed R J, Fine R M, Meltzer H D 1972 Palisaded, encapulated neuromas of the skin. Archives of Dermatology 106: 865–870

Reed R J, Leonard D D 1979 Neurotropic melanoma: A variant of desmoplastic melanoma. American Journal of Surgical Pathology 3: 301–311

Remberger K, Krieg T, Kunze D, Weinmann H-M, Hubner G 1985 Fibromatosis hyalinica multiplex (juvenile hyalin fibromatosis): Light microscopic electron microscopic, immunohistochemical, and biochemical findings. Cancer 56: 614–624

Rentiers P L, Montgomery H 1949 Nodular subepidermal fibrosis (dermatofibroma versus histiocytoma). Archives of Dermatology and Syphilology 59: 568–583

Reye R D K 1956 A consideration of certain subdermal 'fibromatous tumours' of infancy. Journal of Pathology and Bacteriology 72: 149–154

Reye R D K 1965 Recurring digital fibrous tumors of childhood. Archives of Pathology 80: 228–231

Rosai J, Sumner H W, Kostianovsky M, Perez-Mesa C 1976 Angiosarcoma of the skin: a clinicopathologic and fine structural study. Human Pathology 7: 83–109

Rosai J, Gold J, Landy R 1979 The histiocytoid haemangiomas: A unifying concept embracing several previously described entities of skin, soft tissue, large vessels, bone and heart. Human Pathology 10: 707–730

Rosenberg H S, Stenback W A, Spjut H J 1978 The fibromatoses of infancy and childhood. In: Perspectives in pediatric pathology, Vol 4 Year Book Medical Publishers, Chicago p 269–348

Russell W O, Cohen J, Enzinger F M et al 1977 A clinical and pathological staging system for soft tissue sarcomas. Cancer 40: 1562–1570

Salazar H, Totten R S 1970 Leiomyoblastoma of the stomach. An ultrastructural study. Cancer 25: 176–185

Schwartz E E, Rothstein J D 1968 Fibrosarcoma following radiation therapy. Journal of the American Medical Association 203: 296–298

Seemayer T A, Knaack J, Wang N, Ahmed M N 1975 On the ultrastructure of hibernoma. Cancer 36: 1785–1793

Shapiro L 1969 Infantile digital fibromatosis and aponeurotic fibroma. Case reports of two rare pseudosarcomas and review of the literature. Archives of Dermatology 99: 37–42

Shipkey F H, Lieberman P H, Foote F W Jr, Stewart F W 1964 Ultrastructure of alveolar soft part sarcoma. Cancer 17: 821–830

Shmookler B M, Enzinger F M 1981 Pleomorphic lipoma: A benign tumor simulating liposarcoma. A clinicopathologic analysis of 48 cases. Cancer 47: 126–133

Shmookler B M, Enzinger F M 1982 Giant cell fibroblastoma: A peculiar childhood tumor. Laboratory Investigation 46: 76A abstract

Sonoda T, Hashimoto H, Enjoji M 1985 Juvenile xanthogranuloma. Clinicopathologic analysis and immunohistochemical study of 57 patients. Cancer 56: 2280–2286

Sotelo-Avila C, Gonzalez-Crussi F, Demello D et al 1986 Renal and extrarenal rhabdoid tumors in children: a clinicopathologic study of 14 patients. Seminars in Diagnostic Pathology 3: 151–163

Steeper T A, Rosai J 1983 Aggressive angiomyxoma of the female pelvis and perineum. Report of nine cases of a distinctive type of gynecologic soft-tissue neoplasm. American Journal of Surgical Pathology 7: 463–475

Stephens F E, Isaacson A 1959 Hereditary multiple lipomatosis. Journal of Heredity 50: 51–53

Sternberg S S 1954 Pathology of juvenile masopharyngeal angiofibroma — a lesion of adolescent males. Cancer 7: 15–28

Stewart F W, Treves N 1948 Lymphangiosarcoma in postmastectomy lymphedema. A report of six cases in elephantiasis chirurgica. Cancer 1: 64–81

Stout A P 1935a The malignant tumours of the peripheral nerves. American Journal of Cancer 25: 1–36

Stout A P 1935b Tumors of the neuromyo-arterial glomus. American Journal of Cancer 24: 255–272

Stout A P 1937 Solitary cutaneous and subcutaneous leiomyoma. American Journal of Cancer 29: 435–469

Stout A P 1948 Fibrosarcoma. The malignant tumor of fibroblasts. Cancer 1: 30–63

Stout A P 1953 Tumors of the soft tissues. In: Atlas of tumor pathology. Armed Forces Institute of Pathology, section 2, fascicle 5

Stout A P 1954 Juvenile fibromatoses. Cancer 7: 953–978

Stout A P 1962a Bizarre smooth muscle tumours of the stomach. Cancer 15: 400–409

Stout A P 1962b Fibrosarcoma in infants and children. Cancer 15: 1028–1040

Stout A P, Murray M R 1942 Hemangiopericytoma: a vascular tumor featuring Zimmermann's pericytes. Annals of Surgery 116: 26–33

Stout A P, Lattes R 1967 Tumors of the soft tissues. In: Atlas of tumor pathology. Armed Forces Institute of Pathology, 2nd series, fascicle 1

Taxy J B, Gray S R 1979 Cellular angiomas of infancy. An ultrastructural study of two cases. Cancer 43: 2322–2331

Vellios F, Baez J M, Shumacker H B 1958 Lipoblastomatosis: A tumor of fetal fat different from hibernoma. Report of a case, with observations of the embryogenesis of human adipose tissue. American Journal of Pathology 34: 1149–1159

Ward C E, Horton B T 1940 Congenital arteriovenous fistulas in children. Journal of Pediatrics: 16: 746–766

Weiss S W 1976 Ultrastructure of the so-called 'chordoid sarcoma.' Evidence supporting cartilaginous differentiation. Cancer 37: 300–306

Weiss S W, Enzinger F M 1977 Myxoid variant of malignant fibrous histiocytoma. Cancer 39: 1672–1685

Weiss S W, Enzinger F M 1978 Malignant fibrous histiocytoma: An analysis of 200 cases. Cancer 41: 2250–2266

Weiss S W, Enzinger F M 1982 Epithelioid haemangioendothelioma: A vascular tumour often mistaken for a carcinoma. Cancer 50: 970–981

Weiss S W, Enzinger F M 1986 Spindle cell haemangioendothelioma. A low-grade angiosarcoma resembling a cavernous hemangioma and Kaposi's sarcoma. American Journal of Surgical Pathology 10: 521–530

Weiss S W, Ishak K G, Dail D H, Sweet D E, Enzinger F M 1986 Epithelioid hemangioendothelioma and related lesions. Seminars in Diagnostic Pathology 3: 259–287

Wells G C, Whimster I W 1969 Subcutaneous angiolymphoid hyperplasia with eosinophilia. British Journal of Dermatology 81: 1–15

Wirth W A, Lavitt D, Enzinger F M 1971 Multiple intramuscular myxomas. Another extraskeletal manifestation of fibrous dysplasia. Cancer 27: 1167–1173

Wolff M 1973 Lymphangiomyoma: clinicopathologic study and ultrastructural confirmation of its histogenesis. Cancer 31: 988–1007

Woodruff J M, Chernik N L, Smith M C, Millett W B, Foot F W Jr 1973 Peripheral nerve tumors with rhabdomyosarcomatous differentiation (malignant 'Triton' tumors). Cancer 32: 426–439

Woodruff J M 1976 Peripheral nerve tumors showing glandular differentiation (granular schwannomas). Cancer 37: 2399–2413

Woodruff J M, Godwin T A, Erlandson R A, Susin M, Martini N 1981 Cellular schwannoma. A variety of schwannoma sometimes mistaken for a malignant tumour. American Journal of Surgical Pathology 5: 733–744

Woodward A H, Ivins J C, Soule E H 1972 Lymphangiosarcoma arising in chronic lymphedematous extremities. Cancer 30: 562–572

Young S, Gonzalez-Crussi F 1985 Melanocytic neuroectodermal tumor of the foot. Report of a case with multicentric origin. American Journal of Clinical Pathology 84: 371–378

Yunis E J 1986 Ewing's sarcoma and related small round cell neoplasms in children. American Journal of Surgical Pathology 10 (suppl 1): 54–62

5. The biology of the myofibroblast and its relation to the development of soft tissue and epithelial tumours

O. Skalli   G. Gabbiani

THE MYOFIBROBLAST: DEFINITION AND ULTRASTRUCTURAL FEATURES

The study of wound contraction led to the description of the myofibroblast, a cell type with ultrastructural and biological features of fibroblasts and of smooth muscle cells (Gabbiani et al 1971); initially described in rat and human granulation tissue, myofibroblasts were subsequently found in a wide variety of other conditions in animals and humans. Ultrastructurally, myofibroblasts are characterised by:

1. The presence of parallel bundles of microfilaments showing many electron opaque areas (dense bodies)
2. A well developed rough endoplasmic reticulum (Fig. 5.1) (Gabbiani et al 1971).

Other ultrastructural features of myofibroblasts include multiple nuclear indentations or deep folds and cell surface differentiations, such as a contact with a discontinuous basement membrane-like material and gap junctions (Gabbiani et al 1978). Another type of myofibroblastic cell-stroma linkage is the fibronexus, which is a transmembrane complex of intracellular microfilaments in apparent continuity with extracellular fibronectin fibers (Singer 1979, Singer et al 1984). Fibronexuses and gap junctions were postulated to transmit and to synchronise the contracting forces generated by myofibroblasts across the wound space (Gabbiani et al 1978, Singer et al 1984).

DISTRIBUTION OF MYOFIBROBLASTS IN SOFT TISSUE TUMOURS

Myofibroblasts have been described in three groups of pathological situations (for a review see Seemayer et al 1980, Skalli & Gabbiani 1988). These pathological situations can be divided into:

1. Conditions related to inflammation, wound healing and tissue remodelling (such as liver cirrhosis and skin contracture after burns)
2. Fibromatoses (Stiller & Katenkamp 1975, Seemayer et al, 1980, Fletcher et al, 1986)
3. The stromal reaction to neoplasia, or desmoplasia.

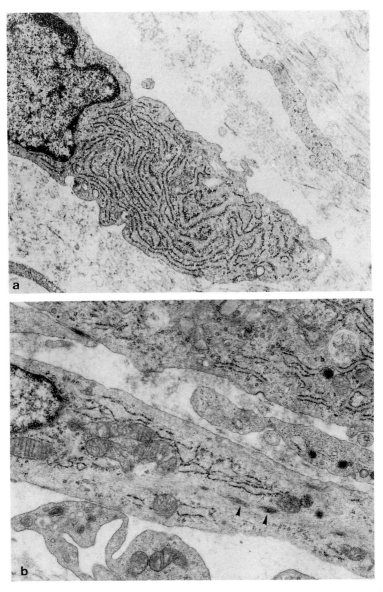

Fig. 5.1 Electron micrographs of a normal rat dermis fibroblast (**a**) and of a rat granulation tissue myofibroblast 7 days after removal of a 4 cm² skin fragment (**b**). The main feature of the fibroblast (**a**) is a regularly arranged rough endoplasmic reticulum. The myofibroblast (**b**) shows still an abundant rough endoplasmic reticulum with dilated cisternae but, in addition, bundles of microfilaments with dense bodies scattered in between (arrowheads). (× 14 000) (Reproduced with permission from Gabbiani & Rungger-Brändle 1981.)

Thus, myofibroblasts are commonly present in the stroma of a wide variety of primary invasive and metastatic carcinomas (Seemayer et al 1980) and their occurrence has been particularly well documented in infiltrating breast carcinomas (Ghosh et al 1980, Harris & Ahmed 1977, Schürch et al 1981, 1982, Seemayer et al 1979, Tremblay 1979).

Myofibroblasts have also been described as one of the cellular components of some benign soft tissue tumours such as dermatofibroma (Katenkamp & Stiller 1975a, Nakanishi et al 1981), digital fibroma of infancy (Bhawan et al 1979), infantile myofibromatosis (Benjamin et al 1977), pigmented villonodular synovitis (Alguacil-Garcia et al 1978), the recently described intranodal myofibroblastoma (Suster & Rosai 1989) and giant cell dermatofibroma (Weathers & Campbell 1974), although this latter case is controversial (Vasudev & Harris 1978). Malignant fibroblastic tumours contain cells with a spectrum of morphology ranging from the typical fibroblast to the myofibroblast; this has been reported in dermatofibrosarcoma protuberans (Hashimoto et al 1974), parosteal osteogenic sarcoma (Vuletin 1977), liposarcoma (Lagacé et al 1980), osteosarcoma (Reddick et al 1980), malignant fibrous histiocytoma (Alguacil-Garcia et al 1978, Churg & Kahn 1977, Fu et al 1975, Harris 1980; Lagacé et al 1979, 1980, Limacher et al 1978, Nakanishi et al 1981, Reddick et al 1979, Taxy & Battifora 1977), myxofibrosarcomas (Kindblom et al 1979) and for some fibrosarcomas (Crocker & Murad 1969, Lagacé et al 1980, Nakanishi et al 1981, Stiller & Katenkamp 1975). However, the presence of myofibroblasts is not a constant feature of fibrosarcomas and malignant fibrous histiocytomas (Fu et al 1975, Hashimoto et al 1974, Jakobiec & Tannenbaum 1974, Lagacé et al 1980, Stiller & Katenkamp 1975). Interestingly, myofibroblasts were observed in an experimental methylchloranthrene-induced sarcoma (Katenkamp & Stiller 1975b).

Sarcomas where myofibroblasts are the major (if not the only) cellular component have also been reported. They include low-grade spindle cell sarcomas (Ghadially et al 1983, Hashimoto et al 1982, Vasudev & Harris 1978), which have been named sarcoma of myofibroblast (Vasudev & Harris 1978) or myofibroblastoma (Ghadially et al 1983); these tumours were locally aggressive but did not metastasise. Recently, a benign tumour of the breast stroma made up mostly of myofibroblasts was also called myofibroblastoma (Wargotz et al 1987). Myofibroblasts have been described in epithelioid sarcoma (Gabbiani et al 1972). Blewitt et al (1983) suggested that this neoplasm consists only of myofibroblasts which may assume a fibroblastic or an epithelioid shape depending on the extent of filament accumulation in the cytoplasm. Finally, there has been a case report of a metastasising sarcoma of the pleura composed almost exclusively of myofibroblasts (Fig. 5.2) (D'Andiran & Gabbiani 1980). To our knowledge this case is the only exception to the general finding that soft tissue tumours composed of myofibroblasts are benign or low-grade tumours.

CYTOSKELETAL COMPOSITION OF MYOFIBROBLASTS IN NON-NEOPLASTIC CONDITIONS

The histogenesis of granulation tissue fibroblasts and of myofibroblasts has been debated for a long time; it is now generally accepted that they stem from local connective tissue cells (Grillo 1963, MacDonald 1959, Ross et al 1970,

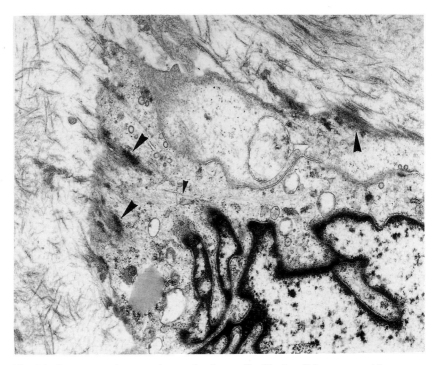

Fig. 5.2 Low power electron micrograph of a myofibroblastic cell in a metastasising sarcoma of the pleura. Note nuclear indentations, bundle of microfilaments with dense bodies scattered in between (large arrowheads), located at the cell periphery. The small arrowhead points at a microtubule. (× 16 800) (Reproduced with permission from D'Andiran & Gabbiani 1980.)

Skalli & Gabbiani 1988). The same probably also holds true for myofibro-blasts from other pathological tissues, although this has not been investigated experimentally. Local connective tissue cells from which myofibroblasts may stem include dermal or subcutaneous fibroblasts, pericytes and smooth muscle cells. A strategy used to clarify this point has been to characterise the cytoskeletal composition of myofibroblasts, since many studies have proven that cytoskeletal proteins, particularly intermediate filament proteins, are good markers of cellular origin (Osborn & Weber 1983, Rungger-Brändle & Gabbiani 1983). Thus, it has been documented in many instances that, in general, neoplastic and fast growing cells maintain the intermediate filament proteins of the cells from which they derive (for review see Osborn & Weber 1983), a condition required for a protein to be considered as a good marker of cellular origin. However, the origin of a mesenchymal cell is difficult to establish unambiguously by means of intermediate filament typing because:

1. Different cells (e.g. endothelial cells and fibroblasts) contain the same intermediate filament protein (vimentin)
2. Vascular smooth muscle cells, although similar ultrastructurally, may express either vimentin alone or vimentin and desmin (Gabbiani et al 1981, Travo et al 1982)

3. Desmin is expressed in some stromal and endothelial cells in different species, including man (Fujimoto & Singer 1986, Skalli et al 1986a, Stamenkovic et al 1986, Toccanier-Pelte et al 1987).

It has been proposed that the evaluation of the actin isoform pattern of a cell population helps in determining its origin (Skalli et al 1987). Although the actin primary sequence has been strongly conserved during evolution, a biochemical microheterogeneity has been observed in actins from different mammalian tissues (Vandekerckhove & Weber 1978a). These tissue (rather than species-specific) differences are mainly located in the 17 aminoterminal amino acids (Vandekerckhove & Weber 1981). In mammals, actin isoforms can be resolved by means of two-dimensional gel electrophoresis as three spots called α, β and γ (Garrels & Gibson 1976, Storti & Rich 1976, Whalen et al 1976). Sequencing studies have led to the recognition of six actin isoforms (Vandekerckhove & Weber 1978a, 1978b); three have an α-electrophoretic mobility: one found in large amounts in striated muscle and in small amounts in the myocardium (α-skeletal actin), one found in large amounts in the myocardium and in minute amounts in the striated muscle (α-cardiac actin) and one specific for smooth muscle (α-smooth muscle actin) (Vandekerckove & Weber 1978b, Vandekerckhove et al 1986). β- and γ-actins correspond to two forms of actin found in every cell and are called 'cytoplasmic'. In addition, a sixth isoform present in smooth muscle migrates with the γ-cytoplasmic actin and is referred to as γ-smooth muscle actin (Vandekerckhove & Weber 1979). Two-dimensional gel electrophoresis of different mesenchymal tissues showed that smooth muscle cells always express α-, β-, γ-actins, although in different proportions, while fibroblastic cells express only β- and γ-actin in a constant ratio (Skalli et al 1987). The pattern of actin isoform expression is modulated in smooth muscle cells during physiological, pathological, and in vitro conditions (Gabbiani et al 1984, Owens et al 1986, Skalli et al 1986b, Skalli et al 1987), but is always characterised by the presence of α- and γ-smooth muscle and of β- and γ-cytoplasmic actins in variable amounts according to the situation.

The distinction between α-smooth muscle actin and the α-sarcomeric actins is an important means by which to evaluate the smooth muscle or striated muscle derivation of neoplasms of mesenchymal origin. This distinction is not possible by two-dimensional gel electrophoresis, but can be done either by protein chemical analysis (Vandeckerckhove & Weber 1981, Vandeckerckhove et al 1986), or by immunohistochemistry with specific antibodies. Thus, a monoclonal antibody specific for α-smooth muscle actin has been obtained by immunisation of mice with the NH_2 terminal peptide of this isoform conjugated to haemocyanin (Skalli et al 1986a); polyclonal and monoclonal antibodies against the α-cardiac and α-skeletal actins have also been obtained (Bulinski et al 1983, Skalli et al 1988). The use of these antibodies on different human and rat tissues (Skalli et al 1986a, 1988) have confirmed, at the histological level, the biochemical data showing that fibroblasts from normal connective tissues never express α-smooth muscle actin nor α-sarcomeric actins, whereas normal smooth muscle cells express α-smooth muscle actin and striated and cardiac cells the sarcomeric actins.

Recently, different reports have focused on the distribution of actin isoforms in mesenchymal tumours. Tumours histologically diagnosed as leiomyosarcomas occasionally expressed α-smooth muscle or α-sarcomeric actins (Fig. 5.3) (Schürch et al 1987). However, most of these neoplasms were stained with an antibody recognising the two smooth muscle and the two striated muscle isoforms of actin (Miettinen et al 1988, Tsukuda et al 1987). Interestingly, this antibody also stained some sarcomas known to contain myofibroblasts such as pleomorphic and spindle cell sarcomas. Rhabdomyosarcomas were consistently positive for this antibody (Miettinen et al 1988, Schmidt et al 1988), a result in agreement with the finding that these neoplasms, even when poorly differentiated, always expressed α-sarcomeric actins, and occasionally also α-smooth muscle actin (Skalli et al 1988). The coexpression of α-smooth muscle and α-sarcomeric actins was also observed in NiS-induced rat rhabdomyosarcomas (Babaï et al 1988). In addition, large amounts of α-cardiac actin were detected in human and experimental rhabdomyosarcomas (Vandekerckhove et al 1987). This demonstrates that the expression of actin isoforms in neoplasms considered of myogenic origin is complex, and possibly reproduces events occurring during normal muscle development. Indeed, it is well documented that α-cardiac actin is transiently expressed during normal myogenesis (Gunning et al 1983, Mayer et al 1984, Minty et al 1982, Vandekeckhove et al 1986, for a review see Alonso 1987), and recently α-smooth muscle actin has been shown to be present temporarily in fetal skeletal muscles (Woodcock-Mitchell et al 1988). These data raise the question as to whether α-smooth muscle actin can reliably be used as a marker of origin in malignant smooth muscle proliferations. One would like to suggest that the use of actin isoforms may be useful to evaluate the degree of differentiation of tumours of myogenic origin, thereby furnishing new criteria for their classification and possibly for the definition of their clinical behaviour. The identification of each individual isoform is important in this regard since it may allow the distinction between tumours with various degrees of differentiation (e.g. rhabdomyosarcomas expressing α-sarcomeric and α-smooth muscle actin versus rhabdomyosarcomas expressing only α-sarcomeric actins).

In contrast to malignant smooth muscle neoplasms, the presence of α-smooth muscle actin in benign soft tissue tumours can be taken as a good clue for smooth muscle derivation since non-neoplastic proliferating smooth muscle cells retain the expression of α-smooth muscle actin, although at a level lower than their quiescent counterpart. This was shown for leiomyomas (Schürch et al 1987, Skalli et al 1987), human and experimental atheroma (Gabbiani et al 1984, Kocher et al 1984, 1986) and for cultured aortic smooth muscle cells (Gabbiani et al 1984, Owens et al 1986, Skalli et al 1986b). This does not apply to smooth muscle myosin since, in non-malignant smooth muscle cell proliferations, the expression of this isoform is replaced by that of

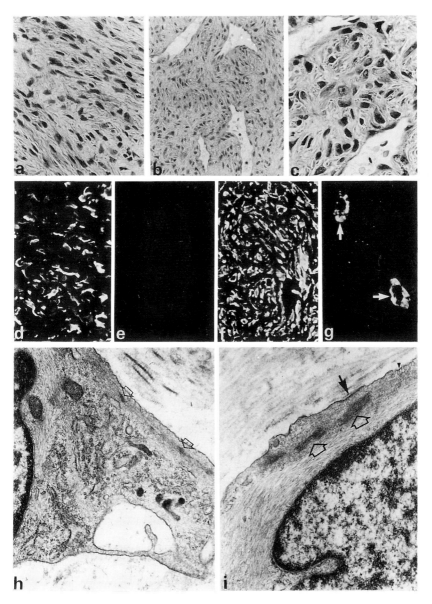

Fig. 5.3   Leiomyosarcoma of the thigh. **a–c** Light micrographs of haematoxylin-phloxine-saffran stained sections reveal fascicles of spindle cells (**a**) and hemangiopericytoma-like pattern (**b** and **c**). **d–e** Double indirect immunofluorescent staining illustrating positive staining for α-striated actin (**d**) and negative staining for desmin (**e**). **f** and **g** Indirect immunofluorescent staining illustrating positive staining for vimentin (**f**) and negative staining for α-smooth muscle actin (**g**); smooth muscle cells of stromal vessels are stained for α-smooth muscle actin (arrows). **h-i** transmission electron micrographs demonstrating smooth muscle differentiation, i.e. cytoplasmic bundles of microfilaments with dense bodies (open arrows), plasmalemmal attachment plaques, remnants of basal lamina (arrow), and pinocytic vesicles (arrowheads). Note the perinuclear bundle of intermediate filaments. (**a, d–g** × 300; **b** × 190, **c** × 480; **h** and **i** × 25 500) (Reproduced with permission from Schürch et al 1987.)

non-muscle myosin, as described for leiomyomas (Donner et al 1983) and for proliferating cultured vascular smooth muscle cells (Benzonana et al 1988, Chamley et al 1977, Larson et al 1984, Rovner et al 1986).

Myofibroblasts from different non-neoplastic pathological situations were found to be heterogeneous in their actin isoform and intermediate filament protein content by means of immunofluorescence using antibodies against α-smooth muscle and α-sarcomeric actins, desmin and vimentin (Skalli et al 1989a). Thus, although myofibroblasts from all conditions examined were positive for vimentin and negative for α-sarcomeric actin, their content of α-smooth muscle actin and desmin was variable; on this basis four distinct cytoskeletal phenotypes could be recognised (Skalli et al 1989a):

1. Phenotype V, positive for vimentin only.
2. Phenotype VAD, positive for vimentin, α-smooth muscle actin and desmin.
3. Phenotype VA, positive for vimentin and α-smooth muscle actin.
4. Phenotype VD, positive for vimentin and desmin.

Accordingly, two categories of myofibroblastic proliferation can be distinguished: the first contains only V-cells and comprises normally healing granulation tissue, eschars and normally healed scars; the second includes hypertrophic scars and fibromatoses (Fig. 5.4). In this latter category, cells with a phenotype V were mixed with various proportions of cells expressing

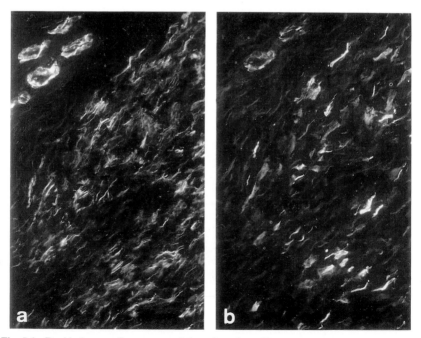

Fig. 5.4 Double immunofluorescent staining of a palmar fibromatosis with anti-α-smooth muscle actin (**a**) and antidesmin (**b**) disclose many cells expressing α-smooth muscle actin, some of which expressing also desmin. (× 400)

cytoskeletal markers of myogenic differentiation, i.e. VAD, VA, VD cells. Stromal cells from different neoplasms also fall in this latter condition (Leoncini et al 1988, Sappino et al 1988, Skalli et al 1986a). A positive reaction for antidesmin or for an antibody to the muscle isoform of actin (i.e. the two smooth muscle and the two striated muscle forms of actin) was also observed in various fibromatoses (Fletcher et al 1987, Miettinen 1988, Shum & McFarlane 1988, Tsukuda et al 1987, Viale et al 1988). Despite their heterogeneity in intermediate filament protein and actin isoform content, myofibroblasts from different settings, including granulation tissue (Benzo-nana et al 1988, Eddy et al 1988), Dupuytren's nodule (Tomasek et al 1986), and hypertrophic scars (Eddy et al 1988) always express only non-muscle myosin. In these conditions, the extracellular matrix around myofibroblasts was strongly stained for antifibronectin but not for antilaminin (Eddy et al 1988, Tomasek et al 1986).

The heterogeneous content of actin isoforms and intermediate filament proteins of myofibroblasts suggest that these cells are either derived from different cell types or that fibroblasts can assume various degrees of differentiation toward a cell type expressing smooth muscle markers. According-ing to the first hypothesis, V cells derive from fibroblasts, whereas VAD and VA cells derive from smooth muscle cells and/or pericytes, since these latter cells have cytoskeletal features similar to those of smooth muscle cells (Fujimoto & Singer 1987, Herman & D'Amore 1985, Joyce et al 1984, 1985a, 1985b, Skalli et al 1989b, Toccanier-Pelte et al 1987). VD-cells could originate from the stromal cells positive for antidesmin and negative for α-smooth muscle actin; these, however, have been found only in various organs, such as spleen (Toccanier-Pelte et al 1987), testis (Skalli et al 1986a), uterus (Glasser & Julian 1986, Skalli et al 1986a) and intestinal submucosa (Skalli et al 1986a). Ultrastructural observations have shown that during pathological and culture conditions fibroblasts and smooth muscle cells acquire morphological features similar to those of myofibroblasts (Chamley-Campbell et al 1979, Kocher et al 1984, 1985, Mosse et al 1985, Olivetti et al 1980, Poole et al 1971). This supports the concept that myofibroblasts may originate from several different cells. Alternatively, myofibroblasts could have a common fibroblastic origin, but the expression of smooth muscle cytoskel-etal proteins may be induced by some yet unknown stimuli. Such a differentiation process has been shown to occur in adult animals, for example in advanced human and experimental atheromatous lesions (Kocher et al 1984, 1986, Osborn et al 1987). However, it should be stressed that, in these subsets of myofibroblasts, smooth muscle differentiation is not complete since they do not express smooth muscle myosin and laminin (Benzonana et al 1988, Eddy et al 1988, Tomasek et al 1986).

THE MYOFIBROBLAST IN DESMOPLASIA

In sarcomas, as well as in the stroma of carcinomas, myofibroblasts have been proposed to be a reactive, rather than an neoplastic component (Seemayer et al 1980). Indeed, some similarities exist between tumour stroma generation and wound healing (Dvorak 1986, Schürch et al 1981, 1982). Thus, it appears more and more clear that local fibrin deposition occurs in tumours as in wounds (Dvorak et al 1979a, 1984a, 1984b). This has been shown by immunohistochemistry in human neoplasms (Dvorak et al 1981, Harris et al 1982) and in an experimental model of tumour stroma formation in which solid tumours are produced after the subcutaneous injection of cells derived from a diethylnitrosamine-induced bile duct carcinoma (Dvorak et al 1979a). However, in wounds, fibrin deposition is due to the coagulation of the fibrinogen extravasated after local vascular injury, whereas in tumours the exudation of fibrinogen and of clotting factors is due to an increase in the permeability of postcapillary venules; this increase is mediated by a factor secreted by tumour cells (Dvorak et al 1979b, Senger et al 1983, 1986). In experimental tumours, the fibrinogen influx and fibrin accumulation remained constantly elevated, but in wounds they declined toward normal a few days after wounding (Brown et al 1988). In the experimental tumour stroma formation model, most of the deposited fibrin was degraded by plasminogen activator secreted by neoplastic cells; the final amount and distribution of stroma deposited was correlated to the final amount and distribution of fibrin (Dvorak et al 1983). It is noteworthy that fibrin gels by themselves induce the formation of granulation tissue even in the absence of platelets or tumour cells (Dvorak et al 1987). However, there is in vitro (Hernandez et al 1985, Merrilees & Finlay 1985, Peres et al 1987) and in vivo (Barsky et al 1982) evidence that neoplastic cells also contribute to the formation of tumour stroma, possibly through the release of some yet undetermined factors.

Ultrastructural observations also support an analogy between tumour stroma formation and wound healing (Schürch et al 1981, 1982, Tamimi & Ahmed 1987). Thus, myofibroblasts of the loose stroma of human invasive breast carcinomas contained a prevalence of secretory organelles, whereas those of the dense stroma of the same neoplasms contained predominantly cytoplastic filaments. Taken together with the results on experimental tumour stroma formation, these findings suggest that myofibroblasts represent, in desmoplastic tissues, a reactive rather than a malignant element.

However, cultured myofibroblasts from Dupuytren's and Peyronie's nodules show some of the properties that characterise neoplastic transformation (Azzarone et al 1983, Somers et al 1982). In cultured myofibroblasts from palmar fibromatosis, these properties were:

1. A growth kinetic intermediate between that of normal fibroblasts and embryonic or virus transformed fibroblasts
2. The formation of colonies in soft agar
3. The secretion of high levels of the urokinase-like species of plasminogen activator
4. The ability to grow in the presence of reduced amounts of fetal calf serum

5. Evidence of karyotypic abnormalities (Azzarone et al 1983, Bowser-Riley et al 1975, Sergovitch et al 1983).

Nevertheless, myofibroblasts from Dupuytren's nodule displayed contact inhibition at the plateau phase and had a limited lifespan. Interestingly, granulation tissue and breast stroma myofibroblasts grew more slowly than control fibroblasts (Vande Berg et al 1984a, 1984b, 1985). Moreover, clonal studies revealed that myofibroblasts originating from the same tissue exhibit different proliferative rates which generally fall into fast and slow categories of growth (Vande Berg & Rudolph 1985). This heterogeneity in the biological behaviour of cultured myofibroblasts is correlated with that observed in their cytoskeletal composition. This further stresses the fact that general conclusions cannot be drawn from studies of myofibroblasts from one location and that more experiments are warranted to examine whether myofibroblasts from desmoplastic tissues and from sarcomas are reactive cells or cells that have undergone benign or malignant transformation.

INFLUENCE OF MYOFIBROBLASTS ON TUMOUR GROWTH AND INVASION

If some light has been shed over the pathogenesis of tumour stroma, the influence of the desmoplastic reaction and of myofibroblasts on tumour growth and invasion remains largely a matter of speculation. Myofibroblasts synthesise components of the extracellular matrix (Barsky et al 1982, 1986), thereby contributing to the fibrotic features of tumour stroma. Several lines of evidence indicate that myofibroblasts probably generate the forces responsible for wound contraction through their actin bundles (for a review see Skalli & Gabbiani 1988). Gap junctions may synchronise these forces, which are probably transduced to the extracellular matrix through fibronexuses (Singer et al 1984). Similarly, myofibroblasts present in the stroma of different neoplasms are considered to be responsible for the clinical and macroscopic features of retraction and rigidity observed in these conditions (Schürch et al 1982). However, myofibroblasts from various sarcomas, although exhibiting a conspicuous contractile apparatus, lack cell to cell coupling and thus may be unable to generate an overall tissue contraction (D'Andiran & Gabbiani 1980). Whether myofibroblasts affect tumour growth and invasion is controversial. Comparison of the biological behaviour of scirrhous and medullary breast carcinoma has suggested that neoplasms with a prominent desmoplastic reaction behave more aggressively than those with a weak reaction (Shimosato et al 1980). However, most authors report that the presence of a prominent stromal reaction is beneficial for the host. Thus, the spontaneous regression of congenital mesenchymal hamartomas (now thought to represent infantile myofibromatosis — Fletcher et al 1987) was attributed to the contractile activity of the numerous myofibroblasts present within this tumour (Benjamin et al 1977). Comparison of two cell lines derived from a bile duct carcinoma showed that the most desmoplastic was the less aggressive (Dvorak et al 1979a). However, it is not clear from these observations whether tumour aggressiveness was related to the intrinsic properties of the different neoplastic cells or to the desmoplastic reaction itself. This issue was addressed in an experimental model where a fibrotic response similar to the human desmo-plastic reaction was elicited in mice after a subcutaneous injection of BL/6 melanoma cells (Barsky & Gopalakrishna 1987). Inhibition of the desmoplas-tic reaction with L-3,4-dehydroproline promoted local invasion of BL/6 cells and increased the incidence of pulmonary metastasis (Barsky & Gopalakrishna 1987), suggesting that the desmoplastic reaction affects tumour aggression (Fig. 5.5).

The distinction between myofibroblasts with different cytoskeletal pheno-types makes it possible to distinguish different types of stromal reactions. Thus, the number of stromal cells expressing α-smooth muscle actin is higher in the desmoplastic reaction associated with breast carcinomas than in non-malignant hyperplastic conditions such as fibrocystic disease and fibroad-enoma (Fig. 5.6) (Sappino et al 1988). In pleomorphic adenomas of salivary and lacrymal glands, stromal cells do not express α-smooth muscle actin whereas the stroma of carcinomas of the same gland is rich in myofibroblasts expressing this smooth muscle marker (Leoncini et al 1988). This suggests that the definition of the cytoskeletal phenotype in stromal cells may be useful for the identification of premalignant or early invasive lesions in different tissues. The mechanisms responsible for the development of stromal cells with different cytoskeletal phenotypes are unknown, as is the effect that these different types of reactions may have on tumour growth and invasiveness.

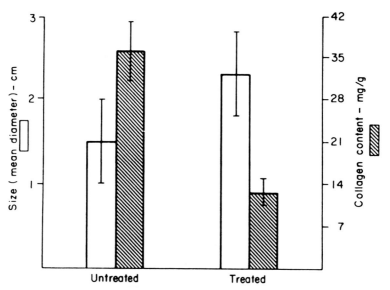

Fig. 5.5 Inverse correlation between collagen content of BL6 tumour nodule and size (mean diameter) is demonstrated. L-3,4 dehydroproline, through inhibition of the desmoplastic response, promotes local invasion of the primary tumour. (Reproduced with permission from Barsky & Gopalakrishna 1987.)

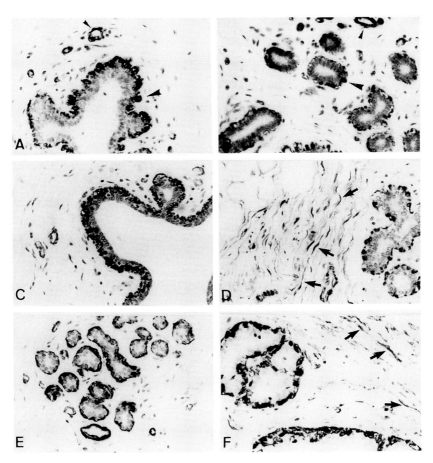

Fig. 5.6 Peroxidase staining of paraffin-embedded breast tissue with anti-α-smooth muscle actin. **A** and **B** Normal breast. A positive reaction is seen in myoepithelial cells (large arrowheads) and the media of small vessels (small arrowheads); stromal cells are negative. **C** and **D** Fibrocystic disease. No immunoreactive stromal cells are seen in association with a cyst (**C**), whereas in another area (**D**) stromal cells positive for anti-α-smooth muscle actin (arrows) are found in the vicinity of a thickened epithelium. **E** and **F** Sclerosing adenosis. Stromal cells present in an area of adenosis are not labelled by anti-α-smooth muscle actin (**E**); scattered immunoreactive stromal cells (arrows) are associated with zones of epithelial proliferation (**F**). (× 400) (Reproduced from Sappino et al 1988.)

How myofibroblasts and the desmoplastic reaction affect tumour growth and progression remains largely hypothetical. It has been proposed that the myofibroblastic stromal response act as a defence against neoplasia by impeding the motility and accessibility of tumour cells to blood vessels (Seemayer et al 1980). Conversely, the stromal reaction may control the access of cells which are potential tumour growth regulators, as suggested by histological evidence showing that inflammatory cells are often confined at the margins of tumours (Dvorak 1986, Dvorak et al 1979a, 1984a, 1984b, Ioachim 1976). Finally, the stromal reaction may influence tumour cell growth, at least for epithelial neoplasms, given the fact that, during development, epithelial growth and differentiation are dependent on mesenchymal support (Adams et al 1988, Kratochwil 1986, Kratochwil & Schwartz 1976, Lee et al 1985, Levine & Stockdale 1985, Li et al 1987, Sakakura 1984).

CONCLUSION

In conclusion, it is not yet clear whether myofibroblasts from most soft tissue tumours represent reactive cells or whether they represent a phenotype of transformed fibroblasts, with true malignant properties. In any event, the data showing an analogy between tumour stroma formation and wound healing make the presence of myofibroblasts in the stroma of several tumours not as surprising as one would have previously thought. In addition, neoplastic cells may secrete factors which could act on stromal cells to affect their proliferation, collagen synthesis and cytoskeletal phenotype. Although the biological implications of desmoplasia on tumour growth and invasiveness are debated, most data presently available point toward a beneficial action for the host. In this respect, the role played by myofibroblasts with different cytoskeletal phenotypes in the tumoral stroma deserves more attention. Our understanding of these questions will certainly benefit from the development of an animal model of tumour stroma formation.

ACKNOWLEDGEMENTS

This work was supported by the Swiss National Science Foundation, Grant Nr 3.108.0-88.

We thank Allan R. Liss (New York), Elsevier North-Holland Biomedical Press (Amsterdam), Masson Publishing USA (New York), The American Journal of Pathology, Cancer Research, Drs S. H. Barsky and R. Gopalakrishna, for having given permission to reproduce Figs 5.1, 5.2, 5.3, 5.5 and 5.6, and Mrs M. M. Rossire for typing the manuscript.

REFERENCES

Adams E F, Newton C J, Tait G H, Braunsberg H, Reed M J, James V H T 1988 Paracrine influence of human breast stromal fibroblasts on breast epithelial cells: secretion of a polypeptide which stimulates reductive 17β-oestradiol dehydrogenase activity. International Journal of Cancer 42: 119–122

Alguacil-Garcia A, Unni K K, Goellner J R 1978 Giant cell tumour of tendon sheath and pigmented villondular synovitis. An ultrastructural study. American Journal of Clinical Pathology 69: 6–17

Alonso S 1987 Coexpression and evolution of the two sarcomeric actin genes in vertebrates. Biochimie 69: 1119–1125

Azzarone B, Failly-Crepin C, Daya-Grosjean L, Chaponnier C, Gabbiani G 1983 Abnormal behavior of cultured fibroblasts from nodule and nonaffected aponeurosis of Dupuytren's disease. Journal of Cellular Physiology 117: 353–361

Babaï F, Skalli O, Schürch W, Seemayer T A, Gabbiani G 1988 Chemically induced rhabdomyosarcomas in rats. Ultrastructural, immunohistochemical, biochemical features and expression of α-actin isoforms. Virchows Archiv B 55: 263–277

Barsky S H, Gopalakrishna R 1987 Increased invasion and spontaneous metastasis of BL6 melanoma with inhibition of the desmoplastic response in C57 BL/6 mice. Cancer Research 47: 1663–1667

Barsky S H, Rao C N, Grotendorst G R, Liotta L A 1982 Increased content of type V collagen in desmoplasia of human breast carcinoma. American Journal of Pathology 108: 276–283

Barksy S H, Huang S J, Bhuta S 1986 The extracellular matrix of pulmonary scar carcinomas is suggestive of a desmoplastic origin. American Journal of Pathology 124: 412–419

Benjamin S P, Mercer R D, Hawk W A 1977 Myofibroblastic contraction in spontaneous regression of multiple congenital mesenchymal hamartomas. Cancer 40: 2343–2352

Benzonana G, Skalli O, Gabbiani G 1988 Correlation between the distribution of smooth muscle or non muscle myosins and α-smooth muscle actin in normal and pathological soft tissues. Cell Motility and the Cytoskeleton 11: 260–274

Bhawan J, Bacchetta C, Joris I, Majno G 1979 A myofibroblastic tumour. Infantile digital fibroma (recurrent digital fibrous tumour of childhood). American Journal of Pathology 94: 19–36

Blewitt R W, Aparicio S G R, Bird C C 1983 Epithelioid sarcoma: a tumour of myofibroblasts. Histopathology 7: 573–584

Bowser-Riley S, Bain A D, Noble J, Lamb D W 1975 Chromosome abnormalities in Dupuytren's disease. Lancet ii: 1282–1283

Brown L F, Van de Water L, Harvey V S, Dvorak H F 1988 Fibrinogen influx and accumulation of cross-linked fibrin in healing wounds and in tumour stroma. American Journal of Pathology 130: 455–465

Bulinski J C, Kumar S, Titani K, Hauschka S D 1983 Peptide antibody specific for the amino terminus of skeletal muscle α-actin. Proceedings of the National Academy of Sciences USA 80: 1506–1510

Chamley J H, Campbell G R, McConnell J D, Gröschel-Steward U 1977 Comparison of vascular smooth muscle cells from adult human, monkey and rabbit in primary culture and subculture. Cell and Tissue Research 177: 503–522

Chamley-Campbell J H, Campbell G R, Ross R 1979 The smooth muscle cell in culture. Physiological Reviews 59: 1–61

Churg A M, Kahn L B 1977 Myofibroblasts and related cells in malignant fibrous and fibrohistiocytic tumours. Human Pathology 8: 205–218

Crocker D.J, Murad T M 1969 Ultrastructure of fibrosarcoma in a male breast. Cancer 23: 891–899

D'Andiran G, Gabbiani G 1980 A metastasizing sarcoma of the pleura composed of myofibroblasts. In: Fenoglio C M, Wolff M (eds) Progress in surgical pathology, vol 2, Masson Publishing USA, New York, p 31–40

Donner L, de Lanerolle P, Costa J 1983 Immunoreactivity of paraffin-embedded normal tissues and mesenchymal tumours for smooth muscle myosin. American Journal of Clinical Pathology 80: 677–681

Dvorak H F 1986 Similarities between tumour stroma generation and wound healing. New England Journal of Medicine 315: 1650–1659

Dvorak H F, Dvorak A M, Manseau E J, Wiberg L, Churchill W H 1979a Fibrin gel investment associated with line 1 and line 10 solid tumour growth, angiogenesis, and fibroplasia in guinea pigs. Role of cellular immunity, myofibroblasts, microvascular damage, and infarction in line 1 tumour regression. Journal of the National Cancer Institute 62: 1459–1472

Dvorak H F, Orenstein N C S, Carvalho A C et al 1979b Induction of a fibrin-gel investment: an early event in line 10 hepatocarcinoma growth mediated by tumour-secreted products. The Journal of Immunology 122: 166–174

Dvorak H F, Dickersin G R, Dvorak A M, Manseau E J, Pyne K 1981 Human breast carcinoma: fibrin deposits and desmoplasia: inflammatory cell type and distribution: microvasculature and infarction. Journal of the National Cancer Institute 67: 335–345

Dvorak H F, Senger D R, Dvorak A M 1983 Fibrin as a component of the tumour stroma: origins and biological significance. Cancer Metastasis Reviews 2: 41–73

Dvorak H F, Harvey V S, McDonagh J 1984a Quantitation of fibrinogen influx and fibrin deposition and turnover in line 1 and line 10 guinea pig carcinomas. Cancer Research 44: 3348–3354

Dvorak H F, Form D M, Manseau E J, Smith B D 1984b Pathogenesis of desmoplasia. I. Immunofluorescence identification and localization of some structural proteins in line 1 and line 10 guinea pig tumours and of healing wounds. Journal of the National Cancer Institute 73: 1195–1205

Dvorak H F, Harvey V S, Estrella P, Brown L F, McDonagh J, Dvorak A M 1987 Fibrin containing gels induce angiogenesis. Implications for tumour stroma generation and wound healing. Laboratory Investigation 57: 673–686

Eddy R J, Petro J A, Tomasek J J 1988 Evidence for the nonmuscle nature of the 'myofibroblast' of granulation tissue and hypertrophic scar. An immunofluorescence study. American Journal of Pathology 130: 252–260

Fletcher C D M, Stirling R W, Smith M A, Pambakian H, McKee P H 1986 Multicentric extra-abdominal 'myofibromatosis': report of a case with ultrastructural findings. Histopathology 10: 713–724

Fletcher C D M, Achu P, Van Noorden S, McKee P H 1987 Infantile myofibromatosis: a light microscopic, histochemical and immunohistochemical study suggesting true smooth muscle differentiation. Histopathology 11: 245–258

Fu Y S, Gabbiani G, Kaye G I, Lattes R 1975 Malignant soft tissue tumours of probable histiocytic origin (malignant fibrous histiocytomas): general considerations and electron microscopic and tissue culture studies. Cancer 35: 176–198

Fujimoto T, Singer S J 1986 Immunocytochemical studies of endothelial cells in vivo. I. The presence of desmin only, or of desmin plus vimentin, or vimentin only, in the endothelial cells of different capillaries of the adult chicken. The Journal of Cell Biology 103: 2775–2786

Fujimoto T, Singer S J 1987 Immunocytochemical studies of desmin and vimentin in pericapillary cells of chicken. Journal of Histochemistry and Cytochemistry 35: 1105–1115

Gabbiani G, Ryan G B, Majno G 1971 Presence of modified fibroblasts in granulation tissue and their possible role in wound contraction. Experientia 27: 549–550

Gabbiani G, Fu Y S, Kaye G I, Lattes R, Majno G 1972 Epithelioid sarcoma. A light and electron microscopic study suggesting a synovial origin. Cancer 30: 486–499

Gabbiani G, Chaponnier C, Hüttner I 1978 Cytoplasmic filaments and gap junctions in epithelial cells and myofibroblasts during wound healing. The Journal of Cell Biology. 76: 561–568

Gabbiani G, Rungger-Brändle E 1981 The fibroblast. In: Glynn L E (ed) Handbook of inflammation, Vol 3: Tissue repair and regeneration. Elsevier/North Holland Biomedical Press, Amsterdam

Gabbiani G, Schmid E, Winter S et al 1981 Vascular smooth muscle cells differ from other smooth muscle cells: predominance of vimentin filaments and a specific α-type actin. Proceedings of the National Academy of Sciences USA 78: 298–302

Gabbiani G, Kocher O, Bloom W S, Vandekerckhove J, Weber K 1984 Actin expression in smooth muscle cells of rat aortic intimal thickening, human atheromatous plaque, and cultured rat aortic media. Journal of Clinical Investigation 73: 148–152

Garrels J I, Gibson W 1976 Identification and characterization of multiple forms of actin. Cell 9: 793–805

Ghadially F N, McNaughton J D, Lalonde J M A 1983 Myofibroblastoma: a tumour of myofibroblasts. Journal of Submicroscopic Cytology 15: 1055–1063

Ghosh L, Ghosh B, Dasgupta T 1980 Ultrastructural study of stroma in human mammary carcinoma. American Journal of Surgery 139: 229–232

Glasser S R, Julian J 1986 Intermediate filament protein as a marker of uterine stromal cell decidualization. Biology of Reproduction 35: 463–474

Grillo H C 1963 Origin of fibroblasts in wound healing: an autoradiographic study of inhibition of cellular proliferation by local X-irradiation. Annals of Surgery 157: 453–467

Gunning P, Ponte P, Blau H, Kedes L 1983 α-Skeletal and α-cardiac actic genes are coexpressed in adult human skeletal muscle and heart. Molecular and Cellular Biology 3: 1985–1995

Harris M 1980 The ultrastructure of benign and malignant fibrous histiocytomas. Histopathology 4: 29–44

Harris M, Ahmed A 1977 The ultrastructure of tubular carcinoma of the breast. Journal of Pathology 123: 79–83

Harris N L, Dvorak A M, Smith J, Dvorak H F 1982 Fibrin deposits in Hodgkin's disease. American Journal of Pathology 108: 119–129

Hashimoto K, Braunstein M H, Jakobiec F A 1974 Dermatofibrosarcoma protuberans: a tumour with perineural and epineural cell features. Archives of Dermatology 110: 874–885

Hashimoto K, Matsui K, Akeho M, Okamoto K, Yumoto T, Endo A 1982 A tumour composed of myofibroblasts. An ultrastructural study. Acta Pathologica Japonica 32: 633–640

Herman I M, D'Amore P A 1985 Microvascular pericytes contain muscle and nonmuscle actins. The Journal of Cell Biology 101: 43–52

Hernandez A D, Hibbs M S, Postlethwaite A E 1985 Establishment of basal cell carcinoma in culture: evidence for a basal cell carcinoma-derived factor(s) which stimulates fibroblasts to proliferate and release collagenase. Journal of Investigative Dermatology 85: 470–475

Ioachim H L 1976 The stromal reaction of tumors: an expression of immune surveillance. Journal of the National Cancer Institute 57: 465–470

Jacobiec F A, Tannenbaum M 1974 The ultrastructure of orbital fibrosarcoma. American Journal of Ophthalmology 77: 899 917

Joyce N C, DeCamilli P, Boyles J 1984 Pericytes, like vascular smooth muscle cells, are immunocytochemically positive for cyclic GMP-dependent protein kinase. Microvascular Research 28: 206–219

Joyce N C, Haire M F, Palade G E 1985a Contractile proteins in pericytes. I. Immunoperoxidase localization of tropomyosin. The Journal of Cell Biology 100: 1379–1386

Joyce N C, Haire M F, Palade G E 1985b Contractile proteins in pericytes. II. Immunocytochemical evidence for the presence of two isomyosins in graded concentrations. The Journal of Cell Biology 100: 1387–1395

Katenkamp D, Stiller D 1975a Cellular composition of the so-called dermatofibroma (histiocytoma cutis). Virchows Archiv A: Pathology, Anatomy and Histology 367: 325–336

Katenkamp D, Stiller D 1975b Structural patterns and histological behavior of experimental sarcoma. II. Ultrastructural cytology. Experimental Pathology 11: 190–196

Kindblom L S, Merck C, Angervall L 1979 The ultrastructure of myxofibrosarcoma. Virchows Archiv A: Pathology, Anatomy and Histology 381: 121–139

Kocher O, Gabbiani G 1986 Cytoskeletal features of normal and atheromatous human arterial smooth muscle cells. Human Pathology 17: 875–880

Kocher O, Skalli O, Bloom W S, Gabbiani G 1984 Cytoskeleton of rat aortic smooth muscle cells. Normal conditions and experimental intimal thickening. Laboratory Investigation 50: 645–652

Kocher O, Skalli O, Cerutti D, Gabbiani F, Gabbiani G 1985 Cytoskeletal features of rat aortic cells during development. An electron microscopic, immunohistochemical, and biochemical study. Circulation Research 56: 829–838

Kratochwil K 1986 The stroma and the control of cell growth. Journal of Pathology 149: 23–24

Kratochwil K, Schwartz P 1976 Tissue interaction in androgen response of embryonic mammary rudiment of mouse: identification of target tissue for testosterone. Proceedings of the National Academy of Sciences USA 73: 4041–4044

Lagacé R, Delage C, Seemayer T A 1979 Myxoid variant of malignant fibrous histiocytoma: ultrastructural observations. Cancer 43: 526–534

Lagacé R, Schürch W, Seemayer T A 1980 Myofibroblasts in soft tissue sarcomas. Virchows Archiv A: Pathology, Anatomy and Histology 389: 1–11

Larson D M, Fujiwara K, Alexander R W, Gimbrone Jr M A 1984 Myosin in cultured vascular smooth muscle cells: immunofluorescence and immunochemical studies of alterations in antigenic expression. The Journal of Cell Biology 99: 1582–1589

Lee E Y H P, Lee W H, Kaetzel C S, Parry G, Bissell M J 1985 Interaction of mouse mammary epithelial cells with collagen substrata: regulation of casein gene expression and secretion. Proceedings of the National Academy of Sciences USA 82: 1419–1423

Leoncini P, Cintorino M, Vindigni et al 1988 Distribution of cytoskeletal and contractile proteins in normal and tumour bearing salivary and lacrimal glands. Virchows Archiv A 412: 329–337

Levine J F, Stockdale F E 1985 Cell-cell interactions promote mammary epithelial cell differentiation. The Journal of Cell Biology 100: 1415–1422

Li M L, Aggeler J, Farson D A, Hatier C, Hassell J, Bissell M J 1987 Influence of a reconstituted basement membrane and its components on casein gene expression and secretion in mouse mammary epithelial cells. Proceedings of the National Academy of Sciences USA 84: 136–140

Limacher J, Delage C, Lagacé R 1978 Malignant fibrous histiocytoma: clinicopathologic and ultrastructural study of 12 cases. American Journal of Surgical Pathology 2: 265–274

MacDonald R A 1959 Origin of fibroblasts in experimental healing wounds: autoradiographic studies using tritiated thymidine. Surgery 46: 376–382

Mayer Y, Czosnek H, Zeelon P E, Yaffe D, Nudel U 1984 Expression of the genes coding for the skeletal muscle and cardiac actins in the heart. Nucleic Acids Research 12: 1087–1100

Merrilees M J, Finlay G J 1985 Human tumour cells in culture stimulate glycosaminoglycan synthesis by human skin fibroblasts. Laboratory Investigation 53: 30–36

Miettinen M 1988 Antibody specific to muscle actins in the diagnosis and classification of soft tissue tumours. American Journal of Pathology 130: 205–215

Minty A J, Alonso S, Caravatti M, Buckingham M E 1982 A fetal skeletal muscle actin mRNA in the mouse and its identity with cardiac actin mRNA. Cell 30: 185–192

Mosse P R L, Campbell G R, Wang Z L, Campbell J H 1985 Smooth muscle phenotypic expression in human carotid arteries. I. Comparison of cells from diffuse intimal thickenings adjacent to atheromatours plaques with those of the media. Laboratory Investigation 53: 556–562

Nakanishi I, Kajikawa K, Okada Y, Eguchi K 1981 Myofibroblasts in fibrous tumours and fibrosis in various organs. Acta Pathologica Japonica 31: 423–437

Olivetti G, Anversa P, Melissari M, Loud A V 1980 Morphometric study of early postnatal development of the thoracic aorta in the rat. Circulation Research 47: 417–424

Osborn M, Weber K 1983 Tumor diagnosis by intermediate filament typing: a novel tool for surgical pathology. Laboratory Investigation 48: 372–394

Osborn M, Caselitz J, Püschel K, Weber K 1987 Intermediate filament expression in human vascular smooth muscle and in arteriosclerotic plaques. Virchows Archiv A: Pathology, Anatomy and Histology 411: 449–458

Owens G K, Loeb A, Gordon D, Thompson M M 1986 Expression of smooth muscle-specific α-iosactin in cultured vascular smooth muscle cells: relationship between growth and cytodifferentiation. The Journal of Cell Biology 102: 343–352

Peres R, Betsholtz C, Westermark B, Heldin C H 1987 Frequent expression of growth factors for mesenchymal cells in human mammary carcinoma cell lines. Cancer Research 47: 3425–3429

Poole J C F, Cromwell S B, Benditt E P 1971 Behavior of smooth muscle cells and formation of extracellular structures in the reaction of arterial wall to injury. American Journal of Pathology 62: 391–414

Reddick R L, Michelitch H, Triche T J 1979 Malignant soft tissue tumours (malignant fibrous histiocytoma, pleomorphic liposarcoma and pleomorphic rhabdomyosarcoma). An electron microscopic study. Human Pathology 10: 327–343

Reddick R L, Michelitch H J, Levine A M, Triche T J 1980 Osteogenic sarcoma. A study of the ultrastructure. Cancer 45: 64–71

Ross R, Everett N B, Tyler R 1970 Wound healing and collagen formation. VI. The origin of the wound fibroblast studied in parabiosis. The Journal of Cell Biology 44: 645–654

Rovner A S, Murphy R A, Owens G K 1986 Expression of smooth muscle and nonmuscle myosin heavy chains in cultured vascular smooth muscle cells. Journal of Biological Chemistry 261: 14740–14745

Rungger-Brändle E, Gabbiani G 1983 The role of cytoskeletal and cytocontractile elements in pathologic processes. American Journal of Pathology 110: 361–392

Sakakura T 1984 Epithelial-mesenchymal interactions in mammary gland development and its perturbation in relation to tumorigenesis. In: Rich M A, Hager J C, Furmanski P (eds). Understanding breast cancer, clinical and laboratory concepts. Marcel Dekker, New York, p 261–283

Sappino A P, Skalli O, Jackson B, Schürch W, Gabbiani G 1988 Smooth-muscle differentiation in stromal cells of malignant and non-malignant breast tissues. International Journal of Cancer 41: 707–712

Schmidt R A, Cone R, Haas J E, Gown A M 1988 Diagnosis of rhabdomyosarcomas with HHF35, a monoclonal antibody directed against muscle actins. American Journal of Pathology 131: 19–28

Schürch W, Seemayer T A, Lagacé R 1981 Stromal myofibroblasts in primary invasive and metastatic carcinomas. A combined immunological, light and electron microscopic study. Virchows Archiv A: Pathology, Anatomy and Histology 391: 125–139

Schürch W, Lagacé R, Seemayer T A 1982 Myofibroblastic stromal reaction in retracted scirrhous carcinoma of the breast. Surgery, Gynecology and Obstetrics 154: 351–359

Schürch W, Skalli O, Seemayer T A, Gabbiani G 1987 Intermediate filament proteins and actin isoforms as markers for soft tissue tumour differentiation and origin. I. Smooth muscle tumours. American Journal of Pathology 128: 91–103

Seemayer T A, Schürch W, Lagacé R, Tremblay G 1979 Myofibroblasts in the stroma of invasive and metastatic carcinoma. American Journal of Surgical Pathology 3: 525–533

Seemayer T A, Lagacé R, Schürch W, Thelmo W L 1980 The myofibroblast: biologic, pathologic, and theoretical considerations. Pathology Annual 15: 443–470

Senger D R, Galli S J, Dvorak A M, Perruzzi C A, Harvey V S, Dvorak H F 1983 Tumour cells secrete a vascular permeability factor that promotes accumulation of ascites fluid. Science 219: 983–985

Senger D R, Perruzzi C A, Feder J, Dvorak H F 1986 A highly conserved vascular permeability factor secreted by a variety of human and rodent tumour cell lines. Cancer Research 46: 5629–5632

Sergovich F R, Botz J S, McFarlane R M 1983 Nonrandom cytogenetic abnormalities in Dupuytren's disease. The New England Journal of Medicine 308: 162–163

Shimosato Y, Hashimoto R, Kodama et al 1980 Prognostic implications of fibrotic focus (scar) in small peripheral lung carcinomas. American Journal of Surgical Pathology 4: 365–373

Shum D T, McFarlane R M, 1988 Histogenesis of Dupuytren's disease; an immunohistochemical study of 30 cases. Journal of Hand Surgery 13A: 61–66

Singer I I 1979 The fibronexus: a transmembrane association of fibronectin-containing fibers and bundles of 5 nm microfilaments in hamster and human fibroblasts. Cell 16: 675–685

Singer I I, Kawka D W, Kazazis D M, Clark R A F 1984 In vivo co-distribution of fibronectin and actin fibers in granulation tissue: immunofluorescence and electron microscope studies of the fibronexus at the myofibroblast surface. The Journal of Cell Biology 98: 2091–2106

Skalli O, Gabbiani G 1988 The biology of the myofibroblast. Relationship to wound contraction and fibrocontractive diseases. In: Clark R A F, Henson P M (eds) The molecular and cellular biology of wound repair. Plenum Publishing Corporation, New York, p 373–402

Skalli O, Ropraz P, Trzeciak A, Benzonana G, Gillessen D, Gabbiani G 1986a A monoclonal antibody against α-smooth muscle actin: a new probe for smooth muscle differentiation. The Journal of Cell Biology 103: 2787–2796

Skalli O, Bloom W S, Ropraz P, Azzarone B, Gabbiani G 1986b Cytoskeletal remodeling of rat aortic smooth muscle cells in vitro: relationships to culture conditions and analogies to in vivo situations. Journal of Submicroscopic Cytology 18: 481–493

Skalli O, Vandekerckhove J, Gabbiani G 1987 Actin isoform pattern as a marker of normal or pathological smooth-muscle and fibroblastic tissues. Differentiation 33: 232–238

Skalli O, Gabbiani G, Babaï F, Seemayer T A, Pizzolato G, Schürch W 1988 Intermediate filament proteins and actin isoforms as markers for soft tissue tumour differentiation and origin. II. Rhabdomyosarcomas. American Journal of Pathology 130: 515–531

Skalli O, Schürch W, Seemayer T et al 1989a Myofibroblasts from diverse pathological settings are heterogeneous in their content of actin isoforms and intermediate filament proteins. Laboratory Investigation 60: 275–285

Skalli O, Pelte M F, Peclet M C et al 1989b α-smooth muscle actin, a differentiation marker of smooth muscle cells, is present in microfilamentous bundles of pericytes. Journal of Histochemistry and Cytochemistry 37: 315–321

Somers K D, Dawson D M, Wright Jr G L et al 1982 Cell culture of Peyronie's disease plaque and normal penile tissue. The Journal of Urology 127: 585–588

Stamenkovic I, Skalli O, Gabbiani G 1986 Distribution of intermediate filament proteins in normal and diseased human glomeruli. American Journal of Pathology 125: 465–475

Stiller D, Katenkamp D 1975 Cellular features in desmoid fibromatosis and well-differentiate fibrosarcomas. An electron microscopic study. Virchows Archiv A: Pathology, Anatomy and Histology 369: 155–164

Storti R V, Rich A 1976 Chick cytoplasmic actin and muscle actin have different structural genes. Proceedings of the National Academy of Sciences USA 73: 2346–2350

Suster S, Rosai J 1989 Intranodal hemorrhagic spindle cell tumour with amianthoid fibers. Report of six cases of a distinctive mesenchymal neoplasm of the inguinal region that simulates Kaposi's sarcoma. American Journal of Surgical Pathology 13: 347–357

Tamimi S O, Ahmed A 1987 Stromal changes in invasive breast carcinoma: an ultrastructural study. Journal of Pathology 153: 163–170

Taxy J B, Battifora H 1977 Malignant fibrous histiocytoma. An electron microscopic study. Cancer 40: 254–267

Toccaniner-Pelte M F, Skalli O, Kapanci Y, Gabbiani G 1987 Characterization of stromal cells with myoid features in lymph nodes and spleen in normal and pathologic conditions. American Journal of Pathology 129: 109–118

Tomasek J J, Schultz R J, Episalla C W, Newman S A 1986 The cytoskeleton and extracellular matrix of the Dupuytren's disease 'myofibroblast': an immunofluorescence study of a nonmuscle cell type. Journal of Hand Surgery 11A: 365-371

Travo P, Weber K, Osborn M 1982 Co-existence of vimentin and desmin type intermediate filaments in a subpopulation of adult rat vascular smooth muscle cells growing in primary culture. Experimental Cell Research 139: 87–94

Tremblay G 1979 Stromal aspects of breast carcinoma. Experimental and Molecular Pathology 31: 218–260

Tsukada T, McNutt M A, Ross R, Gown A M 1987 HHF35, a muscle actin-specific monoclonal antibody. II. Reactivity in normal, reactive, and neoplastic human tissues. American Journal of Pathology 127: 389–402

Vande Berg J S, Rudolph R 1985 Cultured myofibroblasts: a useful model to study wound contraction and pathological contracture. Annals of Plastic Surgery 14: 111–120

Vande Berg J S, Rudolph R, Woodward M 1984a Growth dynamics of cultured myofibroblasts from human breast cancer and nonmalignant contracting tissues. Plastic and Reconstructive Surgery 73: 605–616

Vande Berg J S, Rudolph R, Woodward M 1984b Comparative growth dynamics and morphology between cultured myofibroblasts from granulating wounds and dermal fibroblasts. American Journal of Pathology 114: 187–200

Vandekerkchove J, Weber K 1978a At least six different actins are expressed in a higher mammal: an analysis based on the amino acid sequence of the amino-terminal tryptic peptide. Journal of Molecular Biology 126: 783–802

Vanderkerckhove J, Weber K 1978b Mammalian cytoplasmic actins are the products of at least two genes and differ in primary structure in at least 25 identified positions from skeletal muscle actins. Proceedings of the National Academy of Sciences 75: 1106–1110

Vandkerckhove J, Weber K 1979 The amino acid sequence of actin from chicken skeletal muscle actin and chicken gizzard smooth muscle actin. FEBS Letters 102: 219–222

Vandekerckhove J, Weber K 1981 Actin typing on total cellular extracts. A highly sensitive protein-chemical procedure able to distinguish different actins. European Journal of Biochemistry 113: 595–603

Vandekerckhove J, Bugaisky G, Buckingham M 1986 Simultaneous expression of skeletal muscle and heart actin proteins in various striated muscle tissues and cells. A quantitative determination of the two actin isoforms. The Journal of Biological Chemistry 261: 1838–1843

Vandekerckhove J, Osborn M, Altmannsberger M, Weber K 1987 Actin typing of rhabdomyosarcomas shows the presence of the fetal and adult forms of sarcomeric muscle actin. Differentiation 35: 126–131

Vasude K S, Harris M 1978 A sarcoma of myofibroblasts. An ultrastructural study. Archives of Pathology and Laboratory Medicine 102: 185–188

Viale G, Doglioni C, Iuzzolino et al 1988 Infantile digital fibromatosis-like tumour (inclusion body fibromatosis) of adulthood: report of two cases with ultrastructural and immunocytochemical findings. Histopathology 12: 415–424

Vuletin J C 1977 Myofibroblasts in parosteal osteogenic sarcoma. Archives of Pathology and Laboratory Medicine 101:272

Wargotz E S, Weiss S W, Norris H J 1987 Myofibroblastoma of the breast. Sixteen cases of a distinctive benign mesenchymal tumour. American Journal of Surgical Pathology 11: 493–502

Weathers D R, Campbell W G 1974 Ultrastructure of the giant cell fibroma of the oral mucosa. Oral Surgical Pathology and Medicine 38: 550–561

Whalen R G, Butler-Browne G S, Gros F 1976 Protein synthesis and actin heterogeneity in calf muscle cells in culture. Proceedings of the National Academy of Sciences USA 73: 2018–2022

Woodcock-Mitchell J, Mitchell J J et al 1988 α-smooth muscle actin is transiently expressed in embryonic rat cardiac and skeletal muscles. Differentation 39: 161–166

6. What is a fibrohistiocytic tumour?

R. L. Kempson   M. R. Hendrickson

INTRODUCTION

Some comments on 'histogenesis'

Tumour classification since the 19th century has been shaped by the now familiar approach of trying to establish histogenesis ('cell of origin') and fashioning a classification (and associated set of labels) that reflect this pedigree. Operationally, this amounts to characterising, as completely as possible (using available technology), the phenotype of the constituent cells of a neoplasm and, with this information in hand, to turn to a stock of normal cell phenotype (or their embryonic precursors) in search of a good match. If a successful match is identified then two things occur: first, the histogenetic inference is made that the normal cell gave rise to the class of neoplasms under study and, second, a label is concocted that reflects these beliefs about differentation and histogenesis. It is important to emphasise that histogenetic talk is, by and large, talk about phenotype; the 'looks-like-therefore-came-from' part is an inference (Gould 1986, Fletcher 1987). To paraphrase the oft-quoted comment on paternity: 'phenotype is a matter of fact, histogenesis is a matter of opinion', and opinions abound in soft tissue tumour taxonomy.

This histogenetic research programme has had limited success when applied to neoplasms of the somatic soft tissues, chiefly because a majority of malignant neoplasms and many of the distinctive benign clinicopathological entities that involve these tissues are composed of relatively 'undifferentiated' and nondescript spindled and rounded cells with undistinguished phenotypes. The spirit of the problem is conveyed by the following thought experiment. Consider the set of all somatic soft tissue neoplasms, benign, 'intermediate' and malignant. Then successively remove and set to one side the following groups of neoplasms:

1. Carve out those neoplasms whose constituent cells (possibly a very small subset) exhibit a non-controversial, distinctive phenotype beyond that of the normal fibroblast or myofibroblast. The neoplasms removed would include, among others, such entities as the familiar lipomas, differentiated liposarcomas, nerve sheath neoplasms, smooth muscle neoplasms, and clear cell sarcoma (soft tissue melanoma).

2. Carve out those neoplasms whose constituent cells are all 'undifferentiated' but that so strongly resemble, in other morphologic and clinical respects, neoplasms with a particular differentiated phenotype that they are traditionally grouped with this differentiated type. Under this heading would be the small blue cell tumours of childhood that resemble embryonal rhabdomyosarcoma in terms of architecture and clinical response to current rhabdomyosarcoma therapy.

3. Remove those neoplasms composed predominantly of fibroblasts (or myofibroblasts) that fulfill the (currently) rigid morphological criteria for nodular fasciitis, fibromatoses and fibrosarcoma.

Once these subsets have been removed we are left with a very large heterogenous group of neoplasms that fall roughly into two classes:

1. A small minority of these residual neoplasms have a distinctive architectural pattern or recognizable cytological features that do not unequivocally correspond to a normal cell type. This group would include, among others, granular cell tumour, alveolar soft part sarcoma, epithelioid sarcoma and synovial sarcoma.

2. A large group of neoplasms that are composed of a mixture of spindled, collagen-producing cells intimately admixed with a population of inflammatory cells and rounded cells. The latter typically exhibit phagocytosis of lipid or haemosiderin. Multinucleated giant cells of several types—osteoclastic, Touton, etc—may be prominent. The spindled cells may have a non-distinctive architectural configuration or they may be arranged in a variably pronounced storiform or cartwheel pattern.

It is the taxonomy of this second group that concerns us in this review. It is in part the large size and clinical importance of this group that has occasioned the attention that has been lavished on this topic in the histopathological literature over the past several decades. Indeed, many more or less distinctive benign (or locally recurring) clinicopathological entities, involving not only the soft tissues, but also the skin, bone and joints, fall into this category and (perhaps more importantly) so does the majority of the malignancies of somatic soft tissues.

Historical review

The histogenetic construct 'fibrous histiocytoma' was developed approximately 30 years ago to provide an organising principle and nomenclature for this second group of undifferentiated neoplasms. In particular, there was difference of opinion at that time concerning the taxonomy of the relatively common pleomorphic sarcomas within this group that were composed of a mixture of cells with the H & E morphology of fibroblasts and histiocytes. In addition, these sarcomas often contained large bizarre cells that either possessed foamy cytoplasm, and thus were thought by some to resemble lipoblasts, or were endowed with abundant eosinophilic cytoplasm characteristic of rhabdomyoblasts. Against these interpretations was the absence of the characteristic nuclear indentation by a macrovacuole(s) that identifies lipo-blasts and the absence of demonstrable cross striations in the cells with eosinophilic cytoplasm. The uncertainty about the phenotype of these sarco-mas was reflected in the diverse names applied to them, e.g. 'undifferentiated sarcoma', 'pleomorphic liposarcoma', or 'pleomorphic rhabdomyosarcoma'.

Impressed with the resemblance of many of the tumour cells to fibroblasts and histiocytes, and in the absence of convincing evidence of either lipoblastic or rhabdomyoblastic differentiation, O'Brien and Stout (1964) suggested the name 'malignant fibrous histiocytoma' for this group of sarcomas. Studies were then undertaken to attempt to prove that these neoplastic spindled and rounded cells were indeed histiocytes and fibroblasts. In cell cultures carried out by Ozzello et al (1963), the cells of these neoplasms were reported to assume stellate shapes and to exhibit amoeboid movement and phagocytic activity. These investigators took this as evidence of histiocytic differentiation, an interpretation that was not then, and is not now, universally accepted. As a result of these observations, they proposed that malignant fibrous histiocy-tomas were histiocytic neoplasms in which some of the tumour cells took on the appearance and function of fibroblasts (i.e that they were 'facultative fibroblasts'). Subsequently, questions have been raised as to exactly what neoplasms were grown in the cultures and whether or not cell culture is a useful technique to establish histiocytic differentiation (Wood et al 1986, Krawisz et al 1981, Fletcher 1987). When the electron microscope became widely available in the 1960s, a large number of fibrous histiocytomas, particularly the malignant variants, were examined with this instrument (Alguacil-Garcia et al 1978, Churg & Kahn 1977, Fu et al 1975, Harris 1980, Hoffman & Dickersin 1983, Kim & Goldblatt 1982, Lagace et al 1979, Taxy & Battifora 1977, Tsuneyoshi et al 1981). The main conclusion that can be drawn from the large number of published studies is that the cells in malignant fibrous histiocytomas are no more differentiated when examined with the electron microscope than they are when examined with the light microscope using 19th century techniques. Ultrastructurally, some tumour cells have the features of fibroblasts with elongate nuclei and prominent rough endoplasmic reticulum, while other similar cells contain intermediate filaments and the other subcellular components of myofibroblasts. The cells that resemble histiocytes by light microscopy have oval or round nuclei and contain lysosomes, lipid and phagosomes. Langerhan's granules have rarely been reported. All of these cell types can also be found in other neoplasms and, thus, the ultrastructural features of malignant fibrous histiocytomas are disappointingly non-specific. Interestingly, a fourth type of cell, without any of the above ultrastructural features, was also described in many cases. These have been variously interpreted as 'primitive' or 'intermediate' mesenchymal cells and, of course, it has been theorised that these are the long sought-after 'progenitor' cells that give rise to the fibroblasts, myofibroblasts and the histiocyte-like cells that populate the fibrous histiocytomas. Ultrastructural examination of the benign tumours in the fibrous histiocytoma group generally reveal similarly non-descript features (Harris 1980).

More recently, enzyme histochemical and immunohistochemical techniques have been employed in a search for distinctive fibrous histiocytoma antigens or cell products that would shed light on the differentiation of these tumours. Histiocytes/macrophages synthesise a number of enzymes that can be detected by histochemical or immunohistochemical techniques. Alpha-1-antitrypsin and alpha-1-anti-chymotrypsin are among these and when antibodies against these antigens became available, they were found to be present in the tumour cells of most malignant fibrous histiocytomas. (Chowdhury et al 1980, du Boulay 1982, Kindblom et al 1982, McDonnell et al 1988, Meister & Nathrath 1980, Roholl et al 1985, Wolfe & Palmer 1981). Unfortunately, a large number of non-histiocytic cells, including tumour cells of diverse differentiation, also synthesise these enzymes (Soini & Miettinen 1988, 1989). Macrophages also express lysozyme (muramidase) but this was infrequently detected in the tumour cells of the fibrous histiocytomas (Burgdorf et al 1981, Fletcher 1987, Kindblom et al 1982). This caused considerable consternation among the proponents of the histiocyte theory.

In the early 1970s, monocytes/macrophages were shown to be bone marrow derived (Unanue 1976). During the next decade the antigen expression of these cells was extensively studied and antibodies against many of their antigens have become available. These antibodies have been used to study the antigenic and enzymatic profiles of the constituent cells of the benign and malignant fibrous histiocytomas. With only rare exceptions, investigators have failed to find antigens expressed by bone marrow-derived macrophages in the neoplastic cells of the malignant fibrous histiocytomas (Brecher & Franklin 1986, Kanitakis et al 1984, Lawson et al 1987, Roholl et al 1985, Strauchen & Dimitriu-Bona 1986, Wood et al 1986). The non-neoplastic foam cells often present at the margins of malignant fibrous histiocytomas do express these antigens, indicating that they are histiocytes. A recent study by Wood et al (1988) has shown that the constituent cells in nodular tenosynovitis (giant cell tumour of tendon sheath) do express monocyte/macrophage antigens, but the other fibrous histiocytomas so far tested in our laboratory have not been composed of such cells. Enzyme histochemical studies have been performed and most reports indicate the cells in malignant fibrous histiocytomas do not express the enzymes commonly present in monocytes/macrophages, but rather the tumour cells express the enzymatic profile of fibroblasts, whether such cells morphologically resemble fibroblasts or histiocytes (Roholl et al 1985, Wood et al 1986). A few laboratories have reported somewhat different results suggesting some cells in fibrous histiocytes do express histiocytic enzymes (Enjoji et al 1980).

What are the histiocyte-like cells?

The results of the many ultrastructural, histochemical, and immunohistochemical studies summarised above raise the question: Are any of the neoplastic cells in the benign and malignant fibrous histiocytomas (setting aside nodular tenosynovitis), in fact differentiating as histiocytes? The answer appears to be a resounding No (Fletcher 1987, Lawson et al 1987, Meister 1988, Roholl et al 1985, Wood et al 1986). Most ultrastructural studies of the fibrous histiocytomas reported 'primitive' mesenchymal cells and cells having the ultrastructural features of fibroblasts and myofibroblasts, but these studies have been unconvincing in detecting neoplastic histiocytes in these lesions. Immunohistochemical and enzyme histochemical studies provide strong evidence that the fibrous histiocytomas are neoplastic proliferations of primitive mesenchymal cells differentiating as fibroblasts and myofibroblasts and that the constituent cells are not monocytes/macrophages. This is certainly the conclusion that we have reached on the basis of our studies (Wood et al 1986).

Running in parallel with the early histogenetic studies outlined above were other studies aimed at elucidating the clinicopathology of this large undifferentiated 'fibrous histiocytoma' group. These studies played off traditional light microscopic features against clinical outcome in an attempt to develop clinically relevant histopathological subgroups. Because of their relative frequency among the sarcomas, and because they cause considerable diagnostic difficulty, the pleomorphic malignant fibrous histiocytomas were among the first to be evaluated. In 1972, Kempson and Kyriakos reported 30 pleomorphic tumours composed of fibroblasts and histiocyte-like cells that they labelled fibroxanthosarcoma, a type of malignant fibrous histiocytoma. They described morphological features that were characteristic of this group of neoplasms. These include randomly placed elongate fibroblasts that may be arranged in a whorled or storiform pattern or in bundles or fascicles. Other tumour cells are round and some of these become enlarged and/or multinucleate. The nuclei in the latter are often gigantic and strikingly bizarre. Numerous mitotic figures, often abnormal, are a common feature and foam cells are frequently found at the periphery of the tumour. Weiss and Enzinger (1978) reported 200 more cases and renamed the lesion 'pleomorphic malignant fibrous histiocytoma', the label that is now most often used to identify these sarcomas. Almost as soon as these morphological features were recognised and accepted as identifying a clinically useful group of neoplasms, it became apparent that some pleomorphic malignant fibrous histiocytomas contained variably sized areas of myoxid stroma and that the morphological patterns of some pleomorphic malignant fibrous histiocytomas overlapped with those of the neoplasm that had been previously categorised as high-grade fibrosarcoma. These observations indicated the need for a subclassification of the malignant fibrous histiocytic neoplasms. As a result, the categories of the fibrous and the myxoid types of malignant fibrous histiocytomas were created (Kearney et al 1980, Angervall et al 1977, Weiss & Enzinger 1977, Weiss 1982). Kyriakos and Kempson (1976) reported yet another type of fibrous histiocytoma characterised by a predominance of histiocyte-like cells set in a sea of acute inflammation. They labelled this variant 'inflammatory malignant fibrous histiocytoma'.

Other investigators studied the superficial fibrous histiocytomas (Gonzalez & Duarte 1982). An initial focus of attention were those dermal lesions that were histologically identical to pleomorphic malignant fibrous histiocytoma but, paradoxically, did not metastasise ('atypical fibroxanthoma') (Kempson & McGavran 1964). It was also realised that many common dermal and subcutaneous lesions previously labelled 'dermatofibroma', 'sclerosing hae-mangioma', 'dermal histiocytoma', or 'subepidermal nodular fibrosis' were composed of cells resembling fibroblasts and histiocytes. It rapidly became apparent that these largely reactive lesions could be collected under the fibrous histiocytoma umbrella and more sensibly named 'dermal and subcu-taneous fibrous histiocytomas' (Gonzalez & Duarte 1982, Enzinger & Zhang 1988).

Should the label be changed?

Given the results of the immunohistochemical and enzyme histochemical studies, does the term fibrous histiocytoma accurately reflect what is currently believed about this group of neoplasms? We think not. The evidence is overwhelming that the round neoplastic cells in these neo-plasms mimic histiocytes in terms of their shape, phagocytic characteristics and, to some extent, in their enzyme histochemical profile, but are dis-tinctly unlike histiocytes when subjected to more specific tests of histiocytic differentiation.

Should the name 'fibrous histiocytoma' be changed to reflect these facts? We think not. Names serve many purposes in clinical medicine only one of which is to reflect the latest scientific truth; their primary function must always be to facilitate unambiguous communication between clinicians and pathologists concerning patient management issues. Patient management considerations argue that diseases should have stable names and unless renaming a group of tumours has managerial implications, familiar and accepted names, in our opinion, should stay (Dehner 1988, Fletcher 1987, Weiss 1982). Scientific fashions change but the clinicopathological facts about neoplasms remain much the same.

More important to us than changing the name to fit the latest scientific study is the assurance that pathologists are using a shared set of morpho-logical criteria to diagnose soft tissue neoplasms. The clinicopathology of the many lesions encompased by the term 'fibrous histiocytoma' has been delineated by numerous studies over the last 25 years and an extensive published experience has been accumulated and organised using the clas-sificatory structure suggested by Stout 30 years ago. The remainder of this chapter is devoted to a summary of this experience and a brief presenta-tion of the morphological criteria for each of the more important entities in the fibrous histiocytoma group.

SPECIFIC TYPES OF FIBROUS HISTIOCYTOMAS: MORPHOLOGICAL FEATURES, CLINICAL OUTCOME AND DIFFERENTIAL DIAGNOSIS

Our current definition of the fibrous histiocytomas includes a group of benign lesions, some of which are reactive, one neoplasm considered to be of low malignant potential because it rarely metastasises, and the malignant fibrous histiocytomas. The latter group comprises six morphologically defined groups of neoplasms that have different appearances, but that have as their common theme cells that take on the appearance of fibroblasts and histiocytes.

BENIGN REACTIVE AND LOCALLY RECURRING FIBROUS HISTIOCYTOMAS

The nomenclature we use for the benign and locally recurring fibrohistiocytic tumours is presented in Table 6.1. Almost all of these lesions occur in the skin and subcutaneous tissue.

Dermal and subcutaneous fibrous histiocytomas

The commonly encountered dermal fibrous histiocytomas include dermatofibroma, sclerosing hemangioma, dermal histiocytoma, and fibroxanthoma. These lesions have also been grouped together in the past under the heading of subepidermal nodular fibrosis. We applaud the lumping, but we prefer the label dermal fibrous histiocytoma because these lesions are composed of fibroblasts and histiocytic-appearing cells (Gonzalez & Duarte 1982) (Table 6.1). Indeed, true histiocytes are present in some of the lesions as evidenced by xanthoma cells and multinucleate foam cells. Fibrohistiocytic tumours that share many histological features with the dermal fibrous histiocytomas may be occasionally be encountered in the subcutaneous tissue. We label such lesions as subcutaneous fibrous histiocytoma and we think they should be distinguished from those centred in the dermis because, unlike the dermal

Table 6.1 The soft tissue fibrous histiocytomas: benign, reactive and locally recurring

Old nomenclature	Current suggested nomenclature

Subepidermal nodular fibrosis
  Dermatofibroma
  Sclerosing hemangioma
  Dermal histiocytoma
	Dermal fibrous histiocytoma

No generally accepted diagnostic term	Subcutaneous fibrous histiocytoma (plexiform fibrohistiocytic tumour)
Fibroxanthoma	Dermal fibrous histiocytoma
Xanthoma	Xanthoma
Juvenile xanthogranuloma	Juvenile xanthogranuloma
Reticulohistiocytoma	Reticulohistiocytoma
Nodular tenosynovitis or giant cell tumour of tendon sheath	Tenosynovial giant cell tumour
Atypical fibroxanthoma	Atypical fibroxanthoma

lesions, they can recur. However, recurrences are not aggressive. Recently Enzinger & Zhang (1988) reported 65 cases of a distinctive subgroup of subcutaneous fibrous histiocytomas using the label plexiform fibrohistiocytic tumour to draw attention to the multinodular growth pattern that marks these lesions. Occasionally a superficially situated fibrous histiocytoma overlaps the dermal–subcutaneous junction; is it a dermal or subcutaneous fibrous histiocytoma? As a general rule, we reserve the diagnosis of subcutaneous fibrous histiocytoma for those lesions centred on this interface or centred more deeply in the subcutis. Moreover, patients with the usually multinodular subcutaneous fibrous histiocytomas are younger than patients with the usually single nodular dermal fibrous histiocytomas.

Patients who develop dermal fibrous histiocytomas are most often adults. The lesions occur most commonly on the extremities and appear as white or red nodules, although occasionally they may be blue or black because of haemosiderin deposition. Typically they are small, although they can be of large size. Histologically there is a spectrum of patterns varying from tumours that are predominantly fibroblastic (dermatofibroma) (Figs 6.1 and 6.2), through those that are a mixture of fibroblastic and histiocyte-like cells, to those that are predominantly composed of histiocytes and/or histocyte-like cells with only focal evidence of fibrous differentiation (dermal histiocytoma). Lesions that are composed of equal numbers of fibroblasts and foamy

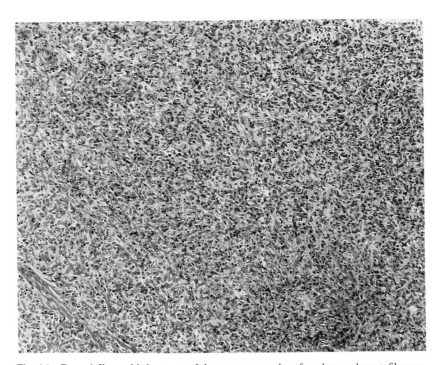

Fig. 6.1 Dermal fibrous histiocytoma of the type commonly referred to as dermatofibroma. This photomicrograph demonstrates the variable cellularity that can be seen in these lesions. A collagenised area on the lower left blends into more cellular areas on the right. × 100.

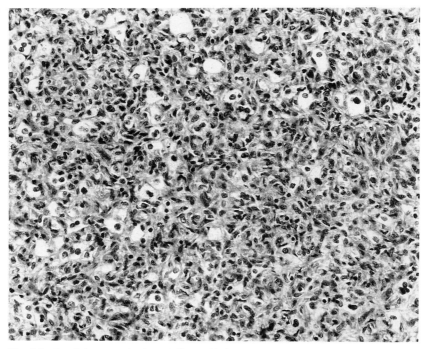

Fig. 6.2 A cellular area of a dermal fibrous histiocytoma (dermatofibroma). Foam cells with clear cytoplasm are present in this example, but are not found in all dermal fibrous histiocytomas. × 200.

macrophages have also been labelled as fibroxanthoma. Pure xanthomas are composed of exclusively foamy histiocytes and, for largely historical reasons, are still labelled as xanthoma. The most commonly encountered pattern is that commonly designated as dermatofibroma, a predominantly fibrous lesion. The constituent fibroblasts are arranged in a more or less random pattern, although they may take on a tufting or storiform arrangement focally (Fig. 6.3) or, rarely, more diffusely. The next most commonly encountered pattern among the dermal fibrous histiocytomas are those with greater numbers of histiocyte-like cells including foam cells. Cells which have phagocytosed haemosiderin and multinucleated giant cells are also common (Leyva & Santa Cruz 1986). Cholesterol clefts may be present. In some dermal fibrous histiocytomas there is sometimes a striking vascular proliferation, which is often associated with haemosiderin deposition (sclerosing haemangioma). Dermal fibrous histiocytomas are completely benign and do not recur unless they are very large. Recurrences are never aggressive.

Subcutaneous plexiform fibrous histiocytomas (Fig. 6.4) develop most frequently on the upper extremities and shoulders, although they can be found in other sites (Enzinger & Zhang 1988). Most of the patients are under 20 years of age and the lesions do occur in children. Subcutaneous fibrous histiocytomas are centred in the subcutaneous tissue, usually near the dermal subcutaneous junction. Architecturally the lesion is characteristically

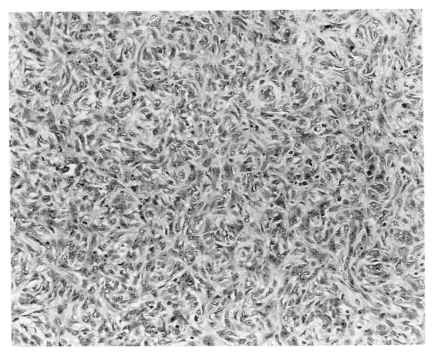

Fig. 6.3 Dermal fibrous histiocytoma with a prominent storiform pattern causing it to resemble dermatofibrosarcoma protuberans. Compare with Figures 6.7 and 6.8. However, the storiform pattern is not as well developed here as it is in DFSP. Haemosiderin, foam cells, and multinucleated giant cells are common in dermal fibrous histiocytomas but not in DFSP. x 200.

multinodular. As with dermal fibrous histiocytomas, the fibrous component may be predominate or there may be a mixture of fibrous and histiocyte-like cells. Often the histological pattern varies from fibrous to fibrohistiocytic within the same tumour. Within some tumours, however, the fibrous tissue predominates and when this occurs, the tumour cells may grow in bundles that extend ray-like into the subcutaneous tissue (Fig. 6.5). This has given rise to the plexiform label used by Enzinger & Zhang (1988). Pleomorphism is minimal in these lesions and mitotic figures are characteristically sparse. Multinucleated giant cells are present in many lesions but foam cells and a storiform pattern are distinctly rare.

  The differential diagnosis of subcutaneous and dermal fibrous histiocytomas is large because many other lesions are composed of similar appearing cells. The main entities to be considered include nodular fasciitis, leiomyosarcoma, neurofibroma, desmoplastic malignant melanoma, fibromatosis, spindle cell carcinoma, haemangiopericytoma, and the other fibrous histiocytomas including juvenile xanthogranuloma and reticulohistiocytoma. It is important to distinguish nodular fasciitis from subcutaneous fibrous histiocytoma, because the latter may recur while nodular fasciitis does not (Fig. 6.6). The two lesions come to resemble one another when the histiocytic

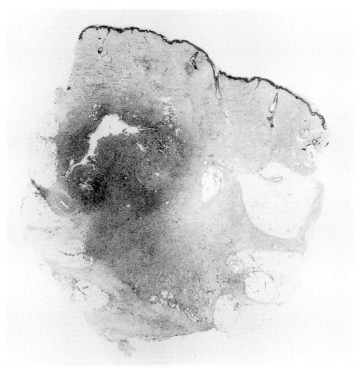

Fig. 6.4 Subcutaneous fibrous histiocytoma. The location is the feature that distinguishes this from dermal fibrous histiocytoma. Note the extension of a more fibrous area into the surrounding subcutaneous tissue from the more cellular nodular mass. This pattern has given rise to the name plexiform fibrous histiocytoma. This histological features of both dermal and subcutaneous fibrous histiocytomas can be identical although the subcutaneous forms are generally more fibrous. × 5.

component of the fibrous histiocytomas is muted. The features we find most helpful in making this distinction are summarised in Table 6.2. The cells in subcutaneous fibrous histiocytoma are predominantly mature fibrocytes rather than the granulation type fibroblasts that make up nodular fasciitis, and the loose background characteristic of nodular fasciitis is largely absent in the subcutaneous fibrous histiocytomas. Most importantly, normal mitotic figures almost always are numerous in nodular fasciitis, while they are typically difficult to find in the subcutaneous fibrous histiocytomas. Whenever there is difficulty in distinguishing between nodular fasciitis and subcutaneous fibrous histiocytoma, this difficulty should be explained to the clinician and the patient warned that the lesion might recur. Neural neoplasms share morphological features with fibrous histiocytomas, particularly the plexiform variety of subcutaneous fibrous histiocytoma, but almost all benign neural tumours express S-100 protein. This is rarely expressed by the cells of fibrous histiocytomas. Smooth muscle tumours are composed of cells with discernible eosinophilic cytoplasm arranged in bundles. The tufting or storiform pattern

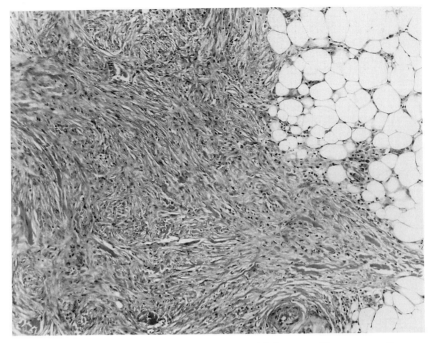

Fig. 6.5   Higher power view of a subcutaneous fibrous histiocytoma. The tumour cells are predominately fibroblastic and are associated with thick bundles of collagen, a feature that helps to distinguish this from nodular fasciitis. × 100.

often found in the dermal fibrous histiocytomas is largely absent, as are foam cells. In addition, smooth muscle cells may express desmin.

Desmoplastic malignant melanoma can easily be mistaken for a dermal fibrous histiocytoma. Whenever a fibrous appearing lesion is encountered in the skin, particularly in the skin of the head and neck of an adult patient, the possibility of desmoplastic malignant melanoma should be considered. There are two features that are particularly useful in identifying desmoplastic melanoma. First, there may be a melanocytic proliferation, usually of the lentigo maligna type, at the dermoepidermal junction. Second, infiltration of nerves by tumour cells, within and at the base of the lesion, is a characteristic feature of desmoplastic melanoma. This causes the nerves to become enlarged. The fibroblastic appearing cells in desmoplastic malignant melanoma are frequently arranged in fascicles and mitotic figures and enlarged melanocytic cells with abnormal nuclei are characteristically mixed among the spindle cells. In most desmoplastic malignant melanomas, at least some of the tumour cells express S-100 protein.

Dermal and subcutaneous fibrous histiocytomas composed predominantly of fibrocytes conceivably could be confused with the desmoid type fibromatosis or a low-grade fibrosarcoma. However, desmoid type fibromatoses and well-differentiated fibrosarcoma do not primarily develop in the dermis, and fibromatoses involving the subcutaneous tissue also infiltrate the underlying

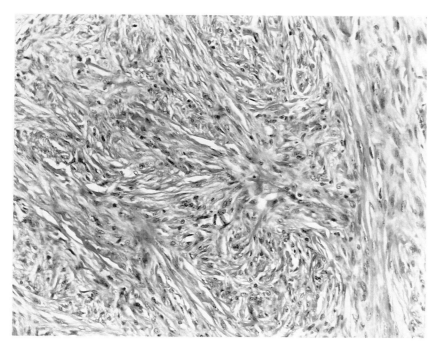

Fig. 6.6 High-power view of a subcutaneous fibrous histiocytoma. The fibroblastic cells have open nuclei closely resembling those found in nodular fasciitis. Table 6.2 presents the features we use to distinguish nodular fasciitis from subcutaneous fibrous histiocytoma. × 200.

muscle. Fibromatoses are large lesions, they lack a histiocytic component and the cells are not arranged in a plexiform pattern. Spindle cell carcinomas are composed of cells with larger nuclei and typically are more cellular with less collagen than the fibrous histiocytomas. Keratin stains should be used for lesions whose appearance raises the possibility of spindle cell carcinoma.

The cells composing haemangiopericytomas share many features with those found in fibrous histiocytomas, and indeed, haemangiopericytoma-like areas can be found in several types of fibrous histiocytoma. Both haemangi-

Table 6.2 Comparison of nodular fasciitis with subcutaneous fibrous histiocytoma

Nodular fasciitis	Subcutaneous fibrous histiocytoma
Constituent fibroblasts are of the granulation type with large open nuclei	Constituent fibroblasts typically are smaller with dense nuclear chromatin
Histiocyte-like cells not a feature	Histiocyte-like cells almost always present at least focally
Granulation tissue-like stroma, often with inflammatory cells and clefts	More collagenous stroma; fibroblasts may be arranged in a plexiform pattern
Not usually multinodular	Often multinodular
Mitotic figures numerous	Mitotic figures variable, but most often sparse
Extravasation of red blood cells often prominent	Extravasation of red blood cells minimal
Orderly vasculature	Disordered vasculature

opericytoma and dermal fibrous histiocytoma may feature cells with a tufted arrangement but the staghorn vessels, typcial of the former, are definitely lacking in the fibrous histiocytomas and haemangiopericytomas lack a histiocyte-like component.

Distinguishing dermal and subcutaneous fibrous histiocytomas from the other types of fibrous histiocytomas is usually not difficult. Juvenile xanthogranuloma is a lesion that occurs almost always in the skin of children and infants, although there may be lesions in other organs. This lesion is predominantly a histiocytic one and the histiocytes have vacuolated or foamy cytoplasm. Touton type giant cells with nuclei in a ring are a hallmark of this lesion, but their numbers vary considerably from area to area within the same tumour and from lesion to lesion. Reticulohistiocytoma is also a predominantly histiocytic lesion that occurs most often in adults. The histiocytes, which may be multinucleated, have glassy eosinophilic cytoplasm. Mitotic figures may be quite numerous and nuclear pleomorphism may be prominent. Atypical fibroxanthoma has a morphological pattern identical to that of pleomorphic malignant fibrous histiocytoma; it is distinguished from the latter on the basis of its location in the dermis. The marked pleomorphism, the anaplasia of the constituent cells, and the presence of abnormal mitotic figures serves to distinguish atypical fibroxanthoma from the other benign fibrous histiocytomas. Dermatofibrosarcoma protuberans is the fibrous histiocytoma most likely to be misinterpreted as a dermal or subcutaneous fibrous histiocytoma. The morphological features of this lesion are described in the next section.

Dermal fibrous histiocytomas are benign lesions and they never recur unless the tumours grow to a rather massive size before the initial excision. Subcutaneous fibrous histiocytomas, on the other hand, do recur in up to 30–40% of cases, but the recurrences are not aggressive. Two patients with the plexiform type have experienced regional lymph node metastasis; however, distant metastases have not been reported. Consequently, we continue to group this lesion with the benign fibrous histiocytomas. Distinguishing subcutaneous fibrous histiocytoma from the dermal variety can be difficult because each can involve both the dermis and subcutaneous tissue. We try to determine where the lesion is centred and consider that the point of origin. If there is any uncertainty about the centre of the lesion, we warn the clinician to watch the patient for possible recurrence, particularly if the lesion is large or if it is multinodular or plexiform.

Atypical fibroxanthoma

Atypical fibroxanthoma is a dermal lesion (Fig 6.7) with the histological features of pleomorphic malignant fibrous histiocytoma malignant fibrous histiocytomas below). It is found most often in the sun-exposed skin of the elderly, where it develops into an ulcerated nodular mass (Dahl 1976, Fretzin & Helwig 1973, Kempson & McGavran 1964). It may, however, occur in other sites, particularly in areas where skin has been traumatised or

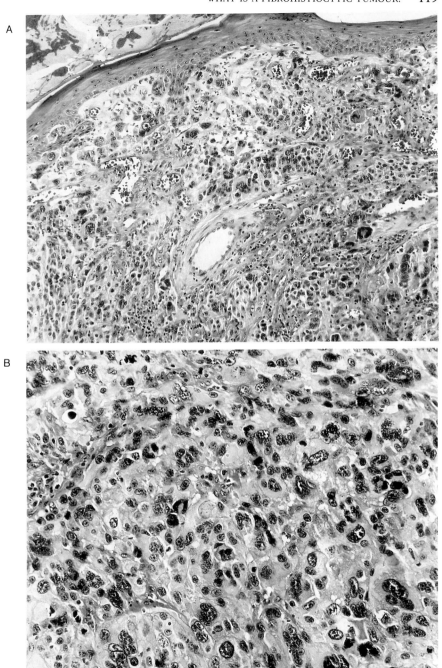

Fig. 6.7 A In this example of atypical fibroxanthoma (AFX), the dermis is infiltrated by multicleated giant cells, many of which have pleomorphic nuclei. There are also histiocyte cells present. The appearance is identical to that of pleomorphic MFH; the distinction from MFH is made on the basis of location. × 100.
B High magnification of AFX. The bizarre nuclei are a common feature. Several different neoplasms can have this appearance and atypical fibroxanthoma is essentially a diagnosis of exclusion, as is discussed in the differential diagnosis section of the text. × 200.

chronically inflamed. Atypical fibroxanthoma can recur; however, recurrences are not aggressive and almost all patients are cured by re-excision. This is the reason we prefer to include atypical fibroxanthoma in the benign fibrous histiocytomas, even though, paradoxically, the histological pattern is that of a malignant neoplasm.

Many lesions can mimic the morphological features of atypical fibroxanthoma (AFX) and, in our view, the diagnosis is one of exclusion. The most important entities to consider in the differential diagnosis of atypical fibroxanthoma are spindle cell and anaplastic squamous cell carcinomas, metastasis, malignant melanoma, leiomyosarcoma, and pleomorphic malignant fibrous histiocytoma (pleomorphic MFH). Whenever faced with a lesion that raises the possibility of atypical fibroxanthoma, we routinely use immunohistochemical stains in an attempt to exclude carcinoma, both primary and metastatic, and malignant melanoma. Since spindle cell squamous cell carcinoma of the skin is also an indolent lesion, distinguishing it from AFX is not of great clinical moment. Likewise, leiomyosarcoma limited to the dermis practically never metastasises. On the other hand, recognising malignant melanoma and metastasis is very important and, fortunately, immunohistochemical stains are often helpful in this regard. By definition, atypical fibroxanthomas are limited to the dermis or at most involve only the superifical subcutaneous tissue. Identical mesenchymal neoplasms involving the subcutaneous tissue metastasise with sufficient frequency to be regarded as malignant and labelled as pleomorphic MFH. The lesions reported by Helwig & May (1986) as 'metastasising atypical fibroxanthoma' extensively involved the subcutaneous tissue or invaded blood vessels and we would label them as pleomorphic malignant fibrous histiocytomas.

Tenosynovial giant cell tumour

Tenosynovial giant cell tumour (giant cell tumour of tendon sheath) is a well-known and easily recognised lesion that we include within the fibrous histiocytoma category for classificatory convenience. Others consider them to be synovial lesions. Recent investigation by Wood et al (1988), at our insitution, provides evidence that the tumour cells are true histiocytes of monocyte/macrophage lineage.

FIBROUS HISTIOCYTOMA OF LOW MALIGNANT POTENTIAL

Dermatofibrosarcoma protuberans (DFSP), a neoplasm characterised by a repetitive storiform or cartwheel pattern (Fig. 6.8) is classified by us as a fibrous histiocytoma of low malignant potential because it frequently recurs, sometimes massively and on rare occasions it metastasises (Burkhardt et al 1966, Fletcher et al 1985, Kahn et al 1978, McPeak et al 1967, Taylor & Helwig 1962). DFSP occurs almost exclusively in the skin and subcutaneous

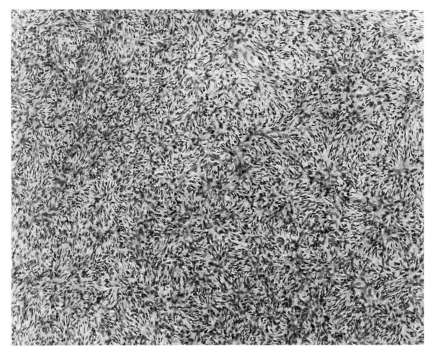

Fig. 6.8   Dermatofibrosarcoma protuberans (DFSP). The characteristic uniform cells with elongate nuclei are arranged in the required repetitive storiform pattern. × 100

tissue as a plaque-like or multinodular mass, but, rarely, morphologically indistinguishable lesions can be found in the deep soft tissues. These are large tumours with an average diameter of 5 cm; it is extremely unusual to encounter a dermatofibrosarcoma protuberans under 2 cm. Microscopically, the tumour cells in DFSP (Fig. 6.9) are monomorphic, uniform, bland fibroblasts, and only rare histiocyte-like cells are present. DFSP is cellular, collagen is usually inconspicuous and foam cells are not present, except occasionally at the edge of the lesion. The morphological definition of DFSP specifically disallows significant anaplasia, or marked pleomorphism, and giant cells are not present. When a tumour is encountered in which the cells form the typical repetitive storiform pattern of DFSP, but also demonstrate anaplasia and/or pleomorphism either focally or diffusely, the proper diagnosis, in our view, is pleomorphic malignant fibrous histiocytoma, or atypical fibroxanthoma, depending on the lesion's location in the subcutaneous tissue or dermis, respectively (see atypical fibroxanthoma above). Photomicrographs of some reported examples of metastasising DFSP reveal pleomorphic and giant cells that would cause us to diagnose the lesions as pleomorphic malignant fibrous histiocytoma. DFSP may very rarely recur as pleomorphic MFH (O'Dowd & Laidler 1988).

Myxoid areas may be found in DFSP and in some tumours they may predominate (Fletcher et al 1985, Frierson & Cooper 1983). Rarely,

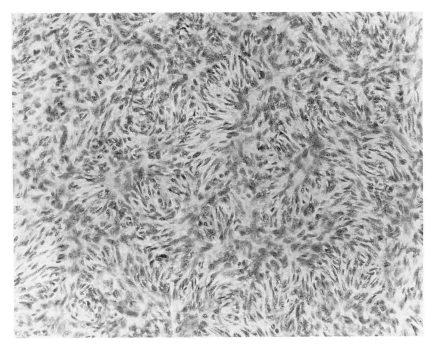

Fig. 6.9   This high power photomicrograph of DFSP displays uniform cells with elongate nuclei arranged in a repetitive storiform pattern. It is the uniformity of the constituent cells, the absence of giant cells and hemosiderin, and the absence of significant pleomorphism that identifies this lesion as DFSP. × 200.

dermatofibrosarcoma protuberans will present as a myxoid neoplasm and only in recurrences will the characteristic storiform pattern be found. Recurrences also may be largely or exclusively myxoid. Rarely, DFSP may contain dendritic cells which produce melanin pigment (Dupree et al 1985, Fletcher et al 1988). The classification of such neoplasms has caused controversy because of the resemblance to pigmented neurofibroma, and because ultrastructural examination does reveal basal lamina around some tumour cells. The pigmented cells synthesise melanosomes and express S-100 protein (Fletcher et al 1988). Because it is unclear whether pigmented DFSP shows biphasic neural and fibrohistiocytic differentiation or is simply colonised by epidermal melanocytes, we keep it in the category of the dermatofibrosarcoma protuberans group. On occasion, fibrosarcoma-like areas are identified in dermatofibrosarcoma protuberans or recurrences feature fibrosarcoma-like regions at least focally (Wrotnowski et al 1988); these are regarded by some as a marker of a more aggressive neoplasm with the potential for metastasis (Enzinger & Weiss 1988).

Neoplasms with histological patterns indistinguishable from DFSP rarely may be encountered in the deep soft tissues. We label them as storiform fibrous histiocytomas. They are unusual enough that accurate information about their behaviour is not available; the storiform fibrous histiocytomas we have encountered have been recurring but not metastasising neoplasms. We have also observed several well-differentiated liposarcomas in the retroperitoneum 'dedifferentiate' into storiform fibrous histiocytoma.

The lesions most likely to be confused with DFSP are the dermal and subcutaneous fibrous histiocytomas, nodular fasciitis, and nerve sheath tumours. The dermal and subcutaneous fibrous histiocytomas are, with noteable exceptions, always under 3 cm whereas DFSP averages 5 cm and is rare under 2 cm. Dermatofibrosarcomas do not contain foam cells and haemosiderin deposits are unusual. Moreover, they have a cellular rather than a collagenous background. A comparison of the histological features of the superficial fibrous histiocytomas and dermatofibrosarcoma protuberans is presented in Table 6.3. Although nodular fasciitis may have a storiform pattern focally, a repetitive storiform pattern is not generally found. Granulation tissue-like stroma, clefting, and cells with enlarged open nuclei, typical of nodular fasciitis, are not features of dermatofibrosarcoma protuberans. Neurofibromas may have a focal storiform pattern and the nuclei can resemble those seen in DFSP. However, a repetitive storiform pattern is most unusual and S-100 expression is typical, indeed almost definitional, for neurofibroma.

Myxoid neoplasms enter into the differential diagnosis because DFSP may have a partially or completely myxoid stroma. DFSP does not contain lipoblasts nor does it have the tubular arborising vascular pattern required for a diagnosis of myxoid liposarcoma. Moreover, myxoid liposarcomas very rarely arise so superficially. Myxoid malignant fibrous histiocytoma and other myxoid lesions are described in more detail in the section devoted to myxoid MFH below. Myxoid DFSP may be indistinguishable from other undifferentiated myxoid lesions unless the repetitive storiform pattern characteristic of DFSP is found. Consequently, myxoid lesions in the skin and subcutaneous tissue should be extensively sampled to be sure that they do not have a focal storiform pattern.

Dermatofibrosarcoma protuberans is a neoplasm with potential for destructive recurrence. The incidence of recurrence seems to be related to the size of the initial lesion and the extent of the primary excision (Roses et al 1986). The metastasis rate for classic DFSP is less than 5% and probably no more than 1% (Fletcher et al 1985). Metastases practically never occur unless the neoplasm has recurred. Some metastasising neoplasms reported as DFSP have contained pleomorphic and anaplastic cells that would cause us to place

Table 6.3 Comparison of histological features of dermal and subcutaneous fibrous histiocytoma and dermatofibrosarcoma protuberans (DFSP)

Dermal and subcutaneous fibrous histiocytoma	DFSP
Usually small (1–2 cm)	Average 5 cm
Variable cellularity with collagenous stroma	Uniformly cellular with minimal collagen
Foam cells and giant cells typical	Foam cells and giant cells rare
Storiform pattern in dermal type, rare in subcutaneous type	Repetitive storiform pattern is definitional feature

the tumour in the category of malignant fibrous histiocytoma. The effect of fibrosarcoma-like patterns in a DFSP is to cause the metastatic rate to rise as the extent of fibrosarcoma increases. We label such neoplasms as DFSP with fibrosarcoma. A high mitotic index also has positively correlated with increased risk of metastasis in some series (McPeak et al 1967).

Because the behaviour of the fibrous histiocytomas depends not only upon morphological features but also upon their location, the diagnostic terms used for histologically identical lesions may differ depending on site in order to reflect this variable behaviour. The nomenclature we use is presented in Table 6.4.

MALIGNANT FIBROUS HISTIOCYTOMAS

Those fibrous histiocytomas that have a significant potential for metastasis vary considerably in their histological patterns. Consequently, the malignant fibrous histiocytomas have been subdivided into the following histological types (Enzinger 1986, Enzinger & Weiss 1988, Lattes 1982, Meister 1988, Weiss 1982):

1. Pleomorphic (fibroxanthosarcoma)
2. Myxoid (myxofibrosarcoma)
3. Inflammatory (xanthosarcoma)
4. Giant cell
5. Fibrous
6. Angiomatoid

Although classic examples of each type of malignant fibrous histiocytoma (MFH) can easily be distinguished one from the other, there is considerable

Table 6.4 Site-specific nomenclature of the fibrous histiocytomas to reflect variable behaviour

Histological pattern	Location		
	Dermis	Subcutaneous	Deep soft tissue
Pleomorphic malignant fibrous histiocytoma	Atypical fibroxanthoma R = low (10%) M = 0	Pleomorphic malignant fibrous histiocytoma R = high M = low	Pleomorphic malignant fibrous histiocytoma R = high M = high
Dermatofibrosarcoma protuberans	Dermatofibrosarcoma protuberans R = high M = very low	Dermatofibrosarcoma protuberans R = high M = very low	Storiform malignant fibrous histiocytoma R = high M = unknown
Dermatofibroma-like lesions	Dermal fibrous histiocytoma R = 0 M = 0	Subcutaneous fibrous histiocytoma R = moderate (30–40%) M = 0	Fibrous histiocytoma of uncertain malignant potential R = unknown M = unknown

R = approximate risk of recurrence   M = approximate risk of metastasis beyond regional lymph nodes overlap of morphological patterns. Consequently, the definitions of the various subtypes may include a quantitation of the extent of a particular feature. For example, greater than 50% of the stroma must be myxoid before a neoplasm is relegated to the myxoid MFH category (Weiss & Enzinger 1977). Partitioning the malignant fibrous histiocytomas into categories has more than just differential disgnostic utility; the myxoid and the angiomatoid variants are less agressive than the other types of malignant fibrous histiocytomas (Enzinger 1979, Weiss & Enzinger 1977).

Pleomorphic malignant fibrous histiocytoma (fibroxanthosarcoma)

The pleomorphic type is the most common malignant fibrous histiocytoma and was among the first to gain acceptance as a useful clinicopathological entity (Enjoji et al 1980, Kearney et al 1980, Kempson & Kyriakos 1972, Weiss & Enzinger 1978). Because the tumour is anaplastic and pleomorphic and because the cells do not demonstrate differentiation beyond spindled fibroblasts, histocyte-like cells and bizzare giant cells, it is important to adhere to a morphological definition of this neoplasm to avoid misplacing other types of anaplastic neoplasms into this category. (Fig. 6.10).

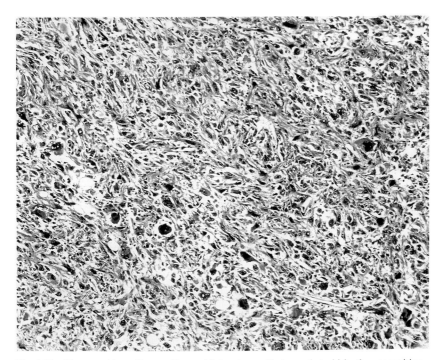

Fig. 6.10 Pleomorphic malignant fibrous histiocytoma. Features that aid in the recognition of this neoplasm are the randomly arranged fibroblasts, the striking pleomorphism, and the giant cells. × 100.

Morphological criteria for the diagnosis of pleomorphic malignant fibrous histiocytoma

1. Mixture of fibroblasts, myofibroblasts, histiocyte-like cells, giant cells and undifferentiated cells in varying proportions
2. Fibroblasts randomly arranged in disorganised bundles or in a storiform pattern
3. Giant cells that may resemble rhabdomyoblasts and lipoblasts
4. Pleomorphism and anaplasia marked
5. Mitotic figures abundant and usually abnormal forms are numerous
6. Xanthoma cells may be present.

We require at least two cell types: one fibroblast or myofibroblast, the other histiocyte-like or giant cells. We include undifferentiated cells in the 'histiocyte-like' designation. The fibroblasts are often randomly arranged, but focally they may grow in small fascicles and bundles. However, the intersecting, organised fascicular arrangement typical of leiomyosarcoma and fibrosarcoma is largely absent. In pleomorphic MFH, it is common for the elongate cells to be arranged in a storiform pattern at least focally, but this pattern is not required for the diagnosis. The histiocyte-like cells vary from those that are small and relatively uniform to those that are large and/or pleomorphic. Some of the latter may be multinucleated and they often have bizarre gigantic nuclei. Anaplasia is typically marked, mitotic figures are frequent and abnormal mitoses are usually easy to find. Xanthoma cells are often present at the periphery of the tumour but they may be scattered within it. Some of the giant cells have strikingly abundant eosinophilic cytoplasm resembling that found in rhabdomyoblasts, others have vacuolated cytoplasm that mimics the cytoplasm of lipoblasts. Haemangiopericytoma-like areas may be encountered. In this circumstance, the diagnosis can only be made when more characteristic patterns are identified elsewhere in the neoplasm. The architectural patterns encountered in pleomorphic malignant fibrous histiocytoma range from a tumour with spindle cells arranged in a repetitive storiform pattern, more typical of DFSP, to neoplasms that are almost exclusively composed of non-spindled anaplastic and pleomorphic cells with only focal fibroblastic or myofibroblastic differentiation. In either case, pleomorphic cells are required for the diagnosis.

Differential diagnosis

It hardly comes as a surprise that the differential diagnosis of the pleomorphic type of malignant fibrous histiocytoma is extensive. The major considerations are:

1. Pleomorphic rhabdomyosarcoma (rhabdomyoblasts)
2. Pleomorphic liposarcoma (lipoblasts)

3. Leiomyosarcoma (evidence of smooth muscle differentiation; fascicular arrangement of cells)
4. Nerve sheath sarcoma (continuity with nerve; neurofibromatosis)
5. Metastasis: malignant melanoma, carcinoma (clinical history; search for melanin, S-100 stain; Keratin stain)
6. Other types of fibrous histiocytomas
7. Hodgkin's disease (clinical history, immunohistochemistry)
8. Large-cell non-Hodgkin's lymphoma (clinical history, immunohistochemistry)

The most critical distinction is to exclude carcinoma and lymphoma. Treatment and outcome for patients with any of the high-grade sarcomas is much the same, so distinguishing between them is not of great importance, except possibly for the pathologist's pride. However, distinguishing metastatic and primary carcinomas from sarcoma is of critical importance. Carcinomas arising in many sites, but most commonly the lung and pancreas, can take on morphological features resembling those of pleomorphic malignant fibrous histiocytoma (Yousem & Hochholzer 1987) (Fig. 6.11). Consequently, the possibility of a carcinoma must always be taken into account whenever a diagnosis of pleomorphic malignant fibrous histiocytoma is contemplated. The use of glycogen, mucin and immunohistochemical stains can be critical

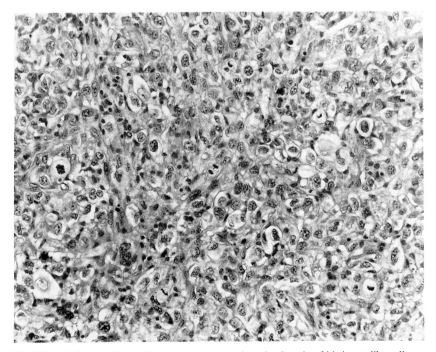

Fig. 6.11 Malignant fibrous histiocytoma composed predominately of histiocyte-like cells. Carcinoma, lymphoma, and melanoma can have a histological appearance very similar to this neoplasm . × 200.

in making this distinction. A point to remember is that rare examples of pleomorphic MFH contain cells that mark with keratin stains (Weiss et al 1988). Clinical correlation is always needed when making the distinction between metastatic carcinoma and pleomorphic MFH.

Pleomorphic rhabdomyosarcoma, by definition, requires that at least some of the tumour cells have unequivocal evidence of skeletal muscle differentiation based either on demonstration of cross striations by light microscopy or thick and thin filaments and/or Z bands by electron microscopy. When these definitional requirements are adhered to, pleomorphic rhabdomyosarcoma becomes a vanishingly rare neoplasm. Immunohistochemical stains for muscle specific actin are of little value in making the distinction between pleomorphic MFH and pleomorphic rhabdomyosarcoma because the myofibroblasts in MFH can express antigens recognised by this antibody, but desmin and myoglobin staining may be useful.

Pleomorphic liposarcoma is distinguished from pleomorphic MFH because lipoblasts define the former and must be a part of the neoplasm before a diagnosis of pleomorphic liposarcoma is made. Therefore, the diagnostic pathologist should have a firm grasp on the definition of a lipoblast before making this distinction. Our definition requires deformation or scalloping of the tumour cell nucleus by the fat vacuole(s). The cells in pleomorphic leiomyosarcoma must demonstrate smooth muscle differentiation by light microscopy, electron microscopy, or immunohistochemical stains. If the patient does not have von Recklinghausen's disease, we think nerve sheath sarcoma should be diagnosed only if the sarcoma is arising from a neurofibroma or from a nerve unless there is ultrastructural evidence of nerve sheath differentiation. S-100 stains are of little help in this regard since several different types of sarcomas express S-100. However, S-100 is rarely expressed by the cells in pleomorphic malignant fibrous histiocytoma.

Since it is of little practical managerial importance to distinguish pleomorphic malignant fibrous histiocytomas from other pleomorphic sarcomas that mimic pleomorphic MFH, spending excessive amounts of pathologists' time and society's resources attempting to make such a distinction makes little sense. On the other hand, distinguishing metastases and lymphomas from pleomorphic sarcomas is of vital importance.

Differentiated sarcomas can evolve into a neoplasm morphologically indistinguishable from pleomorphic MFH (Brooks 1986). If the original sarcoma was high grade, this evolution makes no difference in treatment and patient outcome. If, however, the original sarcoma was low grade, the dedifferentiation to MFH is a warning to expect high-grade sarcoma behaviour, including metastases. For diagnostic purposes we use the differentiated label of the original tumour with the added term 'with evolution to pleomorphic malignant fibrous histiocytoma'.

Malignant melanoma can occasionally mimic pleomorphic MFH because both the spindle cells and the histiocyte-like cells can resemble neoplastic melanocytes. However, the very marked pleomorphism of the usual malignant fibrous histiocytoma is not generally a feature of malignant melanoma. S-100 stains may be helpful in making the distinction between the two neoplasms. Distinguishing pleomorphic MFH from the benign fibrous histiocytomas has been discussed above and separation of pleomorphic MFH from the other types of malignant fibrous histiocytomas is discussed in the following sections. As noted previously, pleomorphic malignant fibrous histiocytoma and atypical fibroxanthoma are morphologically identical and are distinguished one from the other solely on the basis of location. Occasionally large cell lymphomas are so pleomorphic as to be confused with pleomorphic MFH; common leucocyte antigen stains will be critical in this circumstance. Hodgkin's disease also can contain markedly pleomorphic and anaplastic cells; the clinical history as well as immunohistochemical stains may be decisive.

Myxoid malignant fibrous histiocytoma (myxofibrosarcoma)

It is relatively common for pleomorphic malignant fibrous histiocytomas to possess focal areas of myxoid stroma, but when 50% or more of the stroma of such a tumour is myxoid, the term myxoid malignant fibrous histiocytoma or myxofibrosarcoma is applied (Weiss & Enzinger 1977, Merck et al 1983). Such tumours are often grossly mucinous. Microscopically, in easily recognised examples, the myxoid areas contain pleomorphic enlarged cells and the myxoid stroma blends into areas more characteristic of pleomorphic MFH. However, in some myxoid MFHs, the myxoid areas are deceptively bland and pleomorphic cells are difficult to find. We require pleomorphic enlarged cells or areas of pleomorphic MFH before accepting a myxoid neoplasm as myxoid MFH. Moreover, almost all myxoid MFHs contain cells in division and often the mitotic figures are abnormal (Figs. 6.12 and 6.13). Arborising tubular blood vessels may be present in some cases and a storiform pattern can be present in the myxoid areas as well as the pleomorphic areas. Sometimes the tumour cells contain so much mucopolysaccharide that the cytoplasm is vacuolated and they come to resemble lipoblasts. Unlike lipoblasts, however, the nuclei in the cells of myxoid MFH usually are not deformed by the mucin vacuoles. However, such deformation can occur and distinction from lipoblasts then requires the use of acid mucopolysaccharide stains to prove the chemical composition of the vacuoles. We categorise the myxoid malignant fibrous histiocytomas as low grade and high grade, depending on the amount of pleomorphic sarcoma present.

The differential diagnosis of myxoid MFH centres around myxoid liposarcoma, myxoid chondrosarcoma, neural neoplasms, and pleomorphic malignant fibrous histiocytoma as well as metastatic mucinous carcinoma. Pleomorphic malignant fibrous histiocytoma is excluded definitionally by the amount of myxoid stroma in the tumour. The stromal cells in myxoid liposarcoma may be indistinguishable from the stromal cells in the bland areas of myxoid MFH, but myxoid liposarcoma must also contain lipoblasts and the

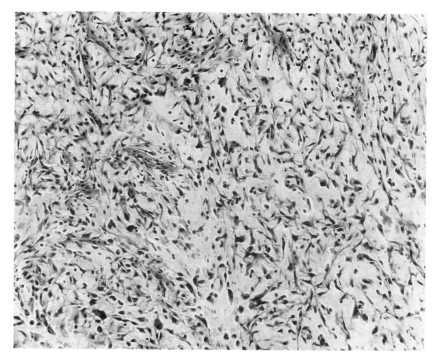

Fig. 6.12 Myxoid MFH is characterised by pleomorphic cells often within large bizarre nuclei, set in a myxoid stroma. Mitotic figures must be present and very often they are abnormal. Occasionally myxoid areas in a myxoid MFH will be more bland, but these blend either into areas similar to the one illustrated in this photomicrograph, or into areas characteristic of pleomorphic malignant fibrous histiocytoma. × 100.

tumour always has a tubular arborising vascular pattern, not often present in myxoid MFH. Pure low-grade liposarcoma very rarely develops in the subcutaneous tissue, a site where myxoid MFH is particularly common. Myxoid liposarcoma can 'dedifferentiate' to round cell liposarcoma or occasionally malignant fibrous histiocytoma and the 'dedifferentiated' areas can demonstrate considerable cellularity, pleomorphism, and mitotic activity. When this occurs the behaviour is that of any high-grade sarcoma. The key to identifying liposarcoma is identifying lipoblasts in the differentiated areas of the tumour. Since the behaviour of pure myxoid liposarcoma and low-grade myxoid MFH without significant areas of pleomorphic MFH is much the same, i.e. usually only local recurrence unless 'dedifferentiation' occurs, distinguishing between the two is of no great importance. High-grade myxoid MFH, on the other hand, can be expected to be much more aggressive. The important thing when making a diagnosis of a low-grade myxoid sarcoma is to be sure that enough sections have been taken to exclude no more than just focal anaplasia or pleomorphism and that large numbers of abnormal mitotic figures are not present.

S-100 stains can help to exclude neural tumours and keratin stains, as well as PAS stains, are sometimes useful in distinguishing metastatic carcinoma

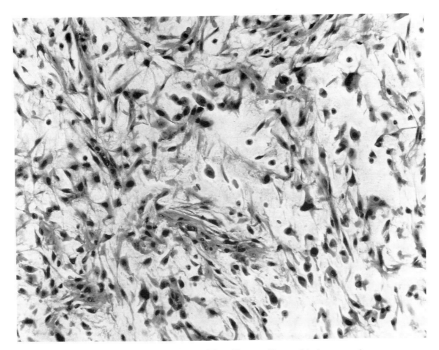

Fig. 6.13   This higher power view of myxoid malignant fibrous histiocytoma better demonstrates the pleomorphism of the tumour cells. × 200.

from myxoid MFH. Malignant melanoma may have a myxoid stroma and the S-100 stain is almost always the key to detecting this neoplasm. Intramuscular myxoma is much less cellular than myxoid MFH, the cells are smaller and they are bland. Myxoid chondrosarcoma has a lobular architecture and the chain-like arrangement of the cell, extending from periphery to the centre of the lobule, is unlike the pattern in myxoid MFH. Moreover, the cells in myxoid chondrosarcoma typically are small and uniform and do not demonstrate the pleomorphism and anaplasia seen at least locally in myxoid MFH.

After these differential diagnostic considerations, there still remains a poorly categorised group of soft tissue neoplasms with a myxoid stroma that do not fit into any of the above named categories. The constituent cells of such tumours are small and bland and they resemble the bland cells in myxoid MFH and myxoid liposarcoma, but lipoblasts and pleomorphic cells are not found. The tumours are usually more cellular than intramuscular myxoma and they rarely develop within a muscle. A tubular arborising vascular pattern may be present. Generally, mitotic figures are sparse and are not abnormal. Such tumours may recur, particularly when they are large or in the deep soft tissues but, in our experience, they do not metastasise unless they 'dedifferentiate' into a more pleomorphic pattern and mitotic activity becomes prominent. We categorise such lesions as myxoid neoplasms without further subclassification (Fig. 6.14) and we point out to clinicians that they

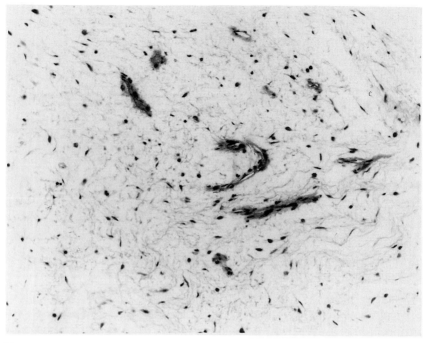

Fig. 6.14 This is a representative photomicrograph of a 15 cm soft tissue mass found in the thigh. Lipoblasts are not present and the pleomorphism required for malignant fibrous histiocytoma is absent. The entire neoplasm had this appearance. We label such lesions as myxoid neoplasm with low-grade recurring potential. We do not think they should be included in the categories of myxoid liposarcoma (there are no lipoblasts) nor in the myxoid MFH category. × 100.

may recur and also point out that they may 'dedifferentiate' into a pleomorphic sarcoma or develop recognisable histological patterns with recurrence. Since the behaviour of these low-grade myxoid neoplasms is the same as for pure low-grade liposarcoma and low-grade myxoid MFH without large areas of pleomorphism, it is no great offence to classify them as either of those entities.

Inflammatory malignant fibrous histiocytoma

This rare malignant neoplasm develops most commonly in the retroperitoneum (Kahn 1973, Kyriakos & Kempson 1976, Merino & LiVolsi 1980) and has also been previously categorised as malignant xanthogranuloma and as xanthosarcoma.

Diagnostic criteria

The diagnostic pathologist should closely adhere to the definitional morphological features because many neoplasms, including pleomorphic MFH and carcinoma, can contain inflammatory cells and cells that look like histiocytes

(Fig. 6.15). Specifically, the tumour is characterised by an accumulation of acute inflammatory cells so numerous as to appear sheet-like or as a 'sea' of polymorphs. These inflammatory cells are punctuated by histiocyte-like cells (Fig. 6.16) which vary from bland xanthoma cells, assuredly reactive histiocytes, to neoplastic cells with foamy cytoplasm and bizarre abnormal nuclei. Abnormal mitotic figures are frequently present and giant cells may also be found. An important diagnostic feature is to find this pattern of the tumour blending into foci of otherwise characteristic pleomorphic MFH.

Differential diagnosis

Many other tumours and inflammatory conditions can take on histological features that closely mimic inflammatory malignant fibrous histiocytoma. Therefore, the differential diagnosis contains many different entities, e.g.

1. Xanthogranulomatous inflammatory conditions
2. Malakoplakia and Whipple's disease (PAS stain)
3. Carcinoma (clinical history; keratin stain)
4. Hodgkin's disease (clinical history; immunohistiochemistry)
5. Other types of fibrous histiocytoma
6. Liposarcoma (lipoblasts)

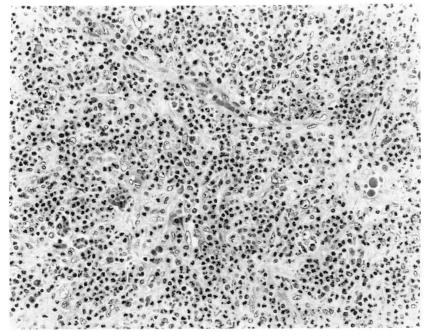

Fig. 6.15 Inflammatory malignant fibrous histiocytoma is characterised by histiocyte-like tumour cells set among large numbers of acute inflammatory cells. As in this case, the tumour cells may be sparse and they can be quite bland. However, somewhere in the tumour either the pattern of pleomorphic MFH, or pleomorphic histiocyte-like cells must be identified. × 100.

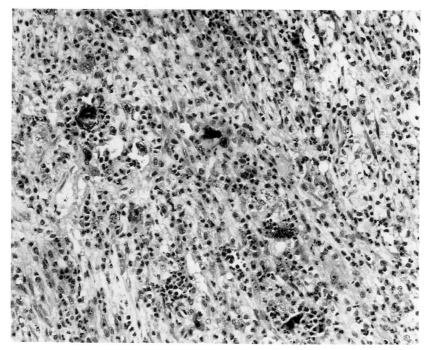

Fig. 6.16 A high-power view of abnormal histiocyte-like cells typically found in inflammatory malignant fibrous histiocytoma. × 200.

Inflammatory conditions that can mimic inflammatory MFH include Whipple's disease, malakoplakia, and extension of xanthogranulomatous pyelonephritis into the retroperitoneum. The cells in malakoplakia and Whipple's disease contain PAS positive material that is diastase resistant. Such material is not abundantly present in the cells of inflammatory MFH. Carcinoma and lymphoma are important entities to exclude and immunohistochemistry is frequently helpful in this regard. Liposarcoma may 'dedifferentiate' into malignant fibrous histiocytoma including inflammatory fibrous histiocytoma. Since the 'dedifferentiated' tumour will behave like the fibrous histiocytoma component, identifying the liposarcoma is not that important for the management of the patient. Lipoblasts identify liposarcoma and are not present in inflammatory fibrous histiocytoma.

Distinguishing other types of fibrous histiocytomas from the inflammatory variant is accomplished by recognising the presence of the large numbers of acute inflammatory cells in the latter. However, the other types of malignant fibrous histiocytoma may contain acute and chronic inflammation focally and necrosis is common in any high-grade malignant fibrous histiocytoma. It is the sheet-like arrangement of the acute, and sometimes chronic, inflammatory cells with interpersed histiocyte-like cells that is the hallmark of the inflammatory variant of MFH. Two observations have been helpful to us when faced with a lesion that may be an inflammatory MFH. Firstly, inflammatory malignant fibrous histiocytoma is an uncommon neoplasm and all of the other possibilities in the differential diagnosis should be carefully excluded before making this diagnosis. Secondly, both neoplastic and inflammatory processes in the retroperitoneum are notoriously treacherous and difficult to diagnose correctly; consequently many sections and liberal use of histochemical and immunohistochemical stains are often rewarding manoeuvres.

Giant cell malignant fibrous histiocytoma

Occasional malignant fibrous histiocytomas contain large number of osteo-clastic type giant cells set in a background characteristic of pleomorphic malignant fibrous histiocytoma (Guccion & Enzinger 1972). These tumours have also been categorised as malignant giant cell sarcoma and giant cell fascial sarcoma. The low-power view typically reveals nodules of tumour cells surrounded by dense fibrous tissue. About half of the neoplasms contain small amounts of metaplastic bone. X-rays are helpful in excluding a primary bone neoplasm. It is the small quantity of the bone that is used to separate giant cell MFH from the rare primary soft tissue osteosarcoma, but occasionally this distinction may be impossible.

Malignant fibrous histiocytoma — fibrous type

Fibrosarcoma is currently defined as a neoplasm composed of uniform spindled cells with scant cytoplasm arranged in fascicles that intersect at acute angles. When such neoplasms develop pleomorphic cells and gaint cells they have been variously labelled as high-grade fibrosarcoma and, more recently, as the fibrous variant of malignant fibrous histiocytoma (Kearney et al 1980) (Fig. 6.17). Our current definition of fibrosarcoma does not allow for significant numbers of pleomorphic cells, and when these are present in a tumour that otherwise meets the criteria of fibrosarcoma, we use the term fibrous variant of malignant fibrous histiocytoma. The need for such a definition arises because of the merging morphological patterns between fibrosarcoma and pleomorphic malignant fibrous histiocytoma. What is observed is a morphologic continuum bounded on one extreme by classic fibrosarcoma and on the other by pleomorphic MFH. Along this continuum there is a gradual loss of the uniform spindle cell population, organised into fascicles characteristic of fibrosarcoma, and a gradual increase in pleomor-phism and anaplasia of the sort found in pleomorphic MFH. In order to distinguish between malignant fibrous histiocytoma and fibrosarcoma, a dividing line needs to be drawn along this continuum. We draw it at the point where pleomorphic and/or giant cells are found in a neoplasm which otherwise meets the criteria of fibrosarcoma. Tumours that contain such cells but still retain the fascicular organisation of their spindle cells are labelled as

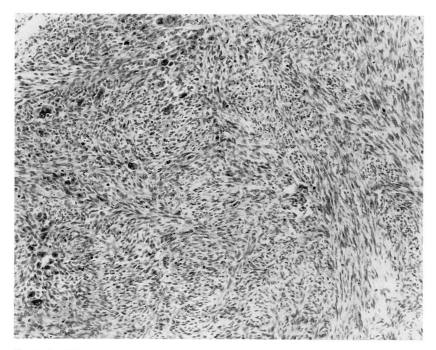

Fig. 6.17   This is the tumour we label as the fibrous variant of malignant fibrous histiocytoma. The features we use to recognise this are the pleomorphic large cells set among spindled tumour cells arranged as in fibrosarcoma. × 100.

the fibrous variant of MFH. When the fascicular organisation of such a neoplasm is largely lost, it should be labelled as pleomorphic MFH. Clinically, all of this line drawing makes little difference since high-grade fibrosarcoma, the fibrous variant of MFH, and pleomorphic MFH all have identical behaviours and all three will be treated in the same way. Mostly, these lines are drawn for classificatory convenience.

Angiomatoid malignant fibrous histiocytoma

Ever since it was first described (Enzinger 1979) questions have been raised as to whether this neoplasm belongs with the rest of the fibrous histiocytomas. Unlike the other malignant fibrous histiocytomas, the majority of the patients with angiomatoid MFH are young and distant metastases occur in less than 15% of patients. The tumour may be associated with globulin and albumin abnormalities and lymph node lesions (Seo et al 1986). These lesions most often involve the dermis or subcutaneous tissue, usually of an extremity. Histologically, angiomatoid MFH is characterised by blood-filled spaces lined by cells that appear to be a cross between histiocytes and myofibroblasts. These cells also grow in sheets. Plasma cells and lymphocytes are prominent and often form a ring around the other cells producing an uncanny resemblance to a lymph node. This mimicry of a lymph node is further enhanced by the organisation of the lymphoid cells into follicular centres. The overall appearance more suggests a vascular or smooth muscle neoplasm in a lymph node than it does a fibrous histiocytoma. Recognition is often enhanced if one remembers to think of this neoplasm when a haemorrhagic structure resembling a lymph node is found in the skin or in an unusual site in the soft tissues. Immunohistochemical and ultrastructural studies have been inconclusive in determining the direction of differentiation of this neoplasm. In any case, it is an important lesion to distinguish from the other malignant fibrous histiocytomas because of its low incidence of mestastases. Because the term malignant fibrous histiocytoma is currently appended to this neoplasm, we point out to clinicians that the behaviour of this tumour is distinctly different than the rest of the malignant fibrous histiocytomas (except low grade myxoid MFH).

CLINICAL PROFILE OF THE MALIGNANT FIBROUS HISTIOCYTOMAS

With the exception of the angiomatoid and low-grade myxoid types, the malignant fibrous histiocytomas have a rather consistent clinical profile (Enzinger & Weiss 1988). Typically, they are neoplasms that develop in middle aged and older individuals. Rarely they develop in children, but one should exercise great caution when making such a diagnosis (Zuppan et al 1987). Most commonly they are found in the extremities and in the retroperitoneum, although the literature is replete with reports of malignant fibrous histiocytomas occurring in almost every conceivable part of the body. Most malignant fibrous histiocytomas are deep soft tissue tumours and less than 10% are reported in the subcutaneous tissue. When malignant fibrous histiocytomas develop in the subcutis, they are reported to have a better prognosis and patients with smaller tumours tend to do better than those with large lesions. As noted in the section devoted to atypical fibroxanthoma, when pleomorphic MFH is limited to the dermis, it does not metastasise. It is common for the deep-seated malignant fibrous histiocytomas to be quite large before they are detected, and haemorrhage and necrosis are common. Local recurrences have been reported to occur in over 50% of cases, but the recurrence rate seems to be related to the adequency of excision. However, in spite of adequate local excision, overall survival seems only to be around 30–40% (Bertoni et al 1985). Essentially, the survival of patients with malignant fibrous histiocytoma is the same as with patients with any other high-grade pleomorphic sarcoma.

Again, leaving aside the low-grade myxoid and angiomatoid variants, malignant fibrous histiocytomas histologically are high-grade tumours and their clinical behaviour parallels their morphological appearance. Therefore, pleomorphic, fibrous, inflammatory and giant cell malignant fibrous histiocytomas usually are not graded because they are high grade by definition. Attempts to find prognostically significant morphological features, such as mitotic activity, extent of pleomorphism, etc. within each of the subtypes of MFH have largely failed (Kearney et al 1980, Kempson & Kyriakos 1972, Weiss & Enzinger 1978). Therefore, prognosis is best judged on the basis of the histological subtype, extent of necrosis, location of the tumour and its size. Our experience indicates that the behaviour of the myxoid variant worsens as the amount of pleomorphic MFH in the tumour increases. We thus designate the myxoid variant as low grade or high grade, depending on the amount of anaplasia and pleomorphic tumour present. With the exception of the angiomatoid type, we then consider all of the other variants to be high-grade sarcomas.

REFERENCES

Alguacil-Garcia A, Unni K K, Goellner J R 1978 Malignant fibrous histiocytoma: An ultrastructural study of six cases. American Journal of Clinical Pathology 69: 121–129

Angervall L, Kindblom L-G, Merck C 1977 Myxofibrosarcoma. A study of 30 cases. Acta Pathologica Microbiologica Scandinavica Section A 85: 127–140

Bertoni F, Capanna R, Biagini R et al 1985. Malignant fibrous histiocytoma of soft tissue. An analysis of 78 cases located and deeply seated in the extremities. Cancer 56: 356–367

Brecher M E, Franklin W A 1986 Absence of mononuclear phagocyte antigens in malignant fibrous histiocytoma. American Journal of Clinical Pathology 86: 344–348

Brooks J J 1986 The significance of double phenotypic patterns and markers in human sarcomas. A new model of mesenchymal differentiation. American Journal of Pathology 125: 113–123

Burgdorf W H C, Duray P, Rosai J 1981 Immunohistochemical identification of lysozyme in cutaneous lesions of alleged histiocytic nature. American Journal of Clinical Pathology 75: 162–167

Burkhardt B R, Soule E H, Winkelmann R K, Ivins J C 1966 Dermatofibrosarcoma protuberans. Study of fifty-six cases. American Journal of Surgery 111: 638–644

Chowdhury L M, Swerdlow M A, Jao W, Kathpalia S, Desser R K 1980 Post-irradiation malignant fibrous histiocytoma of the lung. Demonstration of alpha-I-antitrypsin-like material in neoplastic cells. American Journal of Clinical Pathology 74: 820–826

Churg A M, Kahn L B 1977 Myofibroblasts and related cells in malignant fibrous and fibrohistiocytic tumours. Human Pathology 8: 205–218

Dahl I 1976 Atypical fibroxanthoma of the skin. A clinicopathological study of 57 cases. Acta Pathologica et Microbiologica Scandinavica 84: 183–197

Dehner L P 1988 (editorial) Malignant fibrous histiocytoma. Nonspecific morphologic pattern, specific pathologic entity, or both? Archives of Pathology and Laboratory Medicine 112: 236–237

du Boulay C E H 1982 Demonstration of alpha-I-antitrypsin and alpha-I-antichymotrypsin in fibrous histiocytomas using the immunoperoxidase technique. American Journal of Surgical Pathology 6: 559–564

Dupree W B, Langloss J M, Weiss S M 1985 Pigmented dermatofibrosarcoma protuberans (Bednar tumour). A pathologic, ultrastructural, and immunohistochemistry study. American Journal of Surgical Pathology 9: 630–639

Enjoji M, Hashimoto H, Tsuneyoshi M, Iwasaki H, 1980. Malignant fibrous histiocytoma: A clinicopathologic study of 130 cases. Acta Pathologica Japonica 30: 727–741

Enzinger F M 1979 Angiomatoid malignant fibrous histiocytoma: A distinct fibrohistiocytic tumour of children and young adults simulating a vascular neoplasm. Cancer 44: 2147–2157.

Enzinger F M 1986 Malignant fibrous histiocytoma 20 years after Stout. American Journal of Surgical Pathology 10 (Suppl 1): 43–53

Enzinger F M, Weiss S W 1988 Malignant fibrous histiocytoma. In: Soft Tissue Tumours, 2nd edn. C V Mosby, St Louis, p 170–198

Enzinger F M, Zhang R Y 1988 Plexiform fibrohistiocytic tumour presenting in children and young adults. An analysis of 65 cases. American Journal of Surgical Pathology 12: 818–826

Fletcher C D M 1987 Malignant fibrous histiocytoma? Histopathology 11: 433–437

Fletcher C D M, Evans B J, MacArtney J C, Smith N, Wilson Jones E, McKee P H, 1985 Dermatofibrosarcoma protuberans: a clinicopathological and immunohistochemical study with a review of the literature. Histopathology 9: 921–938

Fletcher C D M, Theaker J M, Flanagan A, Krausz T 1988 Pigmented dermatofibrosarcoma protuberans (Bednar tumour): melanocytic colonisation or neuroectodermal differentiation? A clinicopathological and immunohistochemical study. Histopathology 13: 631–643

Fretzin D F, Helwig E B 1973 Atypical fibroxanthoma of the skin. A clinicopathologic study of 40 cases. Cancer 31: 1541–1552

Frierson H F, Cooper P H 1983 Myxoid variant of dermatofibrosarcoma protuberans. American Journal of Surgical Pathology 7: 445–450

Fu Y-S, Gabbiani G, Kaye G l, Lattes R 1975 Malignant soft tissue tumours of probable histiocytic origin (malignant fibrous histiocytomas): General considerations and electron microscopic and tissue culture studies. Cancer 35: 176–198

Gonzalez S, Duarte I 1982 Benign fibrous histiocytoma of the skin. A morphologic study of 290 cases. Pathology, Research and Practice 174: 379–391

Gould V E 1986 Histogenesis and differentiation: a re-evalution of these concepts as criteria for the classification of tumours. Human Pathology 17: 212–215

Guccion J G, Enzinger F M 1972 Malignant giant cell tumour of soft parts. An analysis of 32 cases. Cancer 29: 1518–1529

Harris M 1980 The ultrastructure of benign and malignant fibrous histiocytomas. Histiopathology 4: 29–44

Helwig E B, May D 1986 Atypical fibroxanthoma of the skin with metastasis. Cancer 57: 368–376

Hoffman M A, Dickersin G R 1983 Malignant fibrous histiocytoma: An ultrastructural study of eleven cases. Human Pathology 14: 913–922

Kahn L B 1973 Retroperitoneal xanthogranuloma and xanthosarcoma (malignant fibrous xanthoma). Cancer 31: 411–422

Kahn L B, Saxe N, Gordon W 1978 Dermatofibrosarcoma protuberans with lymph node and pulmonary metastases. Archives of Dermatology 114: 599–601

Kanitakis J, Schmitt D, Thivolet J 1984 Immunohistiologic study of cellular populations of histiocytofibromas (dermatofibromas) Journal of Cutaneous Pathology 11: 88–94

Kearney M M, Soule E H, Ivins J C 1980 Malignant fibrous histiocytoma: A retrospective analysis of 167 cases. Cancer 45: 167–178

Kempson R L, Kyriakos M 1972 Fibroxanthosarcoma of the soft tissue: A type of malignant fibrous histiocytoma. Cancer 29: 961–976

Kempson R L, McGavran M H 1964 Atypical fibroxanthoma of the skin. Cancer 17: 1463–1471

Kim K, Goldblatt P J 1982 Malignant fibrous histiocytoma. Cytologic, light microscopic and ultrastructural studies. Acta Cytologica 26: 507–511

Kindblom L G, Jacobsen G K, Jacobsen M 1982 Immunohistochemical investigations of tumors of supposed fibroblastic-histiocytic origin. Human Pathology 13: 834–840

Krawisz B R, Florine D L, Scott R E 1981 Differentiation of fibroblast-like cells into macrophages. Cancer Research 41: 2891–2899

Kyriakos M, Kempson R L 1976 Inflammatory fibrous histiocytoma: An aggressive and lethal lesion. Cancer 37: 1584–1606

Lagace R, Delage C, Seemayer T A 1979 Myxoid variant of malignant fibrous histiocytoma: ultrastructural observations. Cancer 43: 526–534

Lattes R 1982 Malignant fibrous histiocytoma. A review article American Journal of Surgical Pathology

Lawson C W, Fisher C, Gatter K C 1987 An immunohistochemical study of differentiation in malignant fibrous histiocytoma. Histopathology 11: 375–383

Leyva W H, Santa Cruz D J 1986 Atypical cutaneous fibrous histiocytoma. American Journal of Dermatopathology 8: 467–71

McDonnell T, Kyriakos M, Roper C, Mazoujian G 1988 Malignant fibrous histiocytoma of the lung. Cancer 61: 137–145

McPeak C J, Cruz T, Nicastri A D 1967 Dermatofibrosarcoma protuberans: an analysis of 86 cases–5 with metastasis. Annals of surgery 166: 803–816

Meister P 1988 Malignant fibrous histiocytoma. History, histology, histogenesis. Pathology, Research and Practice 183: 1–7

Meister P, Nathrath W 1980 Immunohistochemical markers of histiocytic tumors. Human Pathology 11: 300–301

Merck C, Angervall L, Kindblom L-G, Oden A 1983 Myxofibrosarcoma. A malignant soft tissue tumour of fibroblstic-histio-cytic origin. A clinicopathologic and prognostic study of 110 cases using multivariate analysis. Acta Pathologica Microbiologica Scandinavica Section A 91: (supplement 282): 1–40

Merino M J, LiVolsi V A 1980 Inflammatory malignant fibrous histiocytoma. American Journal of Clinical Pathology 73: 276–281

O'Brien J E, Stout A P 1964 Malignant fibrous xanthomas. Cancer 17: 1445–1455

O'Dowd J, Laidler P 1988 Progression of dermatofibrosarcoma protuberans to malignant fibrous histiocytoma: report of a case with implications for tumor histogenesis. Human Pathology 19: 368–370

Ozzello L, Stout A P, Murray M R 1963 Cultural characteristics of malignant histiocytomas and fibrous xanthomas. Cancer 16: 331–344

Roholl P J, Kleijne J, van Basten C D, van der Putte S C, van Unnik J A 1985 A study to analyze the origin of tumor cells in malignant fibrous histiocytomas. A multiparametric characterization. Cancer 56: 2809–2815

Roses D F, Valensi Q, LaTrenta G, Harris M N 1986 Surgical treatment of dermatofibrosarcoma protuberans. Surgery, Gynecology and obstetrics 162: 449–452

Seo I S, Frizzera G, Coates T D, Mirkin L D, Cohen M D 1986 Angiomatoid malignant fibrous histiocytoma with extensive lymphadenopathy simulating Castleman's disease. Pediatric Pathology 6: 233–247

Soini Y, Miettinen M 1988 Widespread immunoreactivity for alpha-1-antichymotrypsin in different types of tumors. American Journal of Clinical Pathology 89: 131–136

Soini Y, Miettinen M 1989 Alpha-1-antitrypsin and lysozyme. Their limited significance in fibrohistiocytic tumors. American Journal of Clinical Pathology 91: 515–521

Strauchen J A, Dimitriu-Bona A 1986 Malignant fibrous histiocytoma. Expression of monocyte/macrophage differentiation antigens detected with monoclonal antibodies. American Journal of Pathology 124: 303–309

Taxy J B, Battifora H 1977 Malignant fibrous histiocytoma: An electron microscopic study. Cancer 40: 254–267

Taylor H B, Helwig E B 1962 Dermatofibrosarcoma protuberans: A study of 115 cases. Cancer 15: 717–728

Tsuneyoshi M, Enjoji M, Shinohara N 1981 Malignant fibrous histiocytoma: A electron microscopic study of 17 cases. Virchows Archiv A Pathology and Anatomy 392: 135–145

Unanue E R 1976 Secretory function of mononuclear phagocytes: A review. American Journal of Pathology 83: 396–417

Weiss S W 1982 Malignant fibrous histiocytoma. A reaffirmation. American Journal of Surgical Pathology 6: 773–784

Weiss S W, Bratthauer G L, Morris P A 1988 Postirradiation malignant fibrous histiocytoma expressing cytokeratin. Implications for the immunodiagnosis of sarcomas. American Journal of Surgical Pathology 12: 554–558

Weiss S W, Enzinger F M 1977 Myxoid variant of malignant fibrous histiocytoma. Cancer 39: 1672–1685

Weiss S W, Enzinger F M 1978 Malignant fibrous histiocytoma: An analysis of 200 cases. Cancer 41: 2250–2266

Wolfe H J, Palmer P E 1981 Alpha-I-antitrypsin: Its immunohistochemical localization and significance in diagnostic pathology. In: DeLellis R A ed Dianostic immunohistochemistry. Masson New York, p 227–238

Wood G S, Beckstead J H, Turner R R, Hendrickson M R, Kempson R L, Warnke R A, 1986 Malignant fibrous histiocytoma tumour cells resemble fibroblasts. American Journal of Surgical Pathology 10: 323–335

Wood G S, Beckstead J H, Medeiros L J, Kempson R L, Warnke R A, 1988 The cells of giant cell tumor of tendon sheath resemble osteoclasts. American Journal of Surgical Pathology 12: 444–452

Wrotnowski U, Cooper P H, Shmookler B M 1988 Fibrosarcomatous change in dermatofibrosarcoma protuberans. American Journal of Surgical Pathology 12: 287–293

Yousem S A, Hochholzer L 1987 Malignant fibrous histiocytoma of the lung. Cancer 60: 2532–2541

Zuppan C W, Mierau G W, Wilson H L 1987 Malignant fibrous histiocytoma in childhood: a report of two cases and review of the literature. Pediatric Pathology 7: 303–318

7. Kaposi's sarcoma or Kaposi's disease? A personal reappraisal

A. C. Bayley   S. B. Lucas

INTRODUCTION

In 1960, Lothe described African Kaposi's sarcoma as 'a dangerous disease of unknown cause, selective with respect to region, race and sex, the nature of which is in doubt and treatment of which is difficult' (Lothe 1960). In a detailed pathological study, he considered the suggestions of early European observers that Kaposi's sarcoma might be due to infection, or an allergic arteritis, but found no support for either theory. At a meeting of clinicians and pathologists with extensive experience of African endemic Kaposi's sarcoma, the debate concluded that it was indeed a malignant tumour, although in several respects it did not behave like a typical sarcoma (Symposium 1962). The arrival of the human immunodeficiency virus (HIV) a few years ago has further complicated the situation.

Since 1981, most clinicians meeting Kaposi's sarcoma for the first time in HIV-infected patients have regarded it as a malignant tumour, with uncommon exceptions (Costa & Rabson 1983). Brooks (1986) summarised the pecularities of its pathology, and proposed that it should be reclassified as a 'benign potentially controllable and reversible hyperplasia'. However, he was unable to identify any factors which might be responsible for a disorder of growth.

In this chapter we review the nature of Kaposi's sarcoma. First we discuss the clinical and pathological features of Kaposi's sarcoma and its cell biology. Most of the clinical observations were made in Lusaka, Zambia. Secondly we interpret these phenomena and propose a hypothesis to explain why patients with HIV-related Kaposi's sarcoma benefit from cytotoxic therapy. Finally we consider the consequences of accepting an unorthodox view that the disease named after Moricz Kaposi (Kaposi 1872) is not a malignant tumour. Hereon the entity is referred to as Kaposi's disease (KD).

DEFINITION

Kaposi's disease cannot be defined clinically since its manifestations are too varied, therefore histopathological criteria are used even though the lesions are histologically polymorphic.

KD is a multifocal process characterised by the appearance of irregular lymphatic or vascular channels, followed chronologically by strands, clumps

141

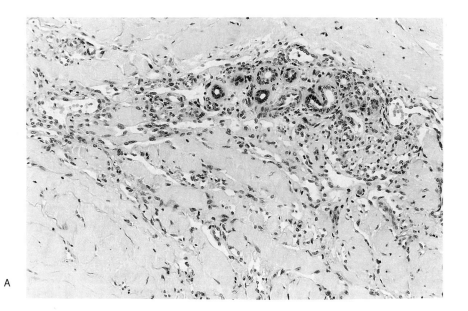

A

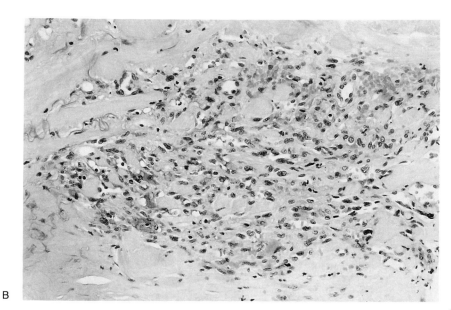

B

Fig. 7.1 Histological sequence of development of Kaposi's disease lesions. **A** Patch/macule: radiating from the vessels associated with a sweat gland, there are irregular dilated thin-walled vascular channels. The nuclei of the endothelial cells in these channels are not enlarged. H & E × 100.
B Plaque/papule: a few jagged thin-walled channels remain, but round-to-spindle cells are proliferating through the dermal collagen. H & E × 200.
C Developed nodule of KD: circumscribed nodule in dermis, H & E × 200.
D Nodule of KD: bands of spindle cells are seen in longitudinal and cross-section, with many slits (holes) in between. A normal mitosis is arrowed. H & E × 400.

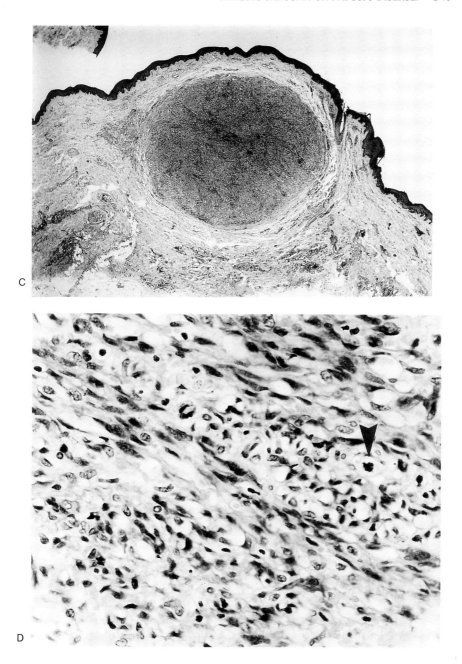

C

D

and nodules of spindle-shaped cells (Ackerman & Gottleib 1988). Fully evolved tissue has a spongy consistency with a mixture of well-developed vessels, spindle cells and slit-like spaces which contain blood (Fig. 7.1). In Africa, this defined a disease which has two distinct but overlapping clinical patterns, both of which are complex.

CLINICAL PATTERNS OF KAPOSI'S DISEASE

Endemic Kaposi's disease

Endemic KD in sub-Saharan Africa affects middle-aged men and rarely children (Taylor et al 1971, Templeton 1972, Olweny et al 1976, Olweny 1981, Bayley 1981). The mean age at presentation is 42 years and the sex ratio is at least 10:1 (male:female). Commonly, the first symptom is intermittent swelling of the feet, followed after months or years by the development of small nodules in or under the skin, often on more than one limb, and almost always on the most distal parts. Some nodules regress spontaneously while new ones appear, tending to spread slowly up the limbs. Rapid growth may occur forming a confluent mass; the overlying skin may ulcerate, leaking copious clear fluid. Progressive thickening and stiffening of the skin proximal to the lesions may lead to crippling contractures of the ankles, knees and hands.

Affected limbs are hot to touch and individual lesions sometimes pulsate. General health is surprisingly well maintained for several years and lymph nodes enlarge only at sites draining much disease. Ultimately, lesions reach the trunk and spread to the viscera (usually gut and pleurae). The patient loses weight and becomes anaemic, but the immediate cause of death is usually difficult to define.

In young children KD is more aggressive, with symmetrical enlargement of all peripheral lymph nodes. Skin lesions are absent or inconspicuous and located on the trunk and proximal limbs, not centrifugally (Slavin et al 1970). Untreated, it spreads to the viscera and death follows within a year of onset.

Atypical African Kaposi's disease (AAKD)

A second disease pattern appeared in Zambia and Uganda around 1982 (Bayley 1984; Serwadda et al 1986). Over 90% of these patients have antibodies to HIV (Bayley et al 1985; Bayley 1988), and their KD resembles Western HIV-related KD though with some differences (Bayley 1987); hereon it is called 'atypical African Kaposi's disease'. It presents with multiple lesions which the patient notices over a short space of time, which is particularly brief if the disease is widely disseminated and aggressive.

Lymphadenopathy

Weight loss is the commonest symptom (76% of patients), but lymph node enlargement is the commonest sign (70% of patients — Bayley 1988). It is bilaterally symmetrical (Fig. 7.2), and the nodes enlarge simultaneously, not in the sequential manner characteristic of malignant lymphoma or metastatic carcinoma.

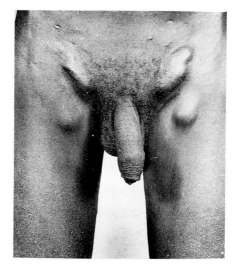

Fig. 7.2 Bilateral inguinal lymphadenopathy due to Kaposi's disease in an HIV-seropositive man.

Oral lesions

Oral lesions are the next commonest sign (58% of patients), starting as flat purple macules which elevate into broad plaques, become nodular and ulcerate (Fig. 7.3). They are most often seen on the hard palate, but are also seen on gums, tonsils and tongue, although they rarely present on buccal mucosa. The whole gingiva may convert into a purple mass of KD. During regression on chemotherapy, oral lesions reverse the stages of their development to leave only a stippling of pigment.

Skin lesions

Whilst in endemic KD, nodules are the characteristic lesions, in AAKD plaques are more common (40% of patients). They are palpably raised, hyperpigmented or purple; the size ranges from a few millimetres to three or four centimetres and the outlines are irregular. The plaques occur at sites such as the head, neck, trunk and proximal parts of the limbs where endemic KD lesions are rarely seen; about 18% of AAKD patients have no skin lesions at all (Bayley 1988). Symmetry of the lesions is common, particularly on the face where the tip of the nose, cheeks and preauricular skin are favoured locations (Fig. 7.4). Occasionally plaques occur at sites of trauma, in scars, or in a distribution suggesting the influence of Lange's lines (Bayley 1984). The medial aspects of both thighs are often involved, but not the upper arms. A hot woody infiltration accompanies plaques on the thighs and lower legs.

On the feet, AAKD plaques or nodules are seen on both insteps, but not on the weight-bearing part of the sole, unlike endemic KD lesions which

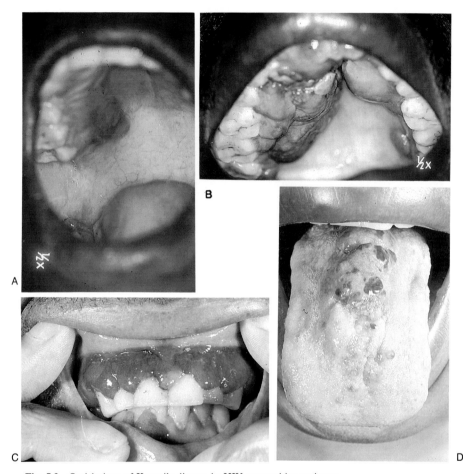

Fig. 7.3 Oral lesions of Kaposi's disease in HIV seropositive patients:
A Early lesion — a dark macule — on the hard palate.
B Nodular lesions on the hard palate.
C Diffuse gingival lesions of KD.
D Plaques and nodules of KD on the tongue.

occur on the sole and may be crippling. We have not seen lesions of AAKD on the pressure areas of the buttocks and elbows, and only rarely on the hairy scalp, although they are quite common on the beard area and occasionally on bald scalps.

Oedema and effusions

Oedema is less common in AAKD than endemic KD. It has a central distribution affecting the face, neck and bikini area, thighs and trunk (Fig. 7.5), but is not always accompanied by skin lesions. Oedema may be marked over enlarged inguinal or iliac lymph nodes without coexisting oedema of the

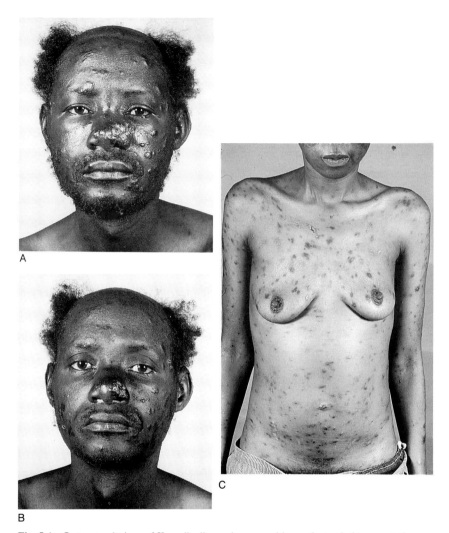

Fig. 7.4 Cutaneous lesions of Kaposi's disease in seropositive patients: **A** At presentation: lesions on nose, cheeks, forehead, with local oedema.
B Same patient after one month of chemotherapy: the lesions have partially regressed, as has the oedema.
C Plaques of KD over the trunk and arms of a female.

external genitalia, so the oedema is not simply a consequence of lymphatic obstruction by KD.

Ulceration of confluent masses of AAKD is less frequent than in endemic KD; but when present the ulcerated KD tissue is extraordinarily wet. No ulcerated carcinoma or sarcoma exudes so much fluid. Pleural effusions are common in AAKD patients and are difficult to manage (Ognibene et al 1985, Fouret et al 1987). Despite aspiration of 1 litre or more of fluid a day, they reaccumulate. Protein-losing enteropathy due to intestinal HIV-related KD

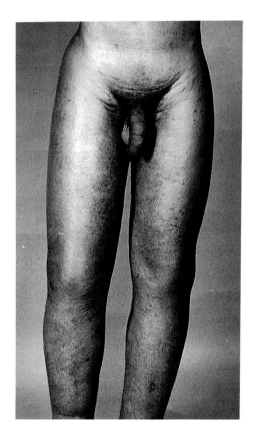

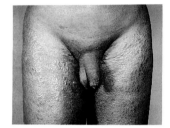

Fig. 7.5   Oedema associated with Kaposi's disease in HIV-seropositive patients: **A** Bilateral leg oedema. **B** Bilateral plaques of KD on the thigh, with oedema.
In neither case are the genitalia oedematous.

has also been described, associated with pleural effusions and hypoalbumin-aemia (Laine et al 1987).

Pulmonary infiltration

Respiratory symptoms and signs occur at presentation in 42% of patients with AAKD in Lusaka. Pulmonary infiltration is even more common than pleural effusions. The patient complains of dry cough, then streak haemoptyses but no sputum, and a chest X-ray shows heavy bronchovasculolymphatic markings. Dyspnoea worsens until the patient is bed-bound after two or three months. Clinical examination reveals symmetrical reduction in air entry to the lung bases, with fine crepitations which do not clear on coughing, suggesting fluid in the alveoli. The chest X-ray now shows a streaky or fluffy infiltrate radiating from the hilum into the mid- and lower zones of the lungs; the lung apices are clear. Serial radiographs show a rapid increase in the extent and density of infiltration over a few weeks, paralleling the worsening dyspnoea (Fig. 7.6). The symptoms, signs and radiographs resemble the spread of breast carcinoma to lung lymphatics.

At autopsy, the volume of macroscopic KD seems insufficient to account for the severity of respiratory failure prior to death. This lung involvement may herald the terminal phase of longterm skin or lymph node AAKD; or it may develop alongside skin and node disease so that death occurs within six months of the first plaque appearing. Although most patients with this

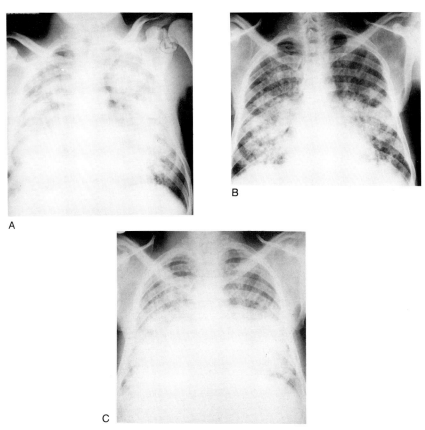

Fig. 7.6 Series of chest X-rays of one patient with pulmonary Kaposi's disease, showing response to chemotherapy but subsequent relapse. **A** Bilateral upper and lower zone fluffy shadowing. **B** After one month of chemotherapy: considerable clearing of the infiltrate. **C** Relapse at three months.

radiological infiltrate have endobronchial plaques of KD on bronchoscopy, we do not have biopsy proof that the infiltrates are KD in the lung parenchyma. However, treatment with cytotoxic drugs is followed by partial or complete disappearance of infiltrates. If the patient survives the first 48 hours of treatment, he usually lives for several weeks, although recurrence of pulmonary KD often leads to death within three months.

RESPONSES TO TREATMENT

Over 90% of patients with endemic KD sustained objective reponses to chemotherapy with actinomycin D and vincristine (Olweny 1981, Bayley 1988), although complete disappearance of disease is rare (Fig. 7.4). The hot limb cools, ulcerated tumours dry up and nodules flatten, leaving mild thickening and some inelasticity of skin, or a depressed scar.

Oral plaques of AAKD regress more quickly than skin lesions. Skin and visceral lesions do not always respond to chemotherapy simultaneously; AAKD may persist on the skin whilst gut lesions regress, and vice versa (Plettenberg et al 1989). Further, in Lusakan patients, there are fluctuations in objective responses which do not relate to interruptions or dose reductions in chemotherapy.

In a multifocal disease which responds to chemotherapy, surgery has a limited role. However, KD behaves differently from sarcoma or melanoma after surgery; instead of recurring vigorously at the operation site within weeks, KD wounds heal quickly and permanently, although remaining KD lesions continue to enlarge (Fig. 7.7).

HISTOPATHOLOGICAL OBSERVATIONS

In carcinomas, such as those of bronchus and cervix, the earliest changes are seen in individual cells which show dyplasia whilst the tissue retains a normal

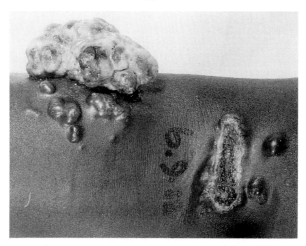

Fig. 7.7 Healing of a Kaposi's disease lesion after surgery. Adjacent nodules continued to enlarge.

organisation. The changes may be reversible, with re-establishment of local regulatory mechanisms. If regression does not take place, the dysplasia persists to in-situ carcinoma, and eventually the cells proliferate into masses which break through the normal epithelial boundaries, infiltrate and metastasise by invading blood vessels and lymphatics.

The histopathology of KD is a chronological sequence of changes relating to vessels, which matches the clinical evolution through the patch, plaque and nodule stages (Ackerman & Gottleib 1988). The earliest form of both patterns of KD is a flat macule/patch. In the upper dermis new vessels appear around existing vascular plexi. These are irregular jagged, dilated spaces with thin endothelial cells without pleomorphism, and very scanty, if any, mitoses. Plasma cells and haemosiderin-laden macrophages are usually present. In addition there may be an increased cellularity around vessels, comprising tiny vascular spaces.

At the later plaque/papule stage, spindle cells and proliferating capillaries appear between the thin-walled spaces, and the lesion occupies more of the dermis. No dysplastic features (i.e. hyperchromasia and hypertrophy of nuclei) are present. The process may go no further, but continued proliferation may produce nodules which are circumscribed and comprise interweaving fascicles of spindle cells (Fig. 7.1). Extravasated erythrocytes are usually plentiful between spindle cells and intracytoplasmic hyaline globules are usually seen. The mitotic rate within spindle cells is variable, but rarely as high as that seen in malignant spindle cell tumours, and the mitoses are not atypical. Also the degree of cell pleomorphism is usually slight. It is notable that intravenous or intra-arterial foci of dysplastic rounded or spindle cells are very rarely seen in KD lesions (Purdy et al 1986, Ackerman & Gottleib 1988), quite unlike other tumours of known malignant nature.

The early classification of KD described three types (Taylor et al 1971); mixed cell, monocellular and anaplastic. These represent variants of nodular lesions, the early patch and plaque stages not being so distinctly recognised then. The 'mixed cell' and 'monocellular' types match the typical nodules, with less erythrocyte extravasation in the latter. The 'anaplastic' pattern is problematical; review of possible anaplastic KD lesions with immunocytochemical techniques in most cases shows them to be malignancies of non-vascular histogenesis. We consider 'anaplastic' KD to be a rare entity; only occasionally does KD progress to a genuine neoplasm (Ziegler 1988).

In lymph nodes that drain a carcinoma, solitary or clumped malignant cells appear in afferent lymphatics and the marginal sinus before deposits appear in the substance of the node. In lymphatic leukaemia, atypical lymphoctyes appear in the nodal mantle or cortical zone. KD follows neither pattern; irregular dilated vessels (like patch stage lesions) appear first in the capsule of nodes and then invade their substance by way of the fibrous trabeculae along the sinuses (Fig. 7.8). There is increased vascularity in the inter- and intrafollicular areas, and plasmacytosis of the medulla. Later, nodular masses of spindle cells evolve and replace the lymphoid tissue.

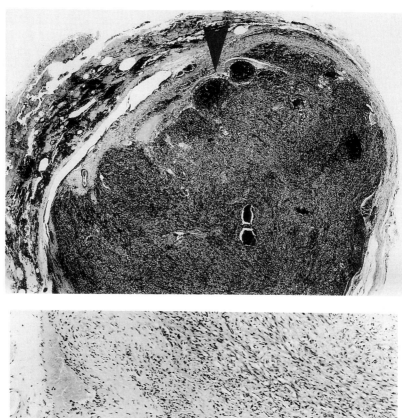

A

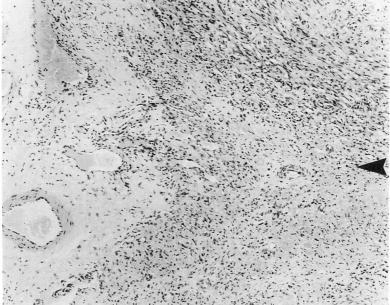

B

Fig. 7.8 Lymph node with Kaposi's disease. **A** KD almost completely replacing the node. Two lymphoid follicles are arrowed. H & E × 20. **B** Capsule of the node (left side) and parasinus fibrous tissue (arrowed) with proliferating capillaries and spindle cells. Slit-forming KD tissue is seen at top right. H & E × 200.

In all organs of the body, the same histopathological sequence of KD lesions is seen. Often there are foci of patch, plaque and nodule stages in adjacent parts of the same tissue. In the lung, KD lesions commence in the pleura, in the connective tissue of secondary lobules, and around bronchial and pulmonary arteries (Fig. 7.9) — all sites where there are lymphatic vessels (Jaffe 1987). They may involve extensive areas of lung in the plaque stage or enlarge to form typical nodules. The pleural effusions, often haemorrhagic, seem to derive from pleural KD lesions at any stage. Thus pulmonary KD is quite unlike classical metastatic malignancies, which present histologically as fully dysplastic foci, but do not recapitulate their development in every secondary deposit.

THE CELL OF ORIGIN OF KAPOSI'S DISEASE.

The cell of origin of KD has puzzled pathologists for decades. With the application of immunocytochemistry to fixed and frozen sections, and the more recent arrival of monoclonal antibodies which may discriminate between various types of endothelial cells, the histogenesis of KD lesions has been widely investigated. There is consensus that the very early jagged slits lined by thin endothelial cells share immunocytochemical reaction patterns with lymphatic endothelium, but not vein or artery endothelium (Beckstead et al 1985, Jones et al 1986, Rutgers et al 1986). About the nodular lesions, there is dispute. The obvious blood vessel structures between the spindle cells have endothelial cells which stain as vascular endothelium. The spindle cells have the immunocytochemical phenotype of vascular endothelium (Rutgers et al 1986) or lymphatic endothelium (Beckstead et al 1985), or both (Jones et al 1986). These apparently disparate results may be resolved; it is agreed that the relevant cells in KD are endothelial; if, in most cases, KD is not a true neoplasm but a hyperplastic proliferation, a consistent single cell phenotype in developed KD lesions need not be anticipated. Dictor & Andersson (1988) have noted that many KD lesions may be traced in development from anatomical connections between the lymphatic and venous system — the lymphaticovenous connections. It is possible that proliferating endothelial cells at these junctions express both lymphatic and vascular markers on immunocytochemistry. The normal distribution of lymphaticovenous connections in the body may hold a key to the puzzling locations and non-locations of KD lesions.

The search for the 'cell of origin' is of more than academic interest. The concept of KD expressed in this paper is that of an endothelial proliferation driven by angiogenic factors of paracrine and possibly autocrine origin. We presume that other vascular proliferations must have a similar underlying mechanism. For example, pyogenic granuloma, epithelioid angiomatosis (Cockerell et al 1987), and angiofollicular lymphoid hyperplasia (Castleman's disease) are all benign vascular proliferative lesions composed of arterioles and capillaries; and the latter two are also associated with HIV infection. Yet

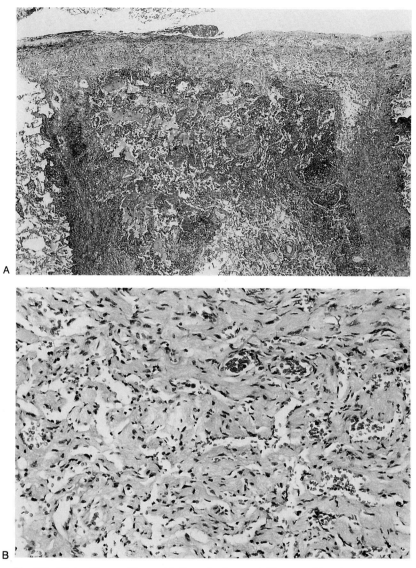

Fig. 7.9 Wedge biopsy of lung with Kaposi's disease: **A** Pleura and interlobular connective tissue thickened by KD. H & E x 25. **B** High-power view of pleura showing irregular proliferating channels of early stage KD. H & E × 200.

KD is an entity histologically distinct from these, particularly in the display of spindle cell aggregates with erythrocytes in slits. Is KD a predominantly lymphatic proliferation, where the relevant cells are induced to form spindle cells, or are there several stimuli that operate on more than one histogenetic type of endothelial cell to produce the complex histology that we recognise as KD?

CYTOGENETIC AND CELL CULTURE STUDIES OF KAPOSI'S DISEASE

Delli Bovi et al (1986) studied 13 cell cultures from 4 AIDS patients with KD. The cultures had a short lifespan in vitro; the cells expressed some endothelial markers, but they were not tumorigenic when injected into nude mice. The chromosome numbers were normal in 11/13 samples. The observed chromosomal rearrangements were often monoclonal within one culture, but differed between cultures, even when from the same biopsied lesion. The authors concluded that KD 'may be polyclonal even within the same lesion'.

A further study of short-term cultures of KD from a male AIDS patient was reported by Saikevych et al (1988). The cells had a predominant karyotype of 48XY on direct preparation, but 46XY in cells from 72-hour cultures, with an increased number of chromosomal abnormalities. 46XY — i.e. normal — has been the commonest karyotype in reports so far published (of only 11 patients) with AIDS-KD.

Before HIV was identified, a study of cultures of over 30 cell lines from biopsies of AIDS-related KD showed the cells to have endothelial characteristics, including production of factor VIII-related antigen and staining with *Ulex europeus* lectin. But the cultures did not grow in soft agar or induce tumours when injected into nude mice (J A Levy, personal commmunication).

Novel growth factors have been detected in culture media from human lymphocytes infected with human retroviruses (Nakamura et al 1988). Lymphocyte cultures infected with HTLV-2 produced the most potent growth-promoting activity; culture media from HIV-1 and HIV-2 infected lymphocytes were less active. Conditioned media from HTLV-2 infected cells (HTLV-2 CM) encouraged longterm in vitro growth of endothelial cells from AIDS-related KD cells in a dose-dependent manner, and the effect was maintained for about 30 passages over 1 year. In contrast, HTLV-2 CM had little effect on normal endothelial cells: human umbilical cord endothelium showed a small proliferative response but cultures survived for less than 2 months. The physicochemical and antigenic characteristics of the growth factor(s) differ from all known cytokines, including fibroblast growth factor. It was concluded that at least two factors are produced by T-cells infected by human retroviruses, one supporting the growth of AIDS-KD cells, the other stimulating normal endothelial cells.

AIDS-KD derived cells in culture produce cytokines which enhance their own growth, and also that of umbilical cord endothelium (Salahuddin et al 1988). Their evidence suggests that, once the abnormal vascular proliferation of KD starts, it may be self-perpetuating through an autocrine loop, which may also function to recruit normal endothelium into the process. The observation that these factors have a greater influence on normal cells than those derived from AIDS-KD cells suggests that they differ from the growth promoters found in HTLV-2 CM.

ANIMAL MODELS OF HIV-RELATED KAPOSI'S DISEASE

In no animal model can tumour be produced that precisely resembles KD in any of its polymorphic stages. However, some interesting histological and molecular biological results have resulted from this line of investigation.

Injection of cultured AIDS-KD derived cells into nude mice produced limited growth for up to six days, with vascular proliferative lesions that were of murine not human cells, i.e. a local angiogenic response. The lesions did include some spindle cells amongst the proliferating capillaries (Salahuddin et al 1988).

The HIV *tat* gene together with its long terminal repeat (LTR) has been introduced transgenically into the germline of mice (Vogel et al 1988). Offspring of these mice carried the LTR-*tat* sequence, but it was expressed only in their skin. At 12–18 months of age, vascular tumours developed in the skin of 15% of male mice; they were not seen in female mice bearing the *tat* gene. The early lesions showed slit-like spaces which were dissimilar to the jagged spaces characteristic in human lesions. The illustrations of the later nodular lesions show rather more nuclear pleomorphism of both endothelial cells and spindle cells compared with human KD; and the nodules lack the human sieve-like pattern with entrapped erythrocytes. The *tat* gene could not be demonstrated in the murine tumour cells, so its role in their genesis is indirect. The specificity for male mice raises intriguing analogies with the sex ratio in endemic KD.

In vitro transfection of NIH/3T3 cells with DNA derived from HIV-related KD cells and their subsequent inoculation into mice results in widespread vascular tumours. Histologically, they comprised sarcomatous spindle cells, vascular channels and erythrocyte extravasation, and the tumours behaved in a metastasising malignant fashion (Lo & Liotta 1985).

Infection of macaques with simian immunodeficiency virus (SIV) causes simian AIDS. The animals often have tumours in the subcutis, retroperitoneum and lymph nodes which histologically resemble fibrous histiocytoma more than human KD. Immunocytochemistry shows positive staining of both vascular endothelium and of spindle cells with factor VIII-related antigen (Giddens et al 1985). There is also an early lesion composed of irregular angiomatoid vessels (A Baskerville & S Lucas, unpublished obervations).

In summary, these animal nodels establish some links with human KD. Some of the animal tumours behave in an unequivocally malignant manner, and none are strictly comparable to human KD.

INTERPRETATIONS

Multiple lesions of atypical African KD appear almost simultaneously on the skin, in the mouth, and in lymph nodes. Furthermore, endoscopically, plaques in the mouth predict multiple mucosal lesions throughout the gastrointestinal tract, and 42% of Lusakan patients already have pulmonary disease at presentation. The process involves a variety of tissues but a single cell type, probably lymphatic endothelium. These phenomena are not the result of mutations occurring simultaneously in hundreds of scattered endothelial cells. The behaviour of AAKD in vitro provides no evidence for an irreversible change in cell behaviour due to the continuous expression of an oncogene. Instead it suggests the importance of essential growth factors, which are not intrinsic to endothelium but may include the growth factor as found in HTLV-2 CM (see above). The failure of human AIDS-related KD cells to grow in nude mice, even though they evoke an angiogenic response by mouse tissues, suggests that at least one component of the KD growth-control system is species-specific.

The symmetry and number of lesions in AAKD indicates a systemic distribution of a growth stimulus. The rapid evolution of signs implies an acute process. Too little attention has been paid to the sites where KD does not develop. There is no lymphatic endothelium in the brain, which may account for the extreme rarity of KD there, but why is AAKD not seen in skeletal muscle, the kidney, suburothelial tissue or the prostate? Why is it rare in the scalp? Leprosy may offer a clue here, for lesions of that disease do not develop in the hairy scalp; the explanation offered is that the temperature there is too high to support multiplication of the bacilli. If KD cell proliferation (or the output of growth-control factors) is in part dependent on temperature, then the immunity of the scalp, and the selection of cool nose and cheeks for KD plaque formation is consistent. However, the effect of temperature obviously must be unimportant in the development of visceral KD lesions.

If the stimulus to begin abnormal vascular growth is widespread in the body, and the target tissue widely distributed, then the stimulus acts, or is activated, only at particular sites. Clinical experience suggests that these sites may be determined by physical factors such as trauma, an absence of pressure, or reduced temperature. If this is so, it may be possible to use physical methods as part of therapy; for example, by heating lesions or applying pressure to them (as in the management of keloids after surgery).

Oedema

Truly obstructive oedema, e.g. due to filariasis, affects an entire anatomical region and feels cool. The oedema of AAKD may envelop both groins while sparing the genitalia (Fig. 7.5) or distend the thigh but spare the foot below it. Children with endemic African KD present with symmetrical lymph node obliteration by KD, yet distal oedema is very rarely seen. In adults with AAKD, oedema may occur in the absence of skin lesions, and we suspect that it identifies sites where the earliest changes of KD are developing in the deep dermis and subcutis. Systematic autopsy studies should resolve this by examination of deep tissues down to the bone in limbs with KD and oedema.

Ulcerated KD exudes clear serous fluid continuously in volumes greater than can be accounted for by drainage of tissue fluid through open lymphatic channels. Could the spindle cells of KD actively secrete fluid into tissue spaces, or — more probably — do they secrete a cytokine which increases the permeability of local capillaries? Alternatively, fluid may leak through gaps in the continuity of KD endothelium (McNutt et al 1983).

Patients with pulmonary infiltration have symptoms and radiographic appearances suggestive of severe pulmonary oedema or lymphangitic spread of carcinoma. Attempts to treat them with diuretics, digoxin or steroids are ineffective, but after injection of actinomycin D and vincristine, dysponea begins to improve within 24 hours, whilst fever often resolves in 48 hours. Is this rapid improvement in respiratory function the result of switching off interstitial secretion of fluid induced by the hyperplastic endothelial cells?

A NEW PERSPECTIVE

Atypical Kaposi's disease fails to behave like a tumour in vivo or in vitro, and fails to grow in nude mice. We do not think that AAKD is a true neoplasm (i.e. a monclonal self-propagating metastasising proliferation). Endemic KD is unlikely to be a neoplasm either, except in the rare case when malignant transformation leads to the evolution of a localised mass with an anaplastic histology.

The evidence assembled by clinicians and basic scientists against KD being neoplastic is so strong that we should explore the consequences of this. If it is not neoplastic, what is it? If it is not a cancer, why and how does cytotoxic chemotherapy benefit patients? If KD tissue consists of metabolically active but untransformed cells, are any of its protein products potentially useful for the treatment of human disease?

THE NATURE OF AAKD

In many respects AAKD behaves like an acute systemic infectious disease, yet there is no microscopic or inoculation evidence for an infective agent. A causative virus, if it exists, is well hidden; invisible to the electron microscope, able to replicate without reverse transcriptase, and undetected by the DNA probes used so far.

The earliest and most characteristic histological change is the proliferation of apparently normal endothelial cells. Levy and Ziegler (1983) suggested that an unidentified product of the immune system's battle with HIV induced or enhanced proliferation of endothelium. This hypothesis deserves more attention.

A revised hypothesis

The distribution of AAKD lesions suggests the interaction of systemic and local factors which permit or promote endothelial cell proliferation. We propose that one local component of the complex control system may be mediated through a direct effect on endothelium of HIV-modified cells. The endothelial cells of AAKD come into contact with lymphocytes, monocytes, tissue macrophages and Langerhans cells (in man, Langerhans cells are a target for HIV infection—Rappersberger et al 1988). In HIV-infected people many of these cells bear HIV gp120 bound to CD4 receptors on their surfaces, with or without integrated HIV in their genome (Lyerly et al 1987). Do endothelial cell membranes include any molecules capable of direct interaction with HIV gp120/CD4 complex? This question may be addressed by observing the effects of soluble gp120/CD4 complexes on the growth of endothelial cell cultures derived from human umbilical cord, adult lymphatics or AIDS-related KD. We propose that physical events — trauma, pressure, stasis due to reduced temperature, or massage due to muscular activity — may influence such interactions.

It is estimated that less than 10% of HIV-infected patients in Africa develop AAKD, thus there must be additional factors operating. The epidemiology of KD in the West, with declining rates in homosexual patients (who are practising safer sex) and very low incidences of KD in haemophiliac HIV-infected patients (who are not repeatedly exposed parenterally to HIV), suggests a sexually transmitted infection. It may not be necessary be postulate a second infectious agent. HIV could be responsible by integration of a whole or part of the HIV genome into critical cells. If the tat-bearing cells in the skin of transgenic mice (see above) are the murine equivalent of Langerhans cells (Vogel et al 1988), they may be inducing vascular cells to proliferate via cytokines. The apparent sexual transmission of a 'KD virus' might be explained by the increased likelihood of integration of the whole or parts of the HIV genome when there are repeated exposures to HIV by heterosexual or homosexual intercourse. The normal migration of Langerhans cells as well as macrophages to lymph nodes suggests a means by which nodes throughout the body may receive angioproliferative stimuli.

CD4 + ve cells become refractory to superinfection with other strains of HIV once gp120 expression results in blocking of membrane receptors, but superinfection is possible soon after the first HIV virion gains entry, as has been demonstrated in vitro (Ikuta et al 1989). Superinfection of a susceptible cell with more than one strain of HIV could result in enhanced viral replication and the expression of a regulatory protein which influences endothelium. The hypothesis, that an interaction between endothelial cells and either gp120-coated lymphoctyes or Langerhans cells carrying the tat gene could switch on a gene coding for a proliferation cytokine, might be tested using nude mice (Fig. 7.10).

What effects do cytotoxic drugs have on Kaposi's disease tissue?

There have been no studies of the histological changes of AAKD lesions following chemotherapy. Biopsies of endemic KD lesions after chemotherapy showed little change in the first few days; then followed reduction in the

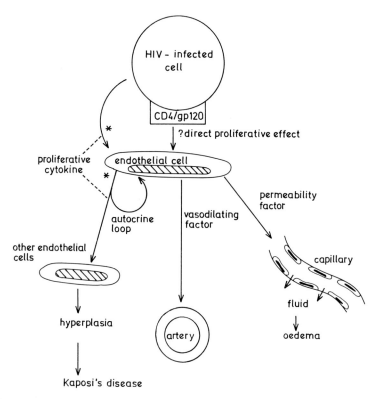

Fig. 7.10 Proposed sequence of events in the development of Kaposi's disease in HIV-infected people. The endothelial cell is crucial, both as responder to and secretor of angioproliferative cytokines.
*Indicates the sites of inhibitory action of α-interferon.

numbers of spindle cells, which became shorter with round hyperchromatic nuclei. Macrophages infiltrated the regressing lesions and the end result was fibrous scars (Cook 1962).

The clinical effects of cytotoxic drugs on AAKD are most obvious in patients with dyspnoea and pulmonary involvement. Oral lesions respond more slowly, and a complete response of skin and nodal lesions is rare, occurring in only 4% of Lusaka patients (Bayley 1988).

Interferon-α (IFN-α) is used as chemotherapy for HIV-related KD in Western countries. In high dosage it produces partial or complete remission of skin lesions in over one third of cases (Real 1987). IFN-α is a potent inhibitor of normal and malignant cell growth, acting as a negative growth regulator, not as a modulator of host immune response (Balkwill 1989). IFN-α also reduces HIV replication (Yamamoto et al 1986). Light and electron microscopic studies of KD lesions after IFN-α therapy show regression of cells, with disorganisation of both cell cytoskeleton and rough endoplasmic reticulum; it suggests that cell secretion is impaired, and the secretion of an autocrine growth factor may thus be reduced (Mayer-da-Silva et al 1987). Experimental models have shown that IFN-α inhibits the angiogenic effect of several different human carcinomas inoculated into mice, an effect that is independent of the antiproliferative effects of IFN. Further, IFN inhibits the vascular response to both allogenic and activated autologous T-lymphocytes, suggesting that IFN modulates angiogenic lymphokine production by T-cells responding to antigen (Sidky & Borden 1987).

All this suggests that chemotherapy switches off excessive production by Kaposi's tissue of angiogenic factors, lymphatic proliferation factors and pyrogen production by interfering with RNA transcription soon after treatment starts. Once growth factor production returns to normal, healing follows by maturation of the Kaposi's lesions into fibrous tissue over a period of weeks, at about the same rate as normal granulation tissue is converted into scar tissue.

Useful products of Kaposi's disease tissue

The molecules synthesised by a tumour have functions that modify the host environment to the tumour's advantage. Is Kaposi's tissue producing substances that could be chemically useful, in particular angiogenic factors? Implantation of KD tissue into rabbit cornea induces proliferation of capillaries, just as AIDS-KD cells do when injected into mouse subcutis. The raised temperature of KD is not confined to the lesions but includes surrounding tissues. The increased blood flow to a limb with KD seems to involve both capillary proliferation in the lesions and an increased blood flow through major supplying vessels, probably with anastomotic channels. Could a capillary angiogenesis factor be harnessed to stimulate growth of healthy granulation tissue in the base of indolent ulcers, or following the separation of burn slough? Could a factor acting on large vessels be used to dilate potential anastomotic channels in the early stages of peripheral vascular disease? If useful molecules are being produced by KD cells, then the relevant genes should be isolated and cloned for beneficial use in man.

CONCLUSION

This review of Kaposi's disease is selective. It has concentrated first on the unique but somewhat neglected clinical features of the disease, which must give clues to its pathobiology. Secondly, we discussed aspects of the cell biology of interactions of HIV with endothelium that may lead to the extraordinary vascular proliferation that comprises Kaposi's disease. Much remains uncertain, including, of course, the aetiology of the non-HIV related endemic Kaposi's disease (Lulat 1989). Nonetheless, the epidemic of HIV has provided the stimulus and opportunity to study the aetiology of this most peculiar vascular hyperplasia. The recent rapid developments in technology for investigating angiogenesis factors and the genes controlling them appear — at the moment — to be the most fruitful way forward.

REFERENCES

Ackerman A B, Gottlieb G J 1988 Atlas of the gross and microscopic features. In: Gottlieb G J, Ackerman A B (eds) Kaposi's sarcoma: a text and atlas. Lea & Febiger, Philadelphia p 26–71

Balkwill F R 1989 Interferons. Lancet i: 1060–1063

Bayley A C 1981 Patterns of disease development in Kaposi's sarcoma. Proceedings of the Association of Surgeons of East Africa 4: 240–244

Bayley A C 1984 Aggressive Kaposi's sarcoma in Zambia. Lancet i: 1318–1320

Bayley A C 1987 Kaposi's sarcoma in Africa. Postgraduate Doctor 9: 147–152

Bayley A C 1988 Atypical Kaposi's sarcoma. In: Giraldo G, Beth-Giraldo E, Clumeck N, Gharbi Md-R, Kyalwazi S K, de The G (eds) AIDS and associated cancers in Africa. Karger, Basel p 152–164

Bayley A C, Chiengsong-Popov R, Dalgleish A G, Downing R G, Tedder R S, Weiss R A 1985 HTLV-III serology distinguishes atypical and endemic Kaposi's sarcoma in Africa. Lancet i: 359–361

Beckstead J H, Wood G S, Fletcher V 1986 Evidence for the origin of Kaposi's sarcoma from lymphatic endothelium. American Journal of Pathology 119: 294–300

Brooks J J 1986 Kaposi's sarcoma: a reversible hyperplasia. Lancet ii: 1309–1311

Cockerell C J, Whitlow M A, Webster G F, Friedman-Klein A E 1987 Epithelioid angiomatosis: a distinct vascular disorder in patients with AIDS or AIDS-related complex. Lancet ii: 654–656

Cook J 1962 The treatment of Kaposi's sarcoma with nitrogen mustard. Acta Unio Internationalis Contra Cancrum 18: 494–501

Costa J, Rabson A S 1983 Generalised Kaposi's sarcoma is not a neoplasm. Lancet ii: 58

Delli Bovi P, Donti E, Knowles I D M et al 1986 Presence of chromosomal abnormalities and lack of AIDS retrovirus DNA sequences in AIDS-associated Kaposi's sarcoma. Cancer Research 46: 6333–6338

Dictor M, Andersson C 1988 Lymphaticovenous differentiation in Kaposi's sarcoma. Cellular phenotypes by stage. American Journal of Pathology 130: 411–417

Fouret P J, Touboul J L, Mayaud C M, Akoun G M, Roland J 1987 Pulmonary Kaposi's sarcoma in patients with acquired immune deficiency syndrome: a clinicopathological study. Thorax 42: 262–268

Giddens W E, Tsai C C, Morton W R, Ochs H D, Knitter G H, Blakely G A 1985 Retroperitoneal fibromatosis and acquired immunodeficiency syndrome in macaques. American Journal of Pathology 119: 253–263

Ikuta K, Yunoki M, Imai H, Miyake S, Hirai K, Kato S 1989 Superinfection with infectious HIV-1 of defective HIV-1 producing cell clones. Abstract Th. C P 56, 5th International Conference on AIDS, Montreal, p 626

Jaffe E A 1987 Biology of endothelial cell. Human Pathology 18: 234–239

Jones R R, Spaull J, Spry C, Jones E W 1986 Histogenesis of Kaposi's sarcoma in patients with and without acquired immune deficiency syndrome (AIDS). Journal of Clinical Pathology 39: 742–749

Kaposi M 1872 Idiopathic multiple pigmented sarcoma of the skin. Archiv für Dermatopathologie und Syphilis 4: 265–273

Laine L, Politoske E J, Parkash G 1987 Protein-losing enteropathy in AIDS due to intestinal Kaposi's sarcoma. Archives of Internal Medicine 147: 174–175

Levy J A, Ziegler J L 1983 Acquired immunodeficiency sydrome is an opportunistic infection and Kaposi's sarcoma results from secondary immune stimulation. Lancet ii: 78–81

Lo S-C, Liotta L A 1985 Vascular tumours produced by NIH/3T3 cells transfected with human AIDS Kaposi's sarcoma DNA. American Journal of Pathology 111: 7–13

Lothe F 1960 Multiple idiopathic haemorrhagic sarcoma of Kaposi in Uganda. Acta Unio Internationalis Contra Cancrum 16: 1447–1451

Lulat A G-M 1989 African Kaposi's sarcoma. Transactions of the Royal Society of Tropical Medicine and Hygiene 83: 1–4

Lyerly H K, Matthews T J, Bolognesi D P, Weinbold K J 1987 Human T-cell lymphotrophic virus III glycoprotein (gp120) bound to CD4 determinants on normal lymphocytes and expressed by infected cells serves as target for immune attack. Proceedings of the National Academy of Sciences 84: 4601–4607

Mayer-de-Silva A, Stadler R, Imcke E, Bratzke B, Orfanos C E 1987 Disseminated Kaposi's sarcoma in AIDS: histogenesis-related populations and influence of long-term treatment with rIFN-α. Journal of Investigative Dermatology 89: 618–624

McNutt N S, Fletcher V, Conant M A 1983 Early lesions of Kaposi's sarcoma in homosexual men; an ultrastructural comparison with other vascular proliferations in skin. American Journal of Pathology 111: 62–77

Nakamura S, Salahuddin S Z, Biberfeld P et al 1988 Kaposi's sarcoma cells: longterm culture with growth factor from retrovirus infected CD4+ T-cells. Science 242: 426–429

Ognibene F P, Steis R G, Macher A M et al 1985 Kaposi's sarcoma causing pulmonary infiltrates and respiratory failure in the acquired immunodeficiency syndrome. Annals of Internal Medicine 102: 471–475

Olweny C L M 1981 Kaposi's sarcoma. Antibiotics and Chemotherapy 29: 88–95

Olweny C L M, Kaddumukasa A, Atine I, Owor R, Magrath I, Ziegler J L 1976 Childhood Kaposi's sarcoma: clinical features and therapy. British Journal of Cancer 33: 555–560

Plettenberg A, Stoehr A, Begemann F, Meigel W 1989 The value of gastrointestinal endoscopy for strategy and control of therapy in epidemics KS. Abstract M.B.P. 234, 5th International AIDS conference, Montreal, p 260

Purdy L J, Colby T V, Yousem S A Battifora H 1986 Pulmonary Kaposi's sarcoma. Premortem histologic diagnosis. American Journal of Surgical Pathology 10: 301–311

Rappersberger K, Gartner S, Schenk P et al 1988 Langerhans' cells are an actual site of HIV-1 replication. Intervirology 29: 185–194

Real F X 1987 Interferon in AIDS-related Kaposi's sarcoma. Clinical Immunology Newsletter 8: 70–72

Rutgers J L, Wieczorek R, Bonetti F, Kaplan K L, Friedman-Kien A E, Knowles D M 1986 The expression of endothelial cell surface antigens by AIDS-associated Kaposi's sarcoma. American Journal of Pathology 122: 493–499

Saikevych I A, Mayer M, White R L, Ho R C S 1988 Cytogenetic study of Kaposi's sarcoma associated with AIDS. Archives of Pathology and Laboratory Medicine 112: 825–828

Salahuddin S Z, Nakamura S, Biberfeld P et al 1988 Angiogenic properties of Kaposi's sarcoma-derived cells after longterm culture in vitro. Science 242: 430–433

Serwadda D, Carswell J W, Ayuko W O, Wamukota W, Madda P, Downing R 1986 Further experience with Kaposi's sarcoma in Uganda. British Journal of Cancer 53: 497–500

Sidky Y A, Borden E C 1987 Inhibition of angiogenesis by interferons: effects on tumour- and lymphocyte-induced vascular responses. Cancer Research 47: 5155–5161

Slavin G, Cameron H M, Forbes C, Mitchell M R 1970 Kaposi's sarcoma in East African children: a report of 51 cases. Journal of Pathology 100: 187–199

Symposium 1962 Symposium on Kaposi's sarcoma (multiple authors). Acta Unio Internationalis Contra Cancrum 18: 330–501

Taylor J L, Templeton A C, Vogel C L, Zielger J L, Kyalwazi S K 1971 Kaposi's sarcoma in Uganda: a clinicopathological study. International Journal of Cancer 8: 122–135

Templeton A C 1972 Studies in Kaposi's sarcoma: postmortem findings and disease pattern in women. Cancer 30: 854–867

Vogel J, Hinrichs S A, Reynolds R K, Luciw P A, Jay G 1988 The HIV *tat* gene induces dermal lesions resembling Kaposi's sarcoma in transgenic mice. Nature 335: 606–611

Yamamoto J K, Barre-Sinousi F, Bolton V, Pedersen N C, Gardner M B 1986 Human alpha and beta interferon but not gamma suppress the in vitro replication of LAV, HTLV-III and ARV-2 Journal of Interferon Research 6: 143–152

Ziegler J L 1988 Etiology: Angiogenesis. In: Ziegler J L, Dorfman R F (eds) Kaposi's sarcoma: pathophysiology and clinical management. Dekker, New York p 151–168

8. Immunohistochemistry of soft tissue tumours

M. Mukai   C. Torikata   H. Iri

It is well known that the histological features of soft tissue tumours show extreme variation, frequently causing difficulty in diagnosis. The biological behaviour of such tumours is also remarkably variable. The prognosis for any given patient is therefore greatly influenced by the framing of an accurate therapeutic policy based on a correct diagnosis; the degree of surgical radicality naturally varies with the type of differential diagnosis arrived at. In the field of soft tissue tumours in which diagnosis is difficult, there has conventionally been a fair proportion of cases in which a final diagnosis is entrusted to very particular specialists. Accordingly, in the absence of objective diagnostic evidence, i.e. persuasive findings facilitating an unequivocal diagnosis, the final decision has been dependent upon the empirical opinions of such specialists.

Since immunocytochemical procedures started to be used in the field of tumour pathology, they have been actively applied in the study of soft tissue tumours as techniques which remove much of the difficulty involved in histological diagnosis and a number of reports are available to show that these procedures have successfully yielded objective findings which allow a universal agreement to be reached in making a diagnosis in many cases. Such is the current state of affairs in the field of soft tissue tumours. Paradoxically, the very fact that immunocytochemical studies in the field of soft tissue tumours are currently one of the most active of all such studies among the various fields of human pathology serves to indicate how difficult diagnosis in this field has been. It is no exaggeration to say that the immunocytochemistry of soft tissue tumours has undergone 'explosive' development, and that its study is now very much in vogue (Roholl et al 1985, Wick et al 1988).

There are a relatively large number of soft tissue tumours in which the histogenesis or pattern of differentiation is unknown or is not yet established because of the existence of various conflicting theories. The use of immunocytochemical procedures has been actively introduced for these tumours, resulting in a considerable number of findings as to their origin and cellular differentiation over the last several years. Accordingly, it can be said from the data obtained using these immunocytochemical procedures that a newly established consensus has already been reached on the histological origin and cellular differentiation of some tumours (e.g. clear cell sarcoma).

The present chapter attempts to describe the progress made in soft tissue tumour immunohistochemistry, placing particular emphasis on the following:

1. Care has been taken to concentrate on those proteins for which a wide consensus has been reached and on those which are thought to show future promise. The reader is no doubt aware of the vast number of proteins which have been described in past reports, many of which are probably rather meaningless or which merely cause confusion.

2. Some proteins have been initially described according to tumour types, while those whose presence extends over several types of cells and tumours have been mentioned in a separate section.

3. Cytoskeletal proteins (microfilaments, intermediate filaments and microtubules) have been described in each section where relevant, and are also summarised in a separate section.

4. Findings regarding tumours of uncertain histogenesis have been described in another section.

Muscular tumours

The use of immunohistochemical staining in the diagnosis of muscular tumours has become widely adopted, and there have been many reports in this field. Among several known markers, myoglobin is a marker, specific for striated muscle (Brooks 1982). Although many markers have been reported to be effective for the diagnosis of striated muscle tumours, myoglobin is the only protein which has strict specificity for striated (skeletal or cardiac) muscle alone, having been examined in many patients and on which a wide consensus has now been reached. Myoglobin, a heme protein involved in the transport and storage of oxygen is an excellent marker of striated muscle differentiation (Mukai et al 1979). In fact, it is also very effective for the diagnosis of tumours which have an element indicating differentiation into striated muscle (Fig. 8.1) (Brooks 1982, Corson & Pinkus 1981, Daimaru et al 1984, Mukai et al 1979, Tsokos et al 1983).

Leiotonin is known to be specific to smooth muscle, but no detailed immunocytochemical examination of this protein has been carried out. Results of future studies are expected to reveal its utility and other aspects of its nature.

Some proteins which are present in large amounts particularly in muscle, are known to be potential markers of muscular differentiation, even though they are inferior to myoglobin in terms of specificity. For example, myosin (Bures et al 1981, Johnson et al 1965, Tsokos et al 1983) and tropomyosin are protein components of cytoskeletal microfilaments, and are also present in tissues other than muscle. However, it is natural that much larger amounts of these proteins are contained in muscles and are therefore effective as markers of muscular tissue. Creatine phosphokinase-MM (CPK-MM), an enzyme which reversibly catalyses the transfer of high-energy phosphates between adenosine triphosphate and creatine, is present in high concentration in

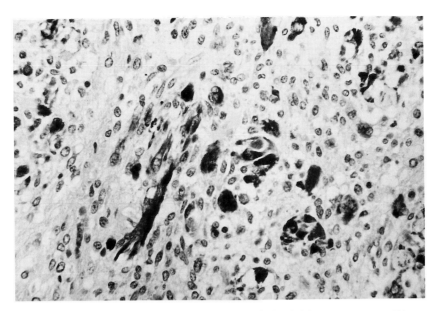

Fig. 8.1   Immunohistochemical localisation of myoglobin in rhabdomyosarcoma. × 180.

skeletal muscle, which suggested the possible use of this enzyme as a marker of such differentiation (Bures et al 1981, Tsokos et al 1983, Wold et al 1981). Desmin has become known as an intermediate filament specific to muscle, being located in both striated and smooth muscle (Denk et al 1983, Gabbiani et al 1981, Miettinen et al 1982b). Z-protein, i.e. a protein present in the Z-band of striated muscle and in dense patches of smooth muscle is, like desmin, a useful marker common to striated and smooth muscle (Mukai et al 1984a). The above-mentioned proteins are inferior to myoglobin in terms of specificity, but can adequately be used in diagnosis if they are always applied with a specific feature in mind. Actually, these proteins have been shown to be localised in tumours of the muscular system with a high incidence, suggesting their diagnostic efficacy (Eusebi et al 1986a, Tsokos 1986). The results of a comparison of the frequency of occurrence of these proteins (including myoglobin) with regard to rhabdomyosarcoma are shown in Table 8.1. It seems worthy of special mention that CPK-MM-positive cells have been found in all cases. All these proteins have been observed at high frequency in large cells enriched with cytoplasm, i.e. highly differentiated

Table 8.1   Immunocytochemistry of rhabdomyosarcoma

Type	Cases	Myoglobin	Myosin	Tropomyosin	CPK-MM	Desmin	Z-protein
Pleomorphic	10	10	10	10	10	10	10
Alveolar	4	4	4	4	4	4	4
Sarcoma botryoides	2	2	2	2	2	1	1
Embryonal	10	6	3	6	10	6	8
Total	26	22	19	22	26	21	23

tumour cells (Mukai et al 1984a), while CPK-MM has also been found even in relatively small-sized undifferentiated cells. This protein is thus very useful for differentiation from other types of small round cell sarcoma (e.g. neuroblastoma, malignant lymphoma, etc.) (De Jong et al 1985).

Reliable identification of smooth muscle tumours is generally more problematic, particularly since 30% or more of leiomyosarcomas fail to express desmin (Evans et al 1983, Schürch et al 1987, Fletcher —unpublished data). Since many of the markers described above do not distinguish between smooth and skeletal muscle, much work is in progress to provide such discriminant antibodies (Eusebi et al 1986b, Osborn et al 1986b, Om & Ghose 1987).

Vascular tumours

Factor-VIII-related antigen is the only protein known to be localised specifically in the vascular endothelium and on which a wide consensus has been reached with regard to its usefulness as a marker in tumour diagnosis. The antigen corresponds to one of the three subunits of factor VIII, a blood coagulation factor, and forms the high-molecular-weight component together with the von Willebrand factor. A previous study using cultured vascular endothelial cells has demonstrated the synthesis of factor VIII-related antigen by these cells (Jaffe et al 1973). Specific localisation of the protein in the vascular endothelium has also been demonstrated immunocytochemically (Burgdorf et al 1981, Hoyer et al 1973, Mukai et al 1980), suggesting its possible application as a marker of vascular endothelial cells. Its localisation at high frequency has also been observed in tumours of the vascular system (Fig. 8.2) (Burgdorf et al 1981, Fortwengler et al 1981, Najdi et al 1981, Sehested & Hou-Jensen 1981), thus showing its diagnostic efficacy. However, the protein shows a marked tendency to be localised only in highly differentiated cells and those involved in the formation of vascular channels (Guarda et al 1982, Ordonez & Batsakis 1984). There are also reports showing that the protein is negative in certain types of benign vascular lesions and angiosarcoma (Burgdorf et al 1981, Holden et al 1987). This should serve as a reminder that there is a degree of limitation to this protein's application to tumour diagnosis.

Although blood group antigens have drawn attention as markers of vascular endothelium (Szulman 1962, Feigl et al 1976), their use has recently decreased, since it has been shown that they do not specifically stain the vascular endothelium, and that they are stained only by the antibody to the antigen corresponding to the patient's blood type. Actin (Mukai et al 1981) and vimentin (Franke et al 1978), among other proteins, show positivity in vascular endothelium. Neither of these proteins is specific to the vascular endothelium, although they do show deep staining with this tissue. Despite the fact that they cannot be used as vascular endothelial markers, they are useful to some degree for determining changes in the vascular endothelium.

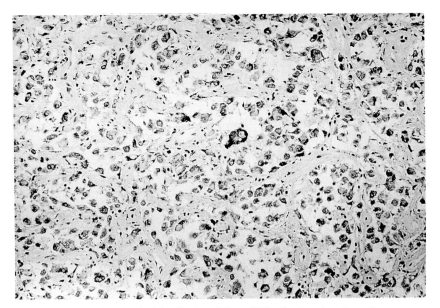

Fig. 8.2 Immunohistochemical localisation of factor VIII-related antigen in angiosarcoma. × 90.

It is widely known that alkaline phosphatase activity is strongly present in vascular endothelium. The activity of this enzyme is observed at a high frequency in tumours of the vascular system. Alkaline phosphatase has several isozymes. If it were shown that the alkaline phosphatase observed in the vascular endothelium is in the form of a specific isozyme, at least different from that present in other soft tissue tumours, then the enzyme could be considered applicable as a relatively effective marker through immunocytochemical staining with a specific antibody for that isozyme. It is strange that no immunohistochemical studies have been undertaken by utilising this feature of the enzyme, despite the fact that the presence of strong alkaline phosphatase activity in the vascular endothelium is widely acknowledged. In preliminary studies, we have observed that the vascular endothelium is satisfactorily stained with an antibody for the intestinal type of isozyme, where as it is not stained with antibodies for the liver, bone or placental types of isozyme (unpublished data). More detailed investigations in the future will probably reveal the efficacy of alkaline phosphatase with regard to its application to tumours of the vascular system which show a negative reaction for factor-VIII-related antigen.

Another alternative, in which the lectin *Ulex europaeus* agglutinin I is applied to tumours negative for factor-VIII-related antigen, has been reported (Miettinen et al 1983), and several other authors have shown this lectin to be more sensitive than factor-VIII-related antigen (Ordonez & Batsakis, 1984, Little et al 1986). However there are significant problems with its specificity (Leader et al 1986). Other markers of possible future use include PAL-E (Holden et al 1986), thrombomodulin and BMA 120 (Alles & Bosslet 1988).

Neurogenic tumours

Since the discovery of S-100 protein as a nervous tissue antigen, a large number of other nervous tissue antigens have been found. Among these antigens, S-100 protein, neuron-specific enolase, neurofilament triplet proteins and myelin-specific antigens have been applied to the immunocytochemical study of soft tissue tumours with various degrees of success.

S-100 protein is a calcium-binding protein, the precise biological role of which remains unknown. One of the sites at which it is localised is in Schwann cells. Providing an effective marker for the diagnosis of Schwannoma, neurofibroma and malignant Schwannoma (Fig. 8.3). There have been many investigations of these types of tumour using S-100 protein (Daimaru et al 1984, Matsunou et al 1985, Mukai 1983, Nakajima et al 1982, Stefansson et al 1982a, Weiss et al 1983), which probably suggests that a wide consensus has been reached with regard to its efficacy (S-100 protein will be discussed later).

Enolase is one of the glycolytic enzymes, possessing α, β and γ subunits. Gamma-enolase (neuron-specific enolase), which is distributed in nerve cells and paraneurons (Kato et al 1982), is a very effective marker in the autonomic and primitive neuroectodermal groups of tumours (including peripheral neuroepithelioma) (Hashimoto et al 1983, Linnoila et al 1986, Osborn et al 1986, Tsokos et al 1984, Vinores et al 1984) (enolase will be described again later).

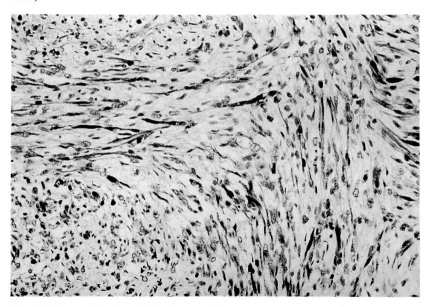

Fig. 8.3 Immunohistochemical localisation of S-100 protein in malignant Schwannoma. × 90.

Neurofilament triplet proteins, which are one of the types of intermediate filament proteins, consist of three kinds with proteins of molecular weights of 200 kD, 150 kD and 68 kD and are distributed in nerve cells and some paraneurons. They are used as an effective marker of the neuroblastoma group and paraganglioma (Lehto et al 1983, Mukai et al 1986b, Osborn et al 1986a, Trojanowski et al 1982, Trojanowski et al 1983) (neurofilament triplet proteins will be discussed again later).

Among the many known myelin-specific antigens, those which have so far proved to be potentially applicable to soft tissue tumours are myelin basic protein, P2 protein and PO protein. Myelin basic protein is a component of both central and peripheral myelin, whereas P2 protein and PO protein are only present in peripheral myelin. All three kinds of proteins are effective markers of cells which phagocytose myelin proteins or produce myelin, and are applicable to neurofibroma, Schwannoma, granular cell tumour, etc. (Mukai 1983, Penneys et al 1983, Penneys et al 1984) (see section of granular cell tumours). However, other authors have since doubted the value of these proteins (Clark et al 1985, Swanson et al 1987).

Of separate interest, it has recently been appreciated that perineurial cells express epithelial membrane antigen (EMA), allowing assessment of the contribution of these cells to neural tumours (Theaker et al 1988, Ariza et al 1988, Theaker & Fletcher 1989).

Fibrohistiocytic tumours

Alpha-1-antitrypsin, α-1-antichymotrypsin and lysozyme have been shown to be histiocytic markers, and it was believed at one time that they were diagnostically useful for malignant fibrous histiocytoma (MFH), etc. (Chowdhury et al 1980, Kindblom et al 1982, Meister & Narthrath 1981). At present, however, such a concept no longer receives wide support, since it has been revealed that these proteins are also observed in many types of soft tissue tumour other than those assigned to be fibrohistiocytic tumour group (Leader et al 1987, Soini & Miettinen 1988, 1989). They have been proved to be localised in synovial sarcoma, epithelioid sarcoma (Fig. 8.4), leiomyosarcoma, etc. (Brooks 1986, Mukai et al 1985). There are various theories as to why these proteins are also found in these other types of tumours: for example, since synovial lining cells essentially possess a histiocytic character (these proteins can, in fact, be observed in synovial lining cells), it seems natural that they should also be observed in synovial sarcoma (Mukai et al 1985); the presence of these proteins in various tumours seems to be the result of the partial appearance of an MFH-like pattern due to tumour dedifferentiation (Brooks 1986). In any case, as these proteins are known to appear in relatively many types of soft tissue tumours and indeed are present in types which are considered to be of issue in the differentiation from MFH (they are well known to appear even in many types of carcinoma), they can never become an effective marker in the diagnosis of fibrohistiocytic tumours. To date, there

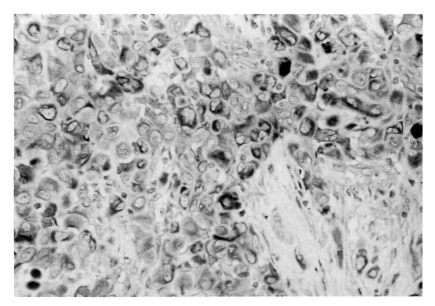

Fig. 8.4 Immunohistochemical localisation of α-1-antichymotrypsin in epithelioid sarcoma. × 90.

is no marker which can be used as an effective tool for the diagnosis of tumours which are classified as being of the fibrohistiocytic type, largely because such neoplasms are not of true monocyte/macrophage lineage (Wood et al 1986, Fletcher 1987, and see Ch. 6).

S-100 protein and enolase

1. S-100 protein

S-100 protein, a dimer consisting of α- and β-chains, has been shown to exist in three forms, i.e. S-100 a_o (α, α), S-100 a (α, β) and S-100 b (β, β). It has also become clear that S-100 protein is also present in tissues other than nervous tissue (Nakajima et al 1982, Stefansson et al 1982a, 1982b), and in terms of soft tissue tumours it should be borne in mind that S-100 protein has been observed in chondrocytes, fat cells and melanocytes, among others. S-100 protein-positive findings are also obtained in chondrosarcoma (Weiss et al 1983, Fletcher et al 1986) (extraskeletal myxoid and extraskeletal mesenchymal types), liposarcoma (Fig. 8.5) (Weiss et al 1983, Hashimoto et al 1984), and clear cell sarcoma of tendons and aponeuroses (Chung & Enzinger 1983, Kindblom et al 1983, Mukai et al 1984b) (the details of which will be described later), suggesting that S-100 protein can be used as an effective marker for the definitive diagnosis of these tumours. Since S-100 protein is observed in various tumours, as described above, it cannot be distinctly recognised as a specific protein. However, it provides a satisfactorily

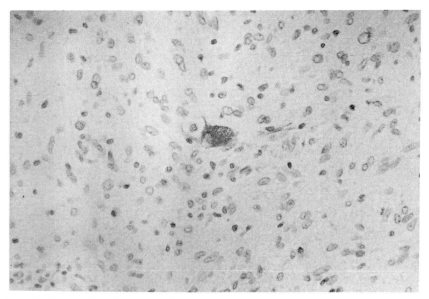

Fig. 8.5   Immunohistochemical localisation of S-100 protein in a lipoblast of liposarcoma.
× 180.

useful diagnostic tool, since malignant Schwannoma, chondrosarcoma, liposarcoma and clear cell sarcoma rarely show any overlapping features in differential diagnosis. Studies using respective specific antibodies for the α- and β-chains have revealed that Schwann cells possess the β-chain alone, whereas chondrocytes and pigment cells possess both the α- and β-chains (Takahashi et al 1984). The application of such a feature should facilitate a more definite differential diagnosis. In fact, the use of subunit-specific antibodies has recently been shown to increase sensitivity in malignant schwannomas (Hayashi et al 1987), a very useful finding since many such undoubted tumours were previously S-100 negative (Matsunou et al 1985, Wick et al 1987). If one problem has to be listed with regard to differential diagnosis, however, the differentiation of extraskeletal myxoid chondrosarcoma from a skin appendage tumour often becomes an issue. It should be kept in mind that S-100 protein is ineffective as a means of differentiation because of the fact that the myoepithelial cells of the sweat glands, for example, also express S-100 protein (Nakajima et al 1982).

2. Enolase

Since the α-subunit of the three (α, β, γ) subunits is distributed throughout almost every organ (Kato et al 1983a), it cannot be used as a specific marker. However, the β-subunit, existing in striated muscle (skeletal muscle and cardiac muscle) (Kato et al 1983a), was expected to become useful as a marker of striated muscle (Kato et al 1983b), and subsequent studies have borne out this assumption and have shown antibodies to β-enolase to be more sensitive than myoglobin in the diagnosis of rhabdomyosarcomas (Ishiguro et al 1987, Royds et al 1985). Although the application of γ-enolase (neuron-specific enolase) to well-differentiated tumours is not so problematic, considerable care should be exercised when it is employed in the study of poorly-differentiated tumours. Gamma-enolase is an antigen expressed at a certain stage of differentiation, so that its chromatic characteristics are markedly reduced in cases of poorly differentiated tumour. Since γ-enolase is one of several isoenzymes, its appearance occasionally depends on 'disdifferentiation'. This seems to be why γ-enolase occasionally appears in tumours other than those of the nervous system (Haimoto et al 1983, Osborn et al 1986a, Schmechel 1985, Tsokos et al 1984, Vinores et al 1984). Unless this aspect is kept in mind, any differential diagnosis will tend to be misleading.

Cytoskeleton

1. Microfilaments

Actin was once believed to have no merit as a specific marker because of the fact that it is seen to be immunocytochemically localised in many kinds of cells (Mukai et al 1981). However, recent advances in immunochemical studies have been breaking down this misconception. It has become known that six kinds of actin exist, each with a slightly different amino acid sequence (Vandekerckhove & Weber 1979): two kinds of striated muscle actin (skeletal muscle and cardiac muscle types), two kinds of smooth muscle actin (visceral smooth muscle and vascular smooth muscular types) and two kinds of non-muscle actin (β and γ) have been demonstrated. It is thus becoming increasingly possible to confirm the cellular differentiation of tumours by preparing the monoclonal antibody for each of these actins and by detecting each of them in tissues specifically (Skalli et al 1986, Schürch et al 1987, Miettinen 1988, Schmidt et al 1988, Skalli et al 1988).

Intermediate filaments

It has become widely known that fibrous components, called intermediate filaments, each of which is 10 nm in diameter, are present in the cell cytoplasm. Although the physiological function of the filaments remains uncertain, they have become increasingly noted in the field of tumour pathology. There are five types of intermediate filaments, each of which has its own particular cell and tissue specificity (Franke et al 1978, Schmid et al 1979), and their trial application for specific tumour diagnosis has been noticeably in vogue in recent years (Gown & Vogel 1984, Miettinen et al 1982a, Miettinen et al 1982b, Osborn & Weber 1983, Altmannsberger et al 1986). As a result, it has become clear that they do not show such strict cell or tissue specificity as was originally considered at the outset (Gould 1985). Even so, these filaments are still effective from the viewpoint of pathological application.

Keratin This protein was believed to be specific to epithelial cells and the mesothelium. It has many subtypes, which show minute differences from each other according to the types and sites of epithelial cells to which they belong. In spite of its apparent specificity to epithelial cells and mesothelium, it has become known that it is also present in such tumours as synovial sarcoma (Fig. 8.6) and epithelioid sarcoma (Chase et al 1984, Corson et al 1983, Daimaru et al 1987, Miettinen et al 1982c, Mukai et al 1985), in addition to mesothelioma. There is thus a tendency for the presence of keratin to be recognised as the expression of an epithelioid character of cells, rather than being specific to epithelial cells. Although it is occasionally effective for the differentiation of epithelial tumours from non-epithelial tumours, considerable attention is therefore required. Of particular concern is the recent demonstration of cytokeratin in a significant proportion of smooth muscle tumours (Brown et al 1987, Norton et al 1987) and in some rhabdomyosarcoma (Miettinen & Rapola 1989). Only a few analyses of the keratin subtypes present in soft tissue tumours have been conducted (Daimaru et al 1987), and this remains a subject for future study.

Vimentin This protein was believed to be specific to mesenchymal cells, and is therefore widely present in soft tissue tumours regardless of type (Fig. 8.7) (Miettinen et al 1982a). It has also become clear that vimentin appears in many poorly differentiated carcinomas (Ramaekers et al 1983), necessitating

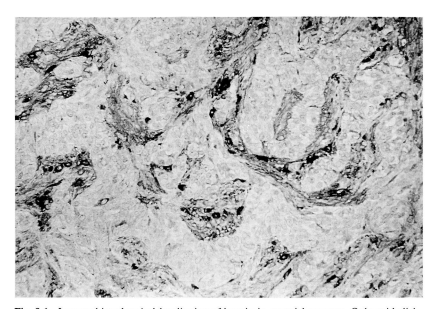

Fig. 8.6 Immunohistochemical localisation of keratin in synovial sarcoma. Only epithelial cells of the glandular structures are stained. × 90.

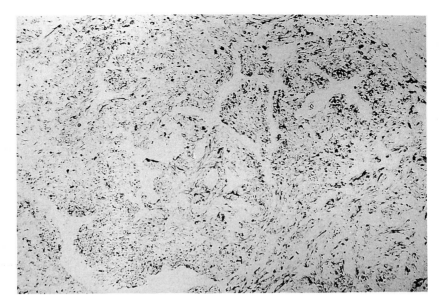

Fig. 8.7 Immunohistochemical localisation of vimentin in synovial sarcoma. Only fibroblastic cells surrounding the glandular structures are stained. × 45.

adequate care in the differentiation of carcinoma from sarcoma. A proportion of lymphomas are also vimentin-positive.

Desmin This protein is specific to muscle (both smooth and striated) acting as an effective marker in the diagnosis of tumours of the muscular system (Denk et al 1983, Gabbiani et al 1981, Miettinen et al 1982b, Dias et al 1987). However, there have been reports demonstrating the appearance of desmin in other cases (e.g. MFH) in addition to muscular tumours (Miettinen et al 1982a). There are thus some problems with regard to specificity, but even so, desmin can still be a very effective marker in most cases.

Neurofilament triplet proteins These are believed to be specific to nervous tissue, and are localised in nerve cells, ganglion cells, paraganglionic cells and neuroendocrine cells. They are also localised in tumours originating from these cells at a high incidence (Lehto et al 1983, Mukai et al 1986b, Osborn et al 1986, Trojanowski et al 1982, Trojanowski et al 1983). These proteins can thus be used as satisfactory markers of the primitive neuroectodermal and autonomic groups of soft tissue tumours (Fig. 8.8). Neurofilament contains three components with different molecular weights (200 kD, 150kD and 68 kD). Among these components, the 68-kD subunit is the most effective marker, often being localised even in cases where the 150-kD or 200-kD subunit is absent, such as in relatively poorly differentiated tumours of the nervous system (Mukai et al 1986b). Although there is a report on the presence of neurofilament triplet protein in other tumours (e.g. rhabdomyosarcoma (Sasaki et al 1985), these proteins are, in fact, adequately applicable as markers in the diagnosis of nervous system tumours.

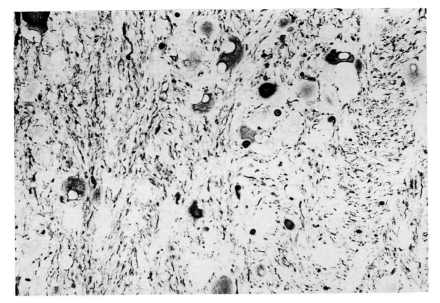

Fig. 8.8   Immunohistochemical localisation of neurofilament protein (68 kDa) in ganglioneuroblastoma. × 90.

Glial fibrillary acidic protein   This is specific to glial cells, and is less applicable to soft tissue tumours with the exception of nasal glioma (Fletcher, unpublished data).

Microtubules

Microtubules, composed of tubulin, microtuble-associated proteins, etc., play an important role in the intracellular transport of materials and in cytokinesis, being present in all cells. From a quantitative viewpoint, however, the amount of this substance present in nervous tissue is extremely large. Microtubular protein is therefore expected to play a role as a diagnostic marker of neurogenic tumours on the basis of this feature, although this has not yet been studied in detail.

IMMUNOHISTOCHEMISTRY OF TUMOURS OF UNCERTAIN HISTOGENESIS

Tumours of uncertain histogenesis have been analysed more actively than ever before since the advent of immunohistochemical techniques. Immuno-chemical procedures, combined with biochemical and electron microscopic studies, also serve to make such analysis more certain, and have already been employed. However, the descriptions below are confined only to immuno-histochemical data.

Granular cell tumour

This type of tumour has conventionally been known as granular cell myoblastoma, and its origin was believed to be striated muscle by some investigators. However, immunohistochemical analysis has revealed an absence of myoglobin (Mukai 1983), but the presence of S-100 protein, neuron-specific enolase myelin basic protein, P2 protein and P0 protein (Mukai 1983, Penneys et al 1983, Buley et al 1988). This tumour is at present widely believed to be of neuroectodermal origin, although actual proof of Schwann cell origin is lacking.

Clear cell sarcoma of tendons and aponeuroses

This form of sarcoma was at first suggested to be of synovial origin. However, since the appearance of a report on a patient with this sarcoma associated with melanin, a concept of the existence of two types of sarcoma, synovial type and melanotic type, has been suggested. Immunohistochemical analysis has revealed that this tumour is positive for S-100 protein regardless of the presence or absence of melanin (Chung & Enzinger 1983, Kindblom et al 1983, Mukai et al 1984b). Therefore, at present, a wide degree of consensus has been reached that the tumour is of neural crest origin. The term malignant melanoma of soft parts has been introduced as a more appropriate name (Chung & Enzinger 1983), and this has been supported by positive immunohistochemical staining for melanoma-specific antigens such as HMB45 (Swanson & Wick 1989).

Alveolar soft part sarcoma

While there have been reports on the immunohistochemical demonstration of desmin, β-enolase, etc, suggesting rhabdomyoblastic differentiation (Denk et al 1983, Mukai et al 1986a, Lieberman et al 1989, Ordonez et al 1989), other reports have shown that the tumour is desmin-negative (Osborn et al 1982, Auerbach & Brooks 1987). No consensus has yet been reached with regard to this tumour, but further recent support for myogenic differentiation has been provided by the detection of skeletal muscle actin in these tumours (Foschini et al 1988).

Epithelioid sarcoma

There have been various theories on the origin of this tumour, including suggestions that it is synovial, fibroblastic or histiocytic. As in synovial sarcoma, keratin (Chase et al 1984, Daimaru et al 1987, Mukai et al 1985), epithelial membrane antigen (EMA) (Wick & Manivel 1986, Fisher 1988), α-1(-antitrypsin and α-1-antichymotrypsin (Mukai et al 1985) have been demonstrated in this tumour, and it is becoming increasingly recognised as being similar in this respect to synovial sarcoma. The histogenesis of both these tumours, however, remains a mystery.

SUMMARY

It can be said that the application of immunohistochemical analysis to soft tissue tumours has already become a routine procedure for many pathologists. Immunohistochemical analysis does offer a number of advances of its own. However, considerable attention should be paid to the use of this procedure, since some proteins which have, at one time, been considered to be very specific have subsequently proved to be less specific than originally thought, and there are always patients who show negative findings for specific proteins. The time now seems to be right for this 'explosive' science of soft tissue tumour immunohistochemistry to enter the 'mature' stage. In the future, a flexible attitude to this type of tumour will be required for all pathologists and in every patient by combining the use of certain specific proteins, at the same time recognising the inherent limits of immunohistochemical techniques. In addition, it is expected that further details of various specific proteins (e.g. actin isoforms, etc.) will be clarified, resulting in an extension of the range of their application.

REFERENCES

Alles J U, Bosslet K 1988 Immunocytochemistry of angiosarcomas. A study of 19 cases with special emphasis on the applicability of endothelial cell specific markers to routinely prepared tissues. American Journal of Clinical Pathology 89: 463–471

Altmannsberger M, Dirk T, Osborn M, Weber K 1986 Immunohistochemistry of cytoskeletal filaments in the diagnosis of soft tissue tumours. Seminars in Diagnostic Pathology 3: 306–316

Ariza A, Bilbao J M, Rosai J 1988 Immunohistochemical detection of epithelial membrane antigen in normal perineurial cells and perineurioma. American Journal of Surgical Pathology 12: 678–683

Auerbach H E, Brooks J J 1987 Alveolar soft part sarcoma. A clinicopathologic and immunohistochemical study. Cancer 60: 66–73

Brooks J J 1982 Immunohistochemistry of soft tissue tumours: myoglobin as a tumour marker of rhabdomyosarcoma. Cancer 50: 1757–1763

Brooks J J 1986 The significance of double phenotypic patterns and markers in human sarcomas. American Journal of Pathology 125: 113–123

Brown D C, Theaker J M, Banks P M, Gatter K C, Mason D Y 1987 Cytokeratin expression in smooth muscle and smooth muscle tumours. Histopathology 11: 477–486

Buley I D, Gatter K C, Kelly P M A, Heryet A, Millard P R 1988 Granular cell tumours revisited. An immunohistological and ultrastructural study. Histopathology 12: 263–274

Bures J C, Barnes L, Mercer D 1981 A comparative study of smooth muscle tumours utilizing light and electron microscopy, immunocytochemical staining and enzymatic assay. Cancer 48: 2420–2426

Burgdorf W H C, Mukai K, Rosai J 1981 Immunohistochemical identification of factor VIII-related antigen in endothelial cells of cutaneous lesions of alleged vascular nature. American Journal of Clinical Pathology 75: 167–171

Chase D R, Enzinger F M, Weiss S W, Langloss J M 1984 Keratin in epithelioid sarcoma. An immunohistochemical study. American Journal of Surgical Pathology 8: 435–441

Chowdhury L N, Swerdlow M A, Jao W, Kathpalia S, Desser R K 1980 Postirradiation malignant fibrous histiocytoma of the lung: Demonstration of alpha-$_1$-antitrypsin-like material in neoplastic cells. American Journal Clinical Pathology 74: 820–826

Chung E B, Enzinger F M 1983 Malignant melanoma of soft parts. A reassessment of clear cell sarcoma. American Journal of Surgical Pathology 7: 405–413

Clark H B, Minesky J J, Agrawal D, Agrawal H C 1985 Myelin basic protein and P2 and myelin basic proteins. American Journal of Pathology 121: 96–101

Corson J M, Pinkus G S 1981 Intracellular myoglobin-A specific marker for skeletal muscle differentiation in soft tissue sarcomas. American Journal of Pathology 103: 384–389

Corson J M, Weiss L M, Banks-Schlegel S, Pinkus G S 1983 Keratin proteins in synovial sarcoma. American Journal of Surgical Pathology 7: 107–109

Daimaru Y, Hashimoto H, Enjoji M 1984 Malignant 'Triton' tumours: A clinicopathologic and immunohistochemical study of nine cases. Human Pathology 15: 768–778

Daimaru Y, Hashimoto H, Tsuneyoshi M, Enjoji M 1987 Epithelial profile of epithelioid sarcoma. An immunohistochemical analysis of eight cases. Cancer 59: 134–141

De Jong A S H, Kessel-Van Vark M V, Albus-Lutter C E, Voute P A 1985 Creatine kinase subunits M and B as markers in the diagnosis of poorly differentiated rhabdomyosarcoma in childhood. Human Pathology 16: 924–928

Denk H, Krepler R, Artlieb V et al 1983 Proteins of intermediate filaments: An immunohistochemical and biochemical approach to the classification of soft tissue tumours. American Journal of Pathology 110: 193–208

Dias P, Kumar P, Marsden H P et al 1987 Evaluation of desmin as a diagnostic and prognostic marker of childhood rhabdomyosarcomas and embryonal sarcomas. British Journal of Cancer 56: 361–365

Eusebi V, Ceccarelli C, Gorza L, Schiaffino S, Bussolati G 1986a Immunocytochemistry of rhabdomyosarcoma. The use of four different markers. American Journal of Surgical Pathology 10: 293–299

Eusebi V, Rilke F, Ceccarelli C, Fedeli F, Schiaffino S, Bussolati G 1986b Fetal heavy chain skeletal myosin. An oncofetal antigen expressed by rhabdomyosarcoma. American Journal of Surgical Pathology 10: 680–686

Evans D J, Lampert I A, Jacobs M 1983, Intermediate filaments in smooth muscle tumours. Journal of Clinical Pathology 36: 57–61

Feigl W, Denk H, Davidovits A, Holzner J H 1976 Blood group isoantigens in human benign and malignant vascular tumours. Virchows Arhiv A Pathological Anatomy and Histology 370: 323–332

Fisher C 1988 Epithelioid sarcoma: the spectrum of ultrastructural differentiation in seven immunohistochemically defined cases. Human Pathology 19: 265–275

Fletcher C D M 1987 Commentary: Malignant fibrous histiocytoma. Histopathology 11: 433–437

Fletcher C D M, Powell G, McKee P H 1986 Extraskeletal myxoid chondrosarcoma: a histochemical and immunohistochemical study. Histopathology 10: 489–499

Fortwengler H P, Jones D, Espinusa E, Tamburro C H 1981 Evidence for endothelial cell origin of vinyl chloride-induced hepatic angiosarcoma. Gastroenterology 80: 1415–1419

Foschini M P, Ceccarelli C, Eusebi V, Skalli O, Gabbiani G 1988 Alveolar soft part sarcoma: immunological evidence of rhabdomyoblastic differentiation. Histopathology 13: 101–108

Franke W W, Schmid E, Osborn M, Weber K 1978 Different intermediate-sized filaments distinguished by immunofluorescence microscopy. Proceedings of the National Academy of Sciences of the USA 75: 5034–5038

Gabbiani G, Kapanci Y, Barazzone P, Franke W W 1981 Immunochemical identification of intermediate-sized filaments in human neoplastic cells-A diagnostic aid for the surgical pathologists. American Journal of Pathology 104: 206–216

Gould V E 1985 The coexpression of distinct classes of intermediate filaments in human neoplasms. Archives of Pathology and Laboratory Medicine 109: 984–985

Gown A M, Vogel A M 1984 Monoclonal antibodies to human intermediate filament proteins: II, Distribution of filament proteins in normal human tissues. American Journal of Pathology 114: 309–321

Guarda L A, Ordonez N G, Smith J L, Hanssen G 1982 Immunoperoxidase localisation of factor VIII in angiosarcoma. Archives of Pathology and Laboratory Medicine 106: 515–516

Hashimoto H, Enjoji M, Nakajima T, Kiryu H, Daimaru Y 1983 Malignant neuroepithelioma (peripheral neuroblastoma). A clinicopathologic study of 15 cases. American Journal of Surgical Pathology 7: 309–318

Hashimoto H, Daimaru Y, Enjoji M 1984 S-100 protein distribution in liposarcoma. An immunoperoxidase study with special reference to the distinction of liposarcoma from myxoid malignant fibrous histiocytoma. Virchows Archiv A (Pathological Anatomy) 405: 1–10

Hayashi K, Takahashi K, Sonobe H, Ohtsuki Y, Taguchi K 1987 The distribution of alpha and beta subunits of S-100 protein in malignant schwannomas arising from neurofibromatosis of von Recklinghausen's disease. Virchows Archiv A (Pathological Anatomy) 411: 515–521

Holden C A, Spaull J, Das A K, McKee P H, Wilson Jones E 1987 The histogenesis of angiosarcoma of the face and scalp: an immunohistochemical and ultrastructural study. Histopathology 11: 37–51

Hoyer L W, De Los Santos R P, Hoyer J R 1973 Antihemophilic factor antigen. Localization in endothelial cells by immunofluorescent microscopy. Journal of Clinical Investigation 52: 2737–2744

Ishiguro Y, Kato K, Ito T, Horisawa M, Nagaya M 1984 Enolase isozymes as markers for differential diagnosis of neuroblastoma, rhabdomyosarcoma, and Wilm's tumour. Japanese Journal of Cancer Research (GANN) 75: 53–60

Jaffe E A, Hoyer L W, Nachman R L 1973 Synthesis of antihemophilic factor antigen by cultured human endothelial cells. Journal of Clinical Investigation 52: 2757–2764

Johnson W, Jurad J, Hiramoto R 1965 Immunohistologic studies of tumours containing myosin. American Journal of Pathology 47: 1139–1155

Kato K, Ishiguro Y, Suzuki F, Ito A, Semba R 1982 Distribution of nervous system-specific forms of enolase in peripheral tissues. Brain Research 237: 441–448

Kato K, Ishiguro Y, Ariyoshi Y 1983a Enolase isozymes and disease markers: Distribution of three enolase subunits (α, β and γ) in various human tissues. Disease Markers 1: 213–220

Kato K, Okagawa Y, Suzuki F, Shimizu A, Mokuno K, Takahashi Y 1983b Immunoassay of human muscle enolase subunit in serum: A novel marker antigen for muscle diseases. Clinica Chimica Acta 131: 75–85

Kindblom L G, Jacobson G K, Jacobson M 1982 Immunohistochemical investigations of tumours of supposed fibroblastic-histiocytic origin. Human Pathology 13: 834–840

Kindblom L G, Lodding P, Angervall L 1983 Clear cell sarcoma of tendons and aponeuroses. An immunohistochemical and electron microscopic analysis indicating neural crest origin. Virchows Archiv A Pathological Anatomy and Histopathology 401: 109–128

Leader M, Collins M, Patel J, Henry K 1986 Staining for factor VIII-related-antigen and Ulex europaeus agglutinin I (UEA-I) in 230 tumours. An assessment of their specificity for angiosarcoma and Kaposi's sarcoma. Histopathology 10: 1153–1162

Leader M, Patel J, Collins M, Henry K 1987 Anti-α antichymotrypsin staining of 194 sarcomas, 38 carcinomas and 17 malignant melanomas. Its lack of specificity as a tumour marker. American Journal of Surgical Pathology 11: 133–139

Lehto V P, Virtanen I, Miettinen M, Dahl D, Kahri A 1983 Neurofilaments in adrenal and extra-adrenal pheochromocytoma. Archives of Pathology and Laboratory Medicine 107: 492–494

Lieberman P H, Brennan M F, Kimmel M, Erlandson R A, Garin-Cjesa P, Flehinger B Y 1989 Alveolar soft part sarcoma. A clinicopathologic study of half a century. Cancer 63: 1–13

Linnoila R I, Tsokos M, Triche T J, Marangos P J, Chandra R S 1986 Evidence for neural origin and PAS-postive variants of the malignant small cell tumour of thoracopulmonary region ('Askin tumour') American Journal of Surgical Pathology 10: 124–133

Little D, Said J W, Siegal R J, Fealy M, Fishbein M C 1986 Endothelial cell markers in vascular neoplasms: an immunohistochemical study comparing factor VIII-related antigen, blood group specific antigens, 6-keto-PGF 1 alpha and Ulex europaneus I lectin. Journal of Pathology 149: 89–95

Matsunou H, Shimoda T, Kakimoto S, Yamashita H, Ishikawa E, Mukai M 1985 Histopathologic and immunohistochemical study of malignant tumours of peripheral nerve sheath (malignant Schwannoma). Cancer 56: 2269–2279

Meister P, Narthrath W 1981 Immunohistochemical characterization of histiocytic tumours. Diagnostic Histopathology 4: 79–87

Miettinen M, 1988 Antibody specific to muscle actins in the diagnosis and classification of soft tissue tumours. American Journal of Pathology 130: 205–215

Miettinen M, Rapola J 1989 Immunohistochemical spectrum of rhabdomyosarcoma and rhabdomyosarcoma-like tumours. Expression of cytokeratin and the 68-kD neurofilament protein. American Journal of Surgical Pathology 13: 120–132

Miettinen M, Lehto V P, Badley R A, Virtanen I 1982a Expression of intermediate filaments in soft tissue sarcomas. International Journal of Cancer 30: 541–546

Miettinen M, Lehto V P, Badley R A, Virtanen I 1982b Alveolar rhabdomyosarcoma: Demonstration of the muscle type of intermediate filament protein, desmin, as a diagnostic aid. American Journal of Pathology 108: 246–251

Miettinen M, Lehto V P, Virtanen I 1982c Keratin in the epithelial-cells of classical biphasic synovial sarcoma. Virchows Archiv B Cell Pathology 40: 157–161

Miettinen M, Holthofer H, Lehto V P, Miettinen A, Virtanen I 1983 Ulex europaeus I lectin as a marker for tumours derived from endothelial cells. American Journal of Clinical Pathology 79: 32–36

Mukai M, 1983 Immunohistochemical localisation of S-100 protein and peripheral nerve myelin proteins (P2 protein, P0 protein) in granular cell tumours. American Journal of Pathology 112: 139–146

Mukai K, Rosai J, Halloway B 1979 Localisation of myoglobin in normal and neoplastic human skeletal muscle cells using immunoperoxidase method. American Journal of Surgical Pathology 3: 373–376

Mukai K, Rosai J, Burgdorf W H C 1980 Localization of factor VIII-related antigen in vascular endothelial cells using an immunoperoxidase method. American Journal of Surgical Pathology 4: 237–276

Mukai K, Schollmeyer J V, Rosai J 1981 Immunohistochemical localization of actin. Application in surgical pathology. American Journal of Surgical Pathology 5: 91–97

Mukai M, Torikaka C, Iri H et al 1983 Alveolar soft part sarcoma. A review on its histogenesis and further studies based on electron microscopy, immunohistochemistry and biochemistry. American Journal of Surgical Pathology 7: 679–689

Mukai M, Iri H, Torikata C, Kageyama K, Morikawa Y, Shimizu K 1984a Immunoperoxidase demonstration of a new muscle protein (z-protein) in myogenic tumours as a diagnostic protein. American Journal of Pathology 114: 164–170

Mukai M, Torikata C, Iri H et al 1984b Histogenesis of clear cell sarcoma of tendons and aponeuroses: An electron-microscopic, biochemical, enzyme histochemical, and immunohistochemical study. American Journal of Pathology 114: 264–272

Mukai M, Torikata C, Iri H et al 1985 Cellular differentiation of epithelioid sarcoma: An electron-microscopic, enzyme-histochemical and immunohistochemical study. American Journal of Pathology 119: 44–56

Mukai M, Torikata C, Iri H et al 1986a Histogenesis of alveolar soft part sarcoma. An immunohistochemical and biochemical study. American Journal of Surgical Pathology 10: 212–218

Mukai M, Torikata C, Iri H et al 1986b Expression of neurofilament triplet proteins in human neural tumours. American Journal of Pathology 122: 28–35

Najdi M, Morales AR, Ziegles-Weissman J, Penneys N S 1981 Kaposi's sarcoma. Immunohistologic evidence for an endothelial origin. Archives of Pathology and Laboratory Medicine 105: 274–275

Nakajima T, Watanabe S, Sato Y, Kameya T, Hirota T, Shimosato Y 1982 An immunoperoxidase study of S-100 protein distribution in normal and neoplastic tissues. American Journal of Surgical Pathology 6: 715–727

Norton A J, Thomas J A, Isaacson P G 1987 Cytokeratin-specific monoclonal antibodies are reactive with tumours of smooth muscle derivation. An immunocytochemical and biochemical study using antibodies to intermediate filament proteins. Histopathology 11: 487–499

Om A, Ghose T 1987 Use of anti-skeletal muscle antibody from myasthenic patients in the diagnosis of childhood rhabdomyosarcoma. American Journal of Surgical Pathology 11: 272–276

Ordonez N G, Batsakis J G 1984 Comparison of Ulex europaeus lectin and factor VIII-related antigen in vascular lesions. Archives of Pathology and Laboratory Medicine 108: 129–132

Ordonez N G, Ro Y G, Mackay B 1989 Alveolar soft part sarcoma. An ultrastructural and immunocytochemical investigation of its histogenesis Cancer 63: 1721–1736

Osborn M, Weber K 1983 Tumour diagnosis by intermediate filament typing: A noval tool for surgical pathology. Laboratory Investigation 48: 372–394

Osborn M, Altmannsberrger M, Shjaw G, Schauer A, Weber K 1982 Various sympathetic derived human tumours differ in neurofilament expression. Virchows Archiv B cell

Pathology 40: 141–156

Osborn M, Käser T D H, Weber K, Altmannsberger M 1986a Immunohistochemical localization of neurofilaments and neuron-specific enolase in 29 cases of neuroblastoma. American Journal of Pathology 122: 433–442

Osborn M, Hill C, Altmannsberger M, Weber K 1986b Monoclonal antibodies to Titin in conjunction with antibodies to desmin separate rhabdomyosarcomas from other tumour types. Laboratory Investigation 55: 101–108

Penneys N S, Adachi K, Ziegels-Weissman J, Najdi M 1983 Granular cell tumours of the skin contain myelin basic protein. Archives of Pathology and Laboratory Medicine 107: 302–303

Penneys N S, Mogollon R, Kowalcyzyk A, Najdi M, Adachi K 1984 A survey of cutaneous neural lesions for the presence of myelin basic protein. An immunohistochemical study. Arhives of Dermatology 120: 210–213

Ramaekers F C S, Haag D, Kant A, Moesker O, Jap P H K, Vooijs G P 1983 Coexpression of keratin- and vimentin-type intermediate filaments in human metastatic carcinoma cells. Proceedings of the National Academy of Sciences of the USA 80: 2618–2622

Roholl P J M, De Jong A S H Ramaekers F C S 1985 Application of markers in the diagnosis of soft tissue tumours. Histopathology 9: 1019–1035

Royds J A, Variend S, Timperley W R, Taylor C B 1985 Comparison of beta enolase and myoglobin as histological markers of rhabdomyosarcoma. Journal of Clinical Pathology 38: 1258–1260

Sasaki A, Hirato J, Nakazato Y, Ishida Y 1985 Immunohistochemical localization of neurofilament protein in rhabdomyosarcoma. Proceedings of the Japanese Cancer Association 44: 396

Schmechel D E 1985 γ-Subunit of the glyolytic enzyme enolase nonspecific or neuron-specific? Laboratory Investigation 52: 239–242

Schmid E, Tapscott S, Bennett G S et al 1979 Different location of different types of intermediate-sized filaments in various tissues of the chick embryo. Differentiation 15: 27–40

Schmidt R A, Cone R, Haas J E, Gown A M, 1988 Diagnosis of rhabdomyosarcomas with HHF 35, a monoclonal antibody directed against muscle actins. American Journal of Pathology 131: 19–28

Schürch W, Skalli O, Seemayer T A, Gabbiani G 1987 Intermediate filament proteins and actin isoforms as markers for soft tissue tumour differentiation and origin. I Smooth muscle tumours. American Journal of Pathology 128: 91–103

Sehested M, Hou-Jensen K 1981 Factor VIII-related antigen as an endothelial cell marker in benign and malignant diseases. Virchows Archiv. A Pathological Anatomy and Histopathology 391: 217–225

Skalli O, Repraz P, Trzeciak A, Benzonana G, Gillessen D, Gabbiani G 1986 A monoclonal antibody against α- smooth muscle actin: A new probe for smooth muscle differentiation. Journal of Cell Biology 103: 2787–2796

Skalli O, Gabbiani G, Babai F, Seemayer T A, Pizzolatto G, Schürch W 1988 Intermediate filament proteins and actin isoforms as markers for soft tissue tumour differentiation and origin II. Rhabdomyosarcomas. American Journal of Pathology 130: 515–531

Soini Y, Miettinen M 1988 Widespread immunoreactivity for alpha-1-antichymotrypsin in different types of tumours. American Journal of Clinical Pathology 89: 131–136

Soini Y, Miettinen M 1989 Alpha-1-antitrypsin and lysozyme. Their limited significance in fibrohistiocytic tumours. American Journal of Clinical Pathology 91: 515–521

Stefansson K, Wollmann R, Jerkovic M 1982a S-100 protein in soft tissue tumours derived from Schwann cells and melanocytes. American Journal of Pathology 106: 261–268

Stefansson K, Wollmann R L, Moore B W 1982b S-100 protein in human chondrocytes. Nature 295: 63–64

Swanson P E, Wick M R 1989 Clear cell sarcoma. An immunohistiochemical analysis of six cases and comparison with other epithelioid neoplasms of soft tissue. Archives of Pathology and Laboratory Medicine 113: 55–60

Swanson P E, Manivel J C, Wick M R 1987 Immunoreactivity for Leu-7 in neurofibrosarcoma and other spindle cell sarcomas of soft tissue. American Journal of Pathology 126: 546–560

Szulman A E 1962 The histological distribution of blood group substances A and B in man. Journal of Experimental Medicine 111: 785–799

Takahashi K, Isobe T, Ohtsuki Y, Agaki T, Sonobe H, Okuyama T 1984

Immunohistochemical study on the distribution of alpha and beta subunits of S-100 protein in human neoplasms and normal tissues. Virchows Archiv B (Cellular Pathology) 45: 385–396

Theaker J M, Gatter K C, Puddle J 1988 Epithelial membrane antigen expression by the perineurium of peripheral nerve and in peripheral nerve tumours. Histopathology 13: 171–179

Theaker J M, Fletcher C D M 1989 Epithelial membrane antigen expression by the perineurial cell: further studies of peripheral nerve lesions. Histopathology 14: 581–592

Trojanowski J Q, Lee V, Pillsbury N, Lee S 1982 Neuronal origin of human esthesioneuroblastoma demonstrated with antineurofilament monoclonal antibodies. New England Journal of Medicine 307: 159–161

Trojanowski J Q, Lee V, Pillsbury N, Lee S 1983 Anti-neurofilament monoclonal antibodies: Reagents for the evaluation of human neoplasm. Acta Neuropathologica 59: 155–158

Tsokos M 1986 The role of immunocytochemistry in the diagnosis of rhabdomyosarcoma. Archives of Pathology and Laboratory Medicine 110: 776–778

Tsokos M, Howard R, Costa J 1983 Immunohistochemical study of alveolar and embryonal rhabdomyosarcoma. Laboratory Investigation 48: 148–155

Tsokos M, Linnoila R J, Chandra R S, Triche T J 1984 Neuron-specific enolase in the diagnosis of neuroblastoma and other small, round cell tumours in children. Human Pathology 15: 575–584

Vandekerckhove J, Weber K 1979 At least six different actins are expressed in a higher mammal: An analysis based on the amino acid sequence of the amino terminal tryptic peptide. Journal of Molecular Biology 126: 783–802

Vinores S A, Bonnin J M Rubinstein L J, Marangos J M 1984 Immunohistochemical demonstration of neuron-specific enolase in neoplasms of the CNS and other tissues. Archives of Pathology and Laboratory Medicine 108: 536–540

Weiss S W, Langloss J M, Enzinger F M 1983 Value of S-100 protein in the diagnosis of soft tissue tumours with particular reference to benign and malignant Schwann cell tumours. Laboratory Investigation 49: 299–308

Wick M R, Manivel J C 1986 Epithelioid sarcoma and isolated necrobiotic granuloma: a comparative immunocytochemical study. Journal of Cutaneous Pathology 13: 253–260

Wick M R, Swanson P E, Manivel J C 1988 Immunohistochemical analysis of soft tissue sarcomas. Comparisons with electron microscopy. Applied Pathology 6: 169–196

Wick M R, Swanson P E, Scheithauer B W, Manivel J C 1987 Malignant peripheral nerve sheath tumour. An immunohistochemical study of 62 cases. American Journal of Clinical Pathology 87: 425–433

Wold L E, Li C Y, Homburger H A 1981 Localization of the B and M polypeptide subunits of creatine kinase in normal and neoplastic human tissues by an immunoperoxidase technic. American Journal of Clinical Pathology 75: 327–332

Wood G S, Beckstead J H, Turner R R, Hendrickson M R, Kempson R L, Warnke R A 1986 Malignant fibrous histiocytoma tumour cells resemble fibroblasts. American Journal of Surgical Pathology 10: 323–335

9. Enzyme histochemistry of soft tissue tumours

O. Myhre-Jensen   K. Bendix-Hansen

In 1965 Jeffree and Price published their study on the distribution of hydrolytic enzymes in osteosarcoma, fibrosarcoma, chondrosarcoma and giant cell tumours of bone, and in 1972 and 1974 Jeffree reported on the enzyme histochemistry of fibroblastic lesions and round cell tumours of bone and soft tissue. Our own investigations were published in 1985 on a broad spectrum of bone and soft tissue tumours examined for some hydrolytic enzymes, with and without the addition of specific inhibitors. Otherwise, enzyme histochemistry — in spite of the availability of simple and reproducible methods based on the diazo technique — seems not to have been applied to any great extent in the classification of soft tissue tumours. As the methods are easily set up in any laboratory, for instance in the cytodiagnostic department performing fine-needle aspirations on soft tissue tumours, a survey of the applicability of enzyme histochemistry in the classification of soft tissue tumours seems justified.

Our studies are performed on cryostat sections of fresh, unfixed tumour specimens and/or cell smears, imprints and cytocentrifuge preparations and are stained for acid phosphatase with and without the addition of tartrate, non-specific esterase with and without the addition of fluoride, and alkaline phosphatase.

STAINING METHODS

Cryostat sections of fresh frozen, unfixed specimens, imprint smears and cytocentrifuge preparations of cell suspensions are air dried. Prior to incubation, the slides are fixed in neutral phosphate buffered formalin with sucrose (75 g/l in 4% formaldehyde solution) for 5 minutes at room temperature and rinsed briefly in tap water. After simultaneous incubation and coupling, sections are rinsed in tap water and counterstained in Mayer's haematoxylin for a few minutes and finally mounted in aqueous medium.

Acid phosphatase (AcP)

Medium : naphthol AS-BI-phosphate (Sigma N 2125) 20 mg in 2 ml N,N dimethylformamide. Coupler: pararosanilin (Sigma P 7632, CI 42500), 4% in

185

2N HCl, 0.6 ml + 0.6 ml sodium nitrite, 4% in water. After 60 seconds addition of 60 ml Michaelis buffer, – pH 5.0. Incubation time 4 hours at room temperature with constant stirring.

Acid phosphatase with tartrate (AcP + T)

As above with the addition of sodium tartrate to a final concentration of 7.5 mg/ml.

Non-specific esterase (NAE)

Medium: alpha-naphthyl acetate (Sigma N 6750) 20 mg in 2 ml acetone with the addition of 0.2M phosphate buffer, 60 ml, and 20 ml distilled water. Coupler: pararosanilin, 4% 2N HC1, 3.2 ml + 3.2 ml sodium nitrite, 4% in water, – pH 7.5. Incubation time 15 minutes at room temperature.

Non-specific esterase with fluoride (NAE + F)

As above with the addition of sodium fluoride to a final concentration of 1.5 mg/ml.

Alkaline phosphatase (AlP)

Medium: naphthol-AS-BI-phosphate, 5 mg in 0.25 ml N,N dimethylformamide. Coupler: Red Violet LB-salt (Difco 8194-13), 30 mg in 25 ml tris buffer and 25 ml distilled water, – pH 8.7. Incubation time 30 minutes at room temperature.

STAINING PATTERNS

Our experience from the study of almost 200 cases is presented in Table 9.1 and can briefly be outlined as follows:

Malignant fibrous histiocytomas

Malignant fibrous histiocytomas were strongly positive for acid phosphatase, usually inhibitable with tartrate. Two malignant fibrous histiocytomas contained areas with weak tartrate-resistant acid phosphatase, mostly due to the presence of osteoclast-like multinucleate giant cells:

the one in a 71-year-old woman located in the left quadriceps, the other in a 15-year-old girl of the upper metaphysis of the left tibia. Otherwise, enzyme reactions and general morphology were typical for malignant fibrous histiocytoma. Alkaline phosphatase activity was confined to vascular endothelium alone.

All cases were strongly positive for non-specific esterase, completely inhibitable with fluoride (Fig. 9.1). Except for a single case all were negative for alkaline phosphatase:

Table 9.1 Histochemical reaction patterns of acid phosphatase (± tartrate), non-specific esterase (± fluoride) and alkaline phosphatase in frozen sections of 184 musculoskeletal tumours according to histogenetic type

Histogenetic type	No	Enzyme histochemical reaction pattern				
		AcP	AcP + T	NAE	NAE + F	AlP
Malignant fibrous histiocytoma	22	+++	0	++/+++	0	**0
Liposarcomas	10	++/+++	0	+/++	0	**0
Fibrous tumours	17	++/+++	0	0/+++	0	0/++
Myogenous tumours	17	+/+++	0	0/++	0	0
Endothelial tumours	23	++/+++	0	++/+++	0	+++
Peripheral nerve sheath tumours	12	+/++	0	0/++	0	0
Osteoblastic tumours	31	++/+++	0/++	+/++	0/+	** +++
Chondroid tumours	21	++/+++	0	+/++	0	0
Other types	20	++/+++	*0/+++	0/+++	0	**0
Metastatic carcinomas	11	+++	0/+	++/+++	0/+	**0

*Giant cell tumours strongly positive; ** a few cases moderately positive (see text).
0 = No reaction; + = weak reaction; ++ = moderate reaction; +++ = strong reaction.

A 77-year-old man had a rapidly growing subcutaneous tumour, 5 cm in diameter, close to the medial aspect of the femur. Tumour was gelatinous and haemorrhagic and microscopically best diagnosed as a high-grade malignant fibrous histiocytoma of myxoid type. Acid phosphatase and non-specific esterase were strongly positive, acid phosphatase being partly tartrate resistant. Alkaline phosphatase, however, was moderately positive. No osteoid or bone formation was detected, neither was any chondroid matrix found, and mucosubstances contained mainly hyaluronic acid. Electron microscopy was compatible with malignant fibrous histiocytoma. Other authors have found a proportion of these tumours to be alkaline phosphatase positive (Wood et al, 1986).

Liposarcomas

Liposarcomas were moderately positive for acid phosphatase and non-specific esterase, completely inhibitable with tartrate and fluoride, respectively. All cases but one, a pleomorphic liposarcoma with a moderately strong reaction, were negative for alkaline phosphatase

A pleomorphic liposarcoma located within the left brachial muscle of a man 60 years old was histologically typical with several uni- and multivacuolated lipoblasts and bizarre tumour giant cells. Alkaline phosphatase was moderately positive within tumour cells. Otherwise, enzyme reactions were as in other liposarcomas.

Fibroblastic tumours

Fibroblastic tumours were all positive for acid phosphatase, completely inhibitable with tartrate, whereas the reaction for non-specific esterase varied from negative to strongly positive, but in all cases was inhibitable with fluoride. Alkaline phosphatase was found in most cases, showing weak to moderately strong reactions and only in some of the tumour cells. Five cases out of 17 studied were completely negative of alkaline phosphatase.

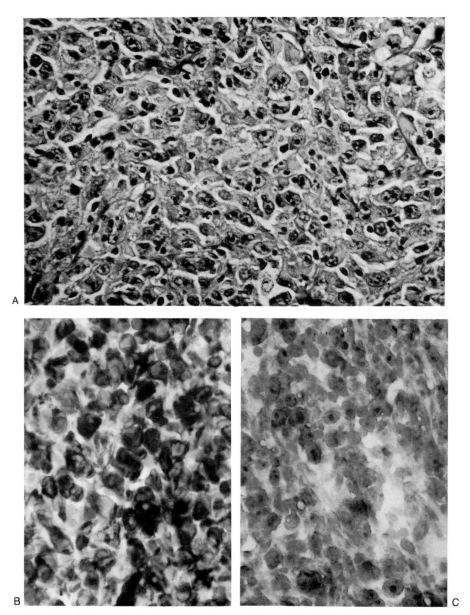

Fig. 9.1 Malignant fibrous histiocytoma pleomorphic type (**A**); with heavy staining for non-specific esterase (**B**), completely inhibitable with fluoride (**C**). Obj. × 25.

Myogenous tumours

Myogenous tumours (including both leiomyosarcomas and rhabdomyosarcomas) were all moderately to strongly positive for acid phosphatase, completely inhibitable with tartrate, and moderately or weakly positive for non-specific esterase, completely inhibitable with fluoride. All cases were negative for alkaline phosphatase.

Vascular tumours

Vascular (endothelial) tumours including haemangiomas and angiosarcomas as well as granulation tissue and a few aneurysmal bone cysts, were all strongly positive for acid phosphatase and non-specific esterase, completely inhibitable with tartrate and fluoride. All cases were strongly positive for alkaline phosphatase

Peripheral nerve sheath tumours

Peripheral nerve sheath tumours, whether benign or malignant, were weakly to moderately positive for acid phosphatase, completely inhibitable with tartrate and moderately positive or completely negative for non-specific esterase, positive cases being completely inhibitable with the addition of fluoride. All cases were negative for alkaline phosphatase.

Osteoblastic tumours

Osteoblastic tumours, including myositis ossificans, osteosarcoma and fibrous dysplasia of bone, were moderately to strongly positive for acid phosphatase and — except for a few cases — partly tartrate resistant (25 out of 31 cases). Most cases were weakly to moderately positive for non-specific esterase, only a few (2 out of 31 cases) being not completely inhibitable with fluoride. All cases were positive for alkaline phosphatase, 24 out of 26 osteosarcomas with a very strong reaction. The remaining two osteosarcomas showed weak and moderately strong reactions for alkaline phosphatase:

The one (Fig. 9.2) in a woman 32 years old was located in the left ilium. The tumour was moderately pleomorphic and contained primitive osteoid matrix. Acid phosphatase and non-specific esterase activities were pronounced and partly resistant to tartrate and fluoride as in most other osteosarcomas.

The other (Fig. 9.3), in a 67-year-old man located in the muscles of the left antebrachium, in most areas resembled a pleomorphic malignant fibrous histiocytoma. Acid phosphatase and non-specific esterase were only moderately or weakly positive, completely inhibitable with tartrate and fluoride. The tumour, however, contained areas with definite malignant osteoid formation.

Chondroid tumours

Chondroid tumours were moderately to strongly positive for acid phosphatase, completely inhibitable with tartrate and weakly to moderately positive for non-specific esterase, completely inhibitable with fluoride. All

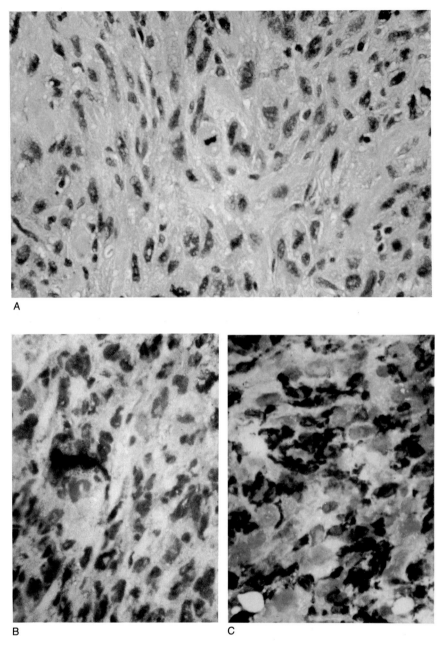

A

B   C

Fig. 9.2 Osteosarcoma containing primitive osteoid matrix (**A**). Weak reaction for alkaline phosphatase (**B**) and moderate to strong reaction for non-specific esterase (**C**). Obj. × 25.

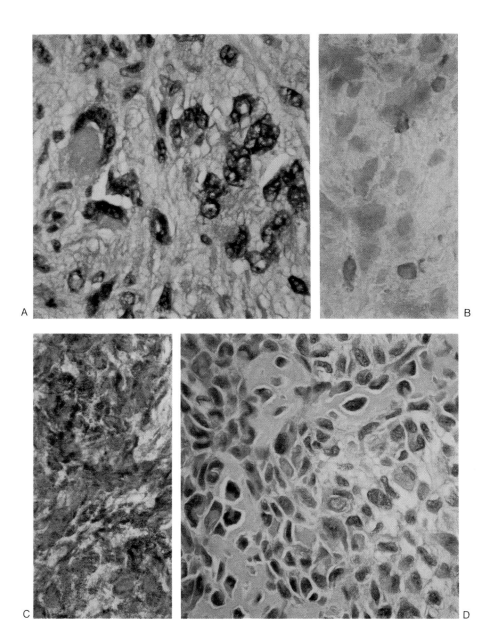

Fig. 9.3   Extraskeletal osteosarcoma, in many fields MFH-like (**A**), but non-specific esterase is confined only to macrophages (**B**). Alkaline phosphatase activity is moderate to strong (**C**), and other fields within tumour show definite osteoid production (**D**). Obj. × 25.

cases were negative for alkaline phosphatase, except when studied in cytocentrifuge preparations in which some cells, probably degenerating cartilage cells, showed a fine granular cytoplasmic staining for alkaline phosphatase (Fig. 9.4).

Other primary musculoskeletal tumours

Other primary musculoskeletal tumours individual types being represented by only a few cases, showed varying patterns of reaction, but all were positive for acid phosphatase. However, many (11 out of 20 cases) showed tartrate resistance, mainly in giant cells (due to the inclusion of 9 giant cell tumours and 3 eosinophilic granulomas of bone). All cases that were positive for non-specific esterase were completely inhibitable with fluoride.

Two cases, a synovial sarcoma and an unclassifiable sarcoma, were moderately positive for alkaline phosphatase. All other cases (18 out of 20) were totally negative. Other authors have also noted alkaline phosphatase positivity in the epithelial component of synovial sarcoma (Pisa et al 1982) and similar results have been published in epithelioid sarcoma (Mukai et al 1985), supporting the proposed relationship between these two tumours.

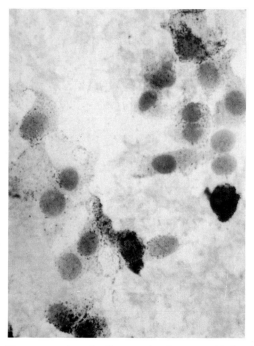

Fig. 9.4 Cytocentrifuge preparation of cell suspension from myxoid chondrosarcoma stained for alkaline phosphatase. Heavy reaction in a few cells and fine granular cytoplasmic reaction in most cells. Obj. × 40.

Carcinomas

Carcinomas, metastatic to the musculoskeletal system, were usually strongly positive for acid phosphatase and non-specific esterase, about half the number being partly resistant to tartrate (5 out of 11) and partly or completely resistant to fluoride (6 out of 11) (Fig. 9.5). One case was strongly positive for alkaline phosphatase and one further case was weakly positive (see below). All the rest (9 out of 11) were totally negative for alkaline phosphatase.

The one tumour located in the soft tissues and bone of the left ileum of a 72-year-old woman was, by subsequent autopsy, proven to be metastatic from a gall bladder carcinoma. The other, located in the soft tissue of the scapular region of a 68-year-old man, was metastatic from a carcinoma of the head of the pancreas.

COMMENTS AND CONCLUDING REMARKS

Our findings are in broad agreement with those of Jeffree, who furthermore showed that reactions for glucuronidase and leucine aminopeptidase somehow seemed to parallel acid phosphatase and non-specific esterase, but tended to be more pronounced in malignant than benign lesions. Additionally, in cases of neuroblastoma, Jeffree (1974) demonstrated moderate to weak reactions for monoamine oxidase, an enzyme of catecholamine metabolism. In other tumours, including Ewing's sarcoma, reactions for monoamine oxidase were negative or only weakly positive, except in some carcinomas.

Histochemical methods more typically used for the study of muscle biopsies, such as staining for nicotinamide adenine dinucleotide tetrazolium reductase, succinate dehydrogenase, myophosphorylase and calcium-mediated adenosine triphosphatase, preincubated at high and low pH, on cryostat sections of fresh frozen specimens from two childhood embryonal rhadomyosarcomas (Sarnat et al 1979), showed that NADH-TR and ATP-ase stainings could contribute to the identification of striated muscle differentiation in rhabdomyosarcomas.

ATP-ase reactions were not performed routinely in our study, but were indicated on rare occasions as the following case illustrates:

An unusual tumour, initially diagnosed as a malignant fibrous histiocytoma (metastatic to an axillary lymph code) based on its pleomorphism and areas with a typical storiform growth pattern, turned out to be only weakly positive for non-specific esterase and moderately positive for alkaline phosphatase. Further investigation revealed heavy staining for ATP-ase and 5'nucleotidase. Electron microscopy showed several desmosome-like junctions, and immunological markers were compatible with a sarcoma derived from dendritic cells of the B-zone of the lymph node (Pallesen & Myhre-Jensen 1987).

The case mentioned above serves to demonstrate the necessity of supplementary investigations, such as electron microscopy and immunohistochemistry, in any tumour with an 'unexpected' enzyme histochemical reaction.

Based on the reports of Jeffree (1972, 1974), and our own experiences, the following guidelines for the use of enzyme histochemistry in the classification of soft tissue tumours can be set up:

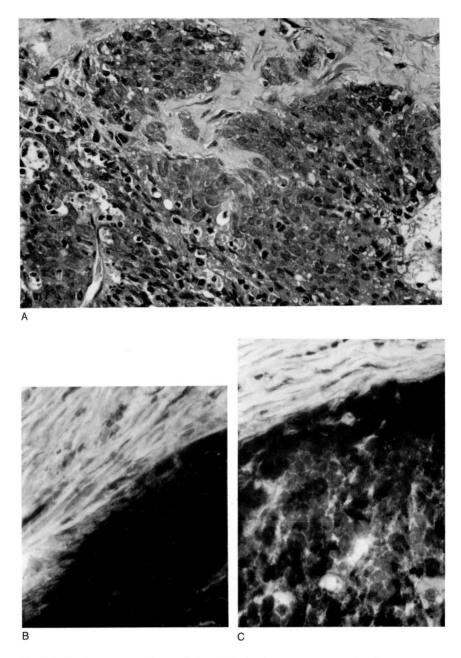

Fig. 9.5 Carcinoma metastatic to soft tissue (**A**), showing very strong reaction for non-specific esterase (**B**), resistant to fluoride (**C**). Obj. × 25.

Alkaline phosphatase

Alkaline phosphatase is the enzyme, among those studied, with the greatest discriminatory power. A strongly positive reaction in a pleomorphic tumour is highly suggestive of osteosarcoma and should prompt a search for osteoid or bone production within the tumour on which a definite diagnosis can be based. A strong reaction for alkaline phosphatase in a spindle cell or round cell tumour points to either osteoblastic or endothelial differentiation if a carcinoma has been excluded. In a pure spindle cell sarcoma a (weak) reaction favours the diagnosis of fibrosarcoma rather than leiomyosarcoma or malignant schwannoma, which are usually completely negative. Synovial sarcomas may be alkaline phosphatase positive in the epithelial component. Other genuine soft tissue tumours are most often completely negative for alkaline phosphatase. The endothelium of normal vessels within a specimen acts as a built-in positive control for this reaction.

Non-specific esterase

Completely inhibitable with fluoride should be positive (together with a strong reaction for acid phosphatase) in a tumour considered to show fibrohistiocytic differentiation. A tumour with a positive reaction for non-specific esterase, which is not complete inhibitable with fluoride, and a tumour which is negative for non-specific esterase is most probably not a malignant fibrous histiocytoma. The occurrence of reactive macrophages (Fig. 9.6), a very common phenomenon in sarcomas and sometimes in such a number that differential diagnosis from malignant fibrous histiocytoma becomes a serious problem, serves as a built-in positive control of the reaction. Reactive mononuclear phagocytes are completely inhibitable with fluoride. The absence of 'histiocytic' enzyme histochemical activity in dermatofibrosarcoma protuberans, albeit in a single case (Nakanishi & Hizawa 1984) would support recent suggestions that this tumour does not belong in the fibrohistiocytic group (Fletcher et al 1985, 1988).

Acid phosphatase

Acid phosphatase is the enzyme with the least discriminatory ability in the differentiation between histogenetic types of soft tissue tumour. Most tumours, including carcinomas, contain acid phosphatase, a feature also noted by Roholl et al (1985). Exceptions are Ewing's sarcoma, which shows no (or rather weak) acid phosphatase activity. The acid phosphatase of most tumour types are completely inhibitable with tartrate. Multinucleate giant cells as in giant cell tumours and some macrophages, especially those having phago-cytosed lipids, are tartrate resistant. Most osteoblastic lesions, as well, have partly tartrate resistant acid phosphatase. As most tumours as well as many normal cells contain acid phosphatase, all specimens, as a built-in positive

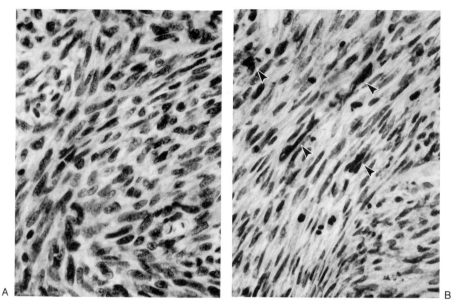

Fig. 9.6 Fibrosarcoma (**A**), being negative for non-specific esterase (**B**). Distinct, brown stained macrophages (marked with arrow-heads) serve as a built-in positive control. Obj. × 40.

control, should contain some positive cells, normal cells being completely inhibitable with tartrate.

Enzyme histochemical reactions, as mentioned above, are easy to perform and reliable whenever unfixed tumour samples are available and can be of great aid in the diagnosis and classification of soft tissue tumours. Characteristic patterns of reaction, especially those of alkaline phosphatase and non-specific esterase are of great value in the distinction between extraskeletal osteosarcoma and malignant fibrous histiocytoma (Fig. 9.7) and in the detection of angiosarcomas, including Kaposi's sarcoma. The addition of specific inhibitors further strengthens the discriminatory powers of enzyme reactions. An elaboration of histochemical methods for alkaline phosphatase including specific inhibitors (Moss 1982, Shephard & Peake 1986 a + b) might, in the future, prove of further value.

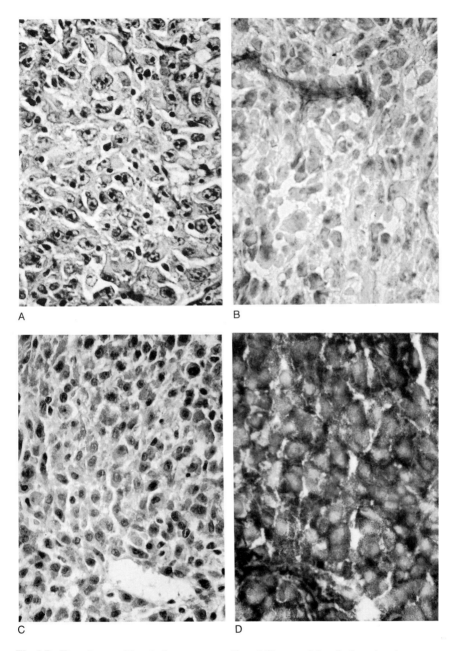

Fig. 9.7   Two pleomorphic soft tissue sarcomas (**A** and **C**), reacted for alkaline phosphatase (**B** and **D**). The malignant fibrous histiocytoma (**A** and **B**) is negative and only the capillary endothelium is positive for alkaline phosphatase. The osteosarcoma (**C** and **D**) stains heavily for alkaline phosphatase. Obj. × 25.

REFERENCES

Bendix-Hansen K, Myhre-Jensen O 1985 Enzyme histochemical investigations on bone and soft tissue tumours. Acta Pathologica Microbiologica et Immunologica Scandinavica Section A93: 73–80

Fletcher C D M, Evans B J, Macartney J C et al 1985 Dermatofibrosarcoma protuberans: a clinicopathological and immunohistochemical study with a review of the literature. Histopathology 9: 921–938

Fletcher C D M, Theaker J M, Flanagan A, Krausz, T 1988 Pigmented dermatofibrosarcoma protuberans (Bednar tumour): melanocytic colonisation or neuroectodermal differentiation? A clinicopathological and immunohistochemical study. Histopathology 13: 631–643

Jeffree G, Price C H G 1965 Bone tumours and their enzymes. Journal of Bone and Joint Surgery 47B: 120–136

Jeffree G M 1972 Enzymes in fibroblastic lesions. Journal of Bone and Joint Surgery 54B: 535–546

Jeffree G M 1974 Enzymes of round cell tumours in bone and soft tissue: A histochemical survey. Journal of Pathology 113: 101–115

Moss D W 1982 Alkaline phosphatase isoenzymes. Clinical Chemistry 28: 2007–2016

Mukai M, Torikata C, Iri H et al 1985 Cellular differentiation of epithelioid sarcoma. An electron microscopic, enzyme histochemical and immunohistochemical study. American Journal of Pathology 119: 44–56

Nakanishi S, Hizawa K 1984 Enzyme histochemical observation of fibrohistiocytic tumours. Acta Pathologica Japonica 34: 1003–1016

Pallesen G, Myhre-Jensen O 1987 Immunophenotypic analysis of neoplastic cells in follicular dendritic cell sarcoma. Leukemia 1: 549–557

Pisa R, Boneth F, Chilosi M, Iannucci A, Menestrina F 1982 Synovial sarcoma. Enzyme histochemistry of a typical case. Virchows Archiv A. (Pathological Anatomy) 398: 67–73

Roholl P J M, Kleijne J, Van Basten C D H, Van Der Putte S C J, Van Unnik J A M 1985 A study to analyze the origin of tumor cells in malignant fibrous histiocytomas. A multiparametric characterization. Cancer 56: 2809–2815

Sarnat H B, deMello D E, Siddiqui S Y 1979 Diagnostic value of histochemistry in embryonal rhabdomyosarcoma. American Journal of Surgical Pathology 3: 177–183

Shephard M D S, Peake M J 1986 Quantitative method for determinating serum alkaline phosphatase isoenzyme activity. A. Guanidine hydrochloride: new reagent for selectively inhibiting major serum isoenzymes of alkaline phosphatase. Journal of Clinical Pathology 39: 1025–1030

Shephard M D S, Peake M J, Walmsley R N 1986 Quantitative method for determinating serum alkaline phosphatase isoenzyme activity. II. Development and clinincal application of method for measuring four alkaline phosphatase isoenzymes. Journal of Clinical Pathology 39: 1031–1038

Wood G S, Beckstead J H, Turner R R et al 1986 Malignant fibrous histiocytoma tumor cells resemble fibroblasts. American Journal of Surgical Pathology 10: 323–33

10. Electron microscopy of soft tissue tumours

B. Mackay

When soft tissue tumours are examined with the electron microscope, a remarkable spectrum of cell structure is revealed. This variety is barely hinted at in paraffin sections, and consequently ultrastructural study can be extremely useful in explaining light microscopic appearances, establishing diagnoses, and enhancing the precision of the subclassification of these neoplasms. Electron microscopy is not extensively used for sarcoma diagnosis, in part because its application in surgical pathology is not routine in many hospitals, and also because clinicians are, as a rule, content to know if their patient's tumour is a soft tissue neoplasm or not and if so, whether it is benign or malignant. Subclassification has traditionally played a minor role in management, although this is gradually changing. There is evidence that the behaviour of soft tissue sarcomas can to some degree be predicted by knowledge of the cell type, and given the increasing complexity of therapeutic modalities, it is reasonable to hope that more correlations between sarcoma type and form of therapy will become established. For this to happen, accuracy in classification is mandatory, and light microscopy alone is often inadequate: perhaps as many as one sarcoma in three can not be firmly subclassified using conventional haematoxylin and eosin stained sections, and uncertainty may even persist over whether a particular tumour is a sarcoma or some other type of neoplasm.

Immunocytochemical screening methods (cytokeratins, S-100 protein, leucocyte common antigen) will often answer the basic question of whether a particular lesion is a sarcoma or a carcinoma, melanoma or lymphoma/leukaemia (Mackay & Ordonez 1986). These stains, however, are not always contributory, and must be interpreted in the light of the clinical and histopathological contexts: for example, keratin-positive soft tissue tumours are recognised, and only about half of malignant Schwann cell neoplasms stain positively with the S-100 antibody while certain other cell types are also immunoreactive.

The aim in this chapter is to briefly review the major ultrastructural features that are seen among the soft tissue neoplasms, and to point out the value of the electron microscope as an adjunct to routine light microscopy and immunocytochemistry in diagnostic evaluation. It must be stressed that ultrastructural study is always complementary to conventional light microscopy and never replaces it. The pattern of the cells in paraffin sections can be as informative as the fine structure of the tumour cells. The contributions of distinguished pathologists who have focussed their attention on the light microscopy of soft tissue neoplasms, from Stout to Enzinger and Weiss, cannot be sufficiently lauded.

When electron microscopy is used as a diagnostic tool, certain basic principles should always be observed. Representative tissue must be obtained promptly following excision and fixed in thin (1 mm) slices in buffered glutaraldehyde. Electron microscopy can be effectively performed on fine needle aspiration biopsies (Mackay et al 1987) but the specimen must be handled and processed carefully in order to harvest enough well-preserved and undistorted tumour cells. The diagnostic study should be performed by a pathologist who is experienced in ultrastructural pathology and aware of the light microscopic appearance of the tumour and the clinical context.

Sarcoma versus other tumour types

Before a soft tissue tumour can be subclassified, it must first be established that the lesion does indeed fall within the broad category of mesenchymal neoplasms, and overlap in morphology with other tumour types makes this a common problem. When light microscopy with clinical correlation is inadequate, selective application of histochemical and immunocytochemical stains may suffice (Mackay & Ordonez 1986). Electron microscopy can be highly effective as a screening procedure to indicate into which major category a problem tumour should be placed, but it is not generally used for this purpose: the expense of the procedure and the limited availability of facilities and experienced pathologist-electron microscopists are the main reasons. Ultrastructural study is generally reserved for tumours that are still diagnostic problems after all the light microscopic studies have been completed. The following paragraphs briefly consider the electron microscopic contribution to the primary classification of malignant tumours.

Sarcoma versus carcinoma

While most carcinomas can become sarcomatoid with dedifferentiation and hence simulate a spindle cell, or less commonly a pleomorphic sarcoma, this type of transformation is seen more often in squamous carcinomas of skin or mucosal surfaces, and renal cell carcinomas. Electron microscopy is of limited value. The frequent desmosomes and cytokeratin filament bundles of a squamous carcinoma, or abundant cytoplasmic glycogen and lipid of a renal cell carcinoma may indicate the diagnosis, but there is a tendency for the cells to assume non-specific or even mesenchymal features with sarcomatoid transformation.

Sarcoma versus mesothelioma

Recent studies (Bolen 1987, Bolen et al 1987) have shown that submesothelial mesenchymal cells possess remarkable structural pliability, being able, when stimulated by an injury to the overlying epithelium, to proliferate, become keratin-positive, and apparently even repair the surface defect by assuming an epithelial configuration. This morphological diversity is reflected in the range of histopathological appearances that can be seen in mesotheliomas, ranging from pure epithelial tumours to spindle cell neoplasms which even by electron microscopy do not show epithelial features. One pleural sarcoma that we have studied was composed of myofibroblasts, and another, a mixed mesothelioma, contained both a differentiated epithelial component and zones of primitive mesenchymal cells.

Sarcoma versus melanoma

It is well known that not all melanomas are of cutaneous origin. Some arise in mucosal surfaces, or the meninges, and a few present as soft tissue masses. The melanocytes from which the tumours derive presumably became misplaced during their embryonic migration from the developing central nervous system, becoming sequestered within soft tissues. Apparently melanocytes with the longest migration route are more prone to become immured within the soft tissues, to judge from the fact that tumours derived from them are more common in the distal part of the lower extremity.

Enzinger described clear cell sarcomas of tendons and aponeuroses in 1965, but demonstration of premelanosomes in the cells, and of melanin by light microscopy, led to the designation being changed to malignant melanoma of soft parts (Chung & Enzinger 1983). Positive immunostaining for S-100 protein facilitates the diagnosis. We have been able to demonstrate premelanosomes in every case we have studied (Benson et al 1985) though they were sometimes sparse and confined to scattered cells, and they persisted in cultured cells from one tumour. A helpful feature by both light and electron microscopy is the large, round, dense nucleoli in many of the cells.

Another variant of melanoma that closely mimics a sarcoma is a spindle cell change accompanied by the assumption of a schwannian appearance. We have used the term neurosarcomatous transformation (DiMaio et al 1982). The cells become markedly elongated, with long slender processes of cytoplasm that contain longitudinally aligned microtubules, and typically several cells are closely apposed within a small bundle. This grouping can often be appreciated by light microscopy. Cytologically, the cells tend to appear rather innocuous and a biopsy may be misinterpreted as an atypical fibroblastic proliferation, but immunostaining for S-100 protein should be positive.

Sarcoma versus lymphoma/leukaemia

We have encountered two situations where lymphomas have closely simulated sarcomas by light microscopy and the ultrastructural features revealed the correct diagnosis.

Granulocytic leukaemia presenting in tissues (granulocytic sarcoma) may have a pseudoalveolar appearance in paraffin sections and be mistaken for an alveolar rhabdomyosarcoma. Electron microscopy will reveal the irregular lysosomes within the cells and this and other features (Mackay et al 1986) will indicate the correct diagnosis. A pleomorphic tumour of transformed lymphocytes or a true histiocytic lymphoma can also simulate a sarcoma (Mackay et al 1986), but neither will closely resemble one of the defined soft tissue sarcomas ultrastructurally. Special stains can confirm the diagnosis in paraffin sections.

Tumours of fibroblasts

The ubiquitous cell of fibrous connective tissue is typically fusiform but it is capable of assuming a variety of sizes and shapes in response to environmental conditions. These changes are reflected in the various proliferative disorders of fibroblasts from reactive lesions to neoplasms.

The structural flexibility of the fibroblast can be strikingly demonstrated in non-neoplastic conditions. Round and often large cells are seen in proliferative myositis and fasciitis, and ultrastructurally these cells have the same profusion of endoplasmic reticulum that characterises spindle-shaped fibroblasts (Fig. 10.1). In nodular fasciitis, many of the spindle cells contain peripheral bundles of myofilaments (Wirman 1976), and anchoring filaments may attach the cell to adjacent collagen: these are features of myofibroblasts.

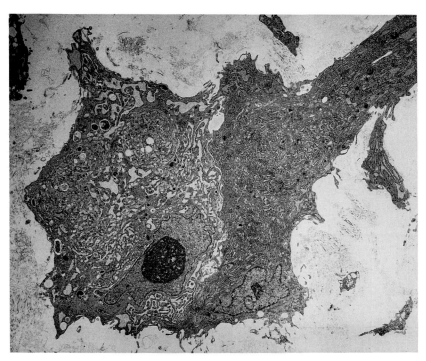

Fig. 10.1 The plump cells of proliferative myositis and fasciitis have the same copious rough endoplasmic reticulum as spindle-shaped fibroblasts. × 4100.

Most cells in the various fibromatoses are spindled fibroblasts or myofibroblasts (Bhawan et al 1979).

In cutaneous atypical fibrous histiocytomas, the cells again are predominantly spindle-shaped fibroblasts, but plumper cells also occur, and the endoplasmic reticulum may contain aggregates of electron-dense material which at low magnification can suggest dense-core granules.

Dermatofibrosarcoma protuberans has been thought to be neural (Hashimoto et al 1974) because of the presence of long, slender cytoplasmic processes, and microtubules in some cells, but it is probable that the cells are fibroblasts with markedly attenuated cytoplasmic extensons. Although the processes superfically simulate perineural cells (Dupree et al 1985), they lack a basal lamina and pinocytotic vesicles.

Fibrosarcoma is no longer a common diagnosis by light microscopy, but by electron microscopy, many sarcomas are seen to be composed of cells with the features of fibroblasts. Myofibroblasts are common in the better differentiated neoplasms (Fig. 10.2). Approximately 5% of sarcomas are composed of cells that resemble fibroblasts but contain only sparse cisternae, and they could be viewed as sarcomas of primitive mesenchymal cells rather than fibrosarcomas.

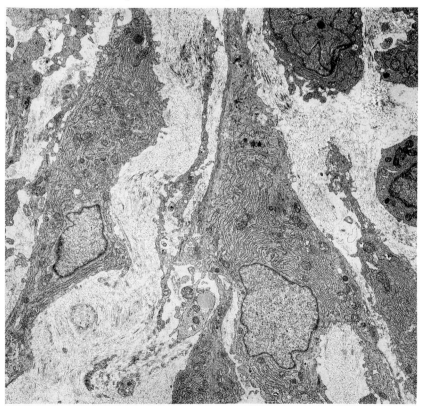

Fig. 10.2 Fibroblasts and myofibroblasts from a well-differentiated congenital fibrosarcoma lie within a collagenous stroma. × 7800.

Cells of the malignant fibrous histicytomas that we have studied, including the large and multinucleated cells, have possessed ultrastructural features that favour their being fibroblasts, and a recent report has supported this view (Wood et al 1988). Some of the spindle cells are myofibroblasts (Churg & Kahn 1977). However, there is a spectrum of ultrastructure within the cells of these tumours (Hoffman & Dickersin 1983, Lagace 1984, Tsuneyoshi et al 1981) and some have less endoplasmic reticulum and contain extensive zones of intermediate filaments (Fig. 10.3). The tumour cells are often closely packed without intervening stroma. Cell junctions occur but they are sparse and confined to mere densities of the apposed cell membranes. Lipid is a common component of neoplastic fibroblasts and is plentiful in some malignant fibrous histiocytomas, but the lipid droplets are small and uniform. Electron-dense material within the endoplasmic reticulum may condense to produce a cribriform network and a similar appearance can be seen in liposarcoma cells (Mackay & Silva 1980).

Tumours of fat cells

The diagnosis of spindle cell, atypical or pleomorphic lipoma is based on light microscopic criteria, and most liposarcomas are also diagnosed and subclassified from their light microscopic appearance. Occasionally, electron microscopy is used to demonstrate the presence of abundant lipid in the cells of a

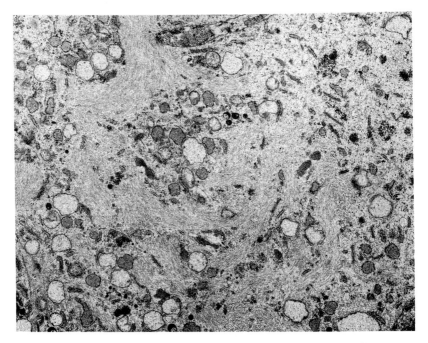

Fig. 10.3   Zones of intermediate filaments are a common finding in malignant fibrous histiocytoma cells. × 9500.

suspected liposarcoma, and this can often be achieved using the thick (light microscopic) sections of the plastic-embedded tissue.

The occurrence of lipid droplets in neoplastic fibroblasts has been mentioned. In contrast, lipomatous tumour cells (Bolen & Thorning 1980) as a rule contain larger numbers of droplets that coalesce with the result that variations in droplet size are typical (Fig. 10.4), the ultimate step being the distinctive signet-ring configuration in which a single large lipid droplet occupies the entire cell save for a thin rim of compressed cytoplasm and nucleus. The lipid droplets in lipoblasts are classically non-membrane-bound (Roussow et al 1986), in contrast to lipid-laden lysosomes.

Tumours of smooth muscle cells

Myofilaments can be distinguished from other intermediate filaments by electron microscopy, rendering the technique suitable for diagnosing myogenic sarcomas. Identical myofilaments occur in certain other neoplasms.

Smooth muscle myofilaments have already been mentioned in myofibroblasts, where they form a band subjacent to the cell membrane. It can be difficult on occasion to decide whether a tumour is composed of myofibroblasts or smooth muscle cells. Intercellular collagen is present in both though apposition of cells is more common in smooth muscle neoplasms. The anchoring filaments of myofibroblasts are unique but they are not always visualised in tumours. Neoplastic smooth muscle cells (Mackay et al 1987b,

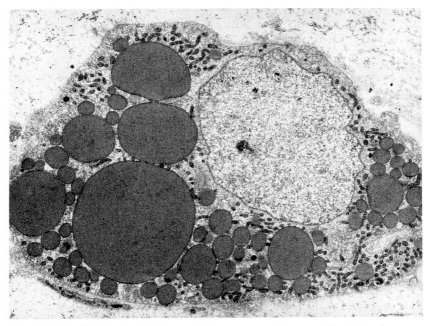

Fig. 10.4 The lipid droplets in this myxoid liposarcoma cell vary considerably in size. × 6900.

Hashimoto et al 1986) may possess peripheral densities, occasionally have pinocytic vesicles, and are sometimes connected by plaque-like junctions. Myofilaments are often sparse in aggressive leiomyosarcomas and it may only be possible to detect them by searching through several areas of a tumour. Paradoxically, some aggressive and metastatic leiomyosarcomas are composed of well-differentiated cells with plentiful myofilaments (Mackay et al 1987b).

A peculiar transformation of neoplastic smooth muscle cells to a spherical form has been designated epithelioid change, and it has principally been studied in tumours of the gut, though it also occurs in uterine and retroperitoneal neoplasms (Floyd et al 1981). We have recently investigated a group of stromal tumors of the gastrointestinal tract using several immuno-staining procedures and electron microscopy (Floyd et al 1981). Among 44 malignant tumours (20 gastric, 14 from small intestine, 10 from large intestine), 9 were S-100 positive and 4 of these showed ultrastructural evidence of Schwann cell differentiation: 1 other was clearly a smooth muscle tumour by electron microscopy. Of the immunostaining procedures used, vimentin was positive in almost every case and consequently was not of value, and desmin was only positive in lesions that contained large numbers of myofilaments (13 tumours). Smooth muscle myosin was somewhat more sensitive, staining 19 tumours including some that did not display fine structural features of smooth muscle differentiation, but failing to stain any of the 16 sarcomas with epithelioid transformation.

Electron microscopy revealed a spectrum of fine structure ranging from differentiated smooth muscle tumours through a small transitional group, in which scattered cells betrayed traces of smooth muscle differentiation, to the largest group (which included all the epithelioid tumours), in which smooth muscle features were totally absent (Fig. 10.5). Among the latter, some tumours contained cells with long filopodia (Fig. 10.6). The prognostic significance of these ultrastructural observations has not yet been determined. There is, of course, no proof that the primitive mesenchymal tumours from the gut are smooth muscle in type, though the impression that they occupy one end of a continous spectrum of ultrastructure extending through the differentiated neoplasms at least suggests that they are composed of cells with latent myogenic potential.

Other tumours containing smooth muscle myofilaments

These neoplasms are often, but not invariably, identified from their light microscopic appearance. Tumours of myofibroblasts have already been mentioned. Smooth muscle myofilaments may occasionally be found in haemangiopericytomas, which are discussed under tumours of vasoformative cells.

Glomus tumours   The round cells of a glomus tumour contain moderate numbers of smooth muscle myofilaments (Tsuneyoshi & Enjoji 1982), and a distinctive feature is the presence of a single row of pinocytotic vesicles

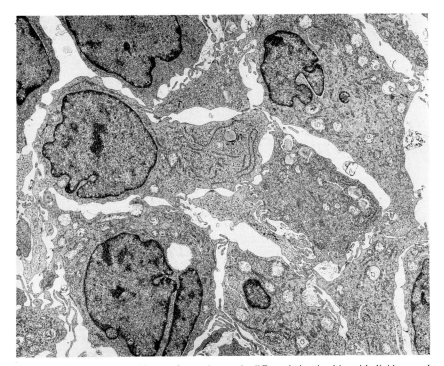

Fig. 10.5 There was no evidence of smooth muscle differentiation in this epithelioid stromal sarcoma from the intestine. × 4800.

subjacent to the cell membrane. Almost all glomus tumours are benign, but we have had the opportunity to examine one malignant example and the electron microscopy was diagnostic (Mackay et al 1981). The cells were similar to those of benign glomus tumours.

Tumours of myoepithelial cells The dual nature of the myoepithelial cell can be expressed in tumours by the copresence of smooth muscle myofilaments, usually in peripheral bands, and denser wavy bands of cytokeratin filaments. Cell junctions are usually present, but they may be scanty and are often primitive in their construction. Myoepithelial cells may be the only cells of a tumour, as in the myoepitheliomas of salivary tissues (Dardick 1985) or breast, or they may coexist with true epithelial cells as in mixed and epithelial-myoepithelial salivary tumours (Luna et al 1985).

Tumours of skeletal muscle cells

Rhabdomyomas are uncommon lesions that are usually recognised without difficulty in light microscopic sections. In contrast, there are often problems identifying rhabdomyosarcomas, even with the assistance of immunostaining methods, and electron microscopy can be helpful (Kahn et al 1983, Mierau & Favara 1980, Schmidt et al 1987).

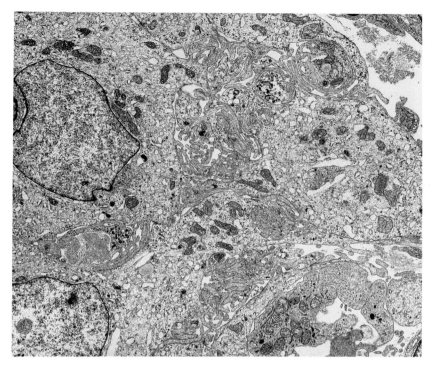

Fig. 10.6   These epithelioid leiomyosarcoma cells have many filopodia. × 12 800.

Among small round cell tumours, convoluted nuclear profiles are suggestive of rhabdomyosarcoma, and the absence of specific features of the other
tumours that enter into the differential diagnosis is also contributory.
However, the truly diagnostic observation is the presence of cytoplasmic
myofilaments (Erlandson 1987). The unique pattern of thick and thin
filaments that characterises striated muscle fibers is often seen in the tumour
cells (Fig. 10.7), but only in a minority of cases are they both sufficiently
abundant and organised as segments of myofibrils in register to produce
cross-striations visible by light microscopy. More frequently, when many
filaments are present, they are haphazardly arranged with patchy Z-band
zones. The very number of the myofilaments may cause the cells to appear
eosinophilic in conventional sections.

When only small numbers of myofilaments are present, it becomes less easy
to identify them as skeletal in type. If they are seen in cross-section, the
unique spatial distribution of the myosin and actin filaments can be visualised.
In oblique or longitudinal section, it may be difficult or impossible to
appreciate that two types are present. A useful observation is the occurrence
of short rows of ribosomes between the filaments towards their ends (Fig.
10.8). If rhabdomyosarcoma is suspected and filaments are not readily
identified, the sections should be scanned at low magnification searching for
cells with denser cytoplasm: closer scrutiny may reveal myofilaments.

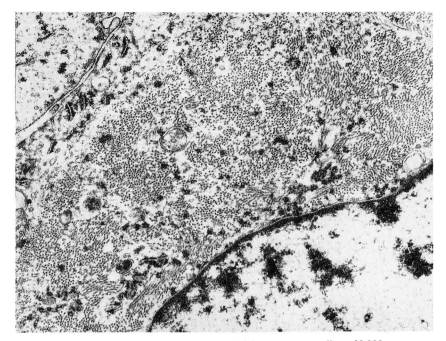

Fig. 10.7 Cross-sectioned myofilaments from a rhabdomyosarcoma cell. × 29 000.

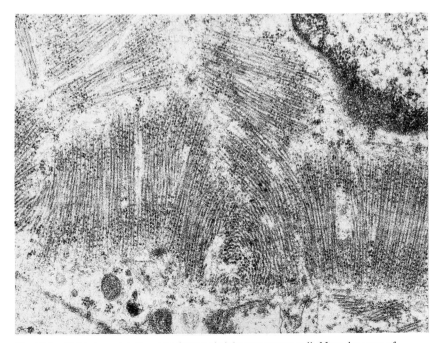

Fig. 10.8 Thick (myosin) filaments from a rhabdomyosarcoma cell. Note the rows of ribosomes along the outer segments of the filaments. × 26 000.

Other tumours containing skeletal muscle myofilaments

Skeletal muscle myofilaments are found in some nephroblastomas (Schmidt et al 1982) and dedifferentiated chondrosarcomas (Tetu et al 1986). Rhabdomyoblasts occur together with schwannian elements in the so-called ectomesenchymoma (Schmidt et al 1982a). These neoplasms are generally recognised without difficulty from the light microscopy and clinical data.

Tumours of vasoformative cells

There are no reliable ultrastructural features that will serve to identify neoplastic endothelial cells. Weibel-Palade bodies are not a consistent finding. The cells sometimes contain considerable numbers of intermediate filaments, and in benign and some differentiated malignant tumours, they display a tendency to form vascular channels (Lagace & Leroy 1987).

The spindle cells of Kaposi's sarcoma look fibroblastic, but they are factor VIII-related antigen positive (Guarda et al 1981), and they aggregate to create crude tubes (Hammar et al 1985) that apparently connect with neighbouring vessels since they contain erythrocytes. However, the poor construction of these primitive channels, which have few cell junctions and initially lack an intact basal lamina, allows the extravasation of red cells through breaches in the vessel wall.

The same attempt to form lumina is often seen in angiosarcomas, and even tumours that appear solid by light microscopy will have irregular clefts within the clusters of neoplastic cells. While these spaces could simply reflect loss of cohesion of neighbouring cells, they occur with sufficient frequency in angiosarcomas to suggest that they represent genuine attempts by the cells to create lumina.

Haemangiopericytoma is a difficult and much abused diagnosis by light microscopy. Foci with an anastomosing vascular pattern are common in sarcomas. However, when haemangiopericytomas are studied with the electron microscope (Nunnery et al 1981), the appearance of the neoplastic cells is, if not distinctive, at least sufficiently different from that of cells of the other defined types of soft tissue tumours to be of some diagnostic value. Haemangiopericytoma-like tumours of the nasal cavity (Compagno & Hyams 1976) ultrastructurally resemble haemangiopericytomas in other locations (Fig. 10.9).

The cells of a haemangiopericytoma may be closely packed within the stroma which intervenes between the many unremarkable vessels, but more commonly the cells are loosely distributed within a collagenous stroma and then slender arms of cytoplasm can be seen extending from one cell to its neighbours. There are tiny membrane densities where the cytoplasmic processes come in contact. The cells range from round or polygonal to short elongated cells which may have a slightly curved or crescentic profile that recalls the normal pericyte. In areas where the cells are compactly grouped, cell junctions are more numerous but still primitive. The organelles may

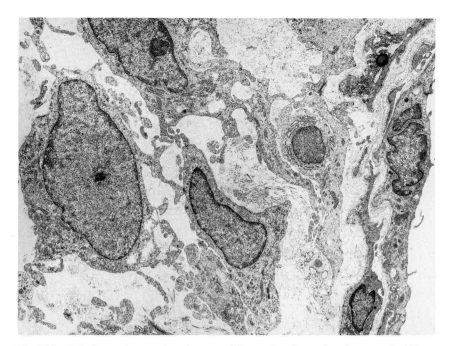

Fig. 10.9 Cells from a haemangiopericytoma of the nasal cavity are loosely grouped within the collagenous stroma. Part of a vessel wall is visible at the right-hand margin of the figure. Slender arms of cytoplasm connect neighbouring tumour cells. × 7900.

include a stack of cisternae of the endoplasmic reticulum, and a few lysosomes or an occasional lipid droplet are sometimes seen. Mitochondria are not usually numerous. It is uncommon to find discrete bundles of smooth muscle myofilaments. More frequently, the filaments are sparse, confined to scattered cells, and nonspecific in their appearance, and most of the tumour cells do not contain groups of filaments.

Tumours of Schwann cells

A broad range of fine structure is seen among tumours of Schwann cells (Erlandson 1985), and it has not been fully defined for the sarcomas. Since S-100 immunostaining is not specific for Schwann cell tumours, and may be negative in as many as half of the sarcomas, electron microscopy is potentially useful in their diagnosis.

Although differences between schwannomas and neurofibromas are described, the neoplastic cells have close ultrastructural similarities. A hallmark is the long cytoplasmic extensions which may be uniform in calibre, but often branch and can create elaborate filigree patterns within the collagenous stroma of a neurofibroma (Fig. 10.10). A basal lamina clothes the processes and the cytoplasm contains intermediate filaments and microtubules. A second feature that reflects the normal Schwann cell is the formation by the

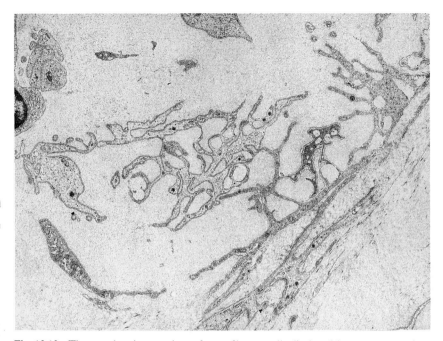

Fig. 10.10 The cytoplasmic extensions of neurofibroma cells display elaborate patterns of branching. × 4400.

neoplastic cells of mesaxon-like structures in which a slender curving tongue of cytoplasm encircles a zone of stroma, possibly including some collagen fibrils, and encloses it in the manner in which a normal Schwann cell envelops an axon. A basal lamina may line the mesaxonal tube.

Similar ultrastructural features serve to identify a sarcoma as a Schwann cell neoplasm, but a wide range of ultrastructural appearances is seen in these tumours (Bruner 1987, Chitale & Dickersin 1983, Dickersin 1987, Erlandson & Woodruff 1982). Processes are often as extensive as in the benign lesions, but the basal lamina disappears as processes become apposed within solid groups of cells. In some sarcomas, large numbers of slender cytoplasmic processes are grouped in bundles (Fig. 10.11). Mesaxon formation is not common in the sarcomas, but when it does occur it is manifested by many of the cells.

Tumours of skeletal cells

The cells of chondrosarcomas and osteosarcomas arising in the soft tissues appear to be similar to those of their intraosseous counterparts. An intriguing finding in some extraskeletal myxoid chondrosarcomas is a profusion of microtubules within the endoplasmic reticulum (DeBlois et al 1986, Suzuki et al, 1988) (Fig. 10.12). The tubules do not show quite the degree of regularity of the parallel tubular arrays seen in melanomas.

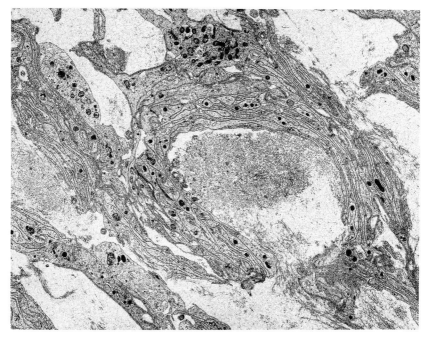

Fig. 10.11   Many slender cytoplasmic processes are intimately apposed in this malignant peripheral nerve sheath tumour. × 13 000.

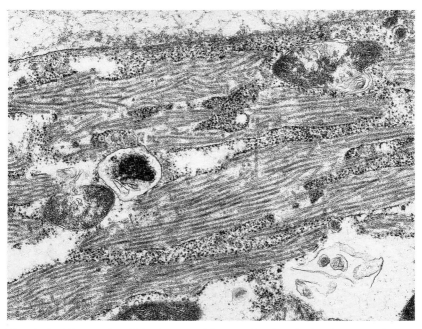

Fig. 10.12   Microtubules within cisternae of the endoplasmic reticulum in an extraskeletal myxoid chondrosarcoma. × 34 000.

The existence of a soft tissue neoplasm resembling Ewing's sarcoma of bone has become widely accepted, though its nature remains as enigmatic as that of the bone tumour. As with other soft tissue neoplasms, there is a relatively typical ultrastructural appearance but also variations on this basic theme (Dickman & Triche 1986, Gillespie et al 1979, Mierau 1985). The smooth cell surfaces are intimately adjoined, but scattered tiny membrane densities are the most one finds in the way of cell contact specialisations. The round nucleus has a uniform profile and fine chromatin and the nucleolus is often small. Organelles are scanty, and glycogen may form diffuse lakes. Variations on the typical theme involve cellular and particularly nuclear pleomorphism, and an increase in the number of organelles, notably mitochondria. In part, Ewing's tumours is distinguished from other small round cell tumors by the absence of specific features seen in these neoplasms (Mierau et al 1985), but there are exceptions and examples of Ewing's tumour of both soft tissue and bone with neuroblastoma-like features have been reported (Schmidt et al 1982b, Shimada et al 1988).

Tumours of uncertain histogenesis

The cell of origin of a number of the named soft tissue tumours has not yet been established, though some plausible hypotheses have been advanced. From the ultrastructural standpoint, the following neoplasms deserve mention.

Synovial sarcoma

Schmidt and Mackay (1982) did not find any close resemblance between the cells of normal synovium or tendon sheath and those of synovial sarcomas. The topic has been addressed recently by Ghadially (1987). This discrepancy between the normal and neoplastic cells, coupled with the frequent occurrence of synovial sarcomas some distance from the nearest joint, has suggested that the designation may be a misnomer. The description of an apparent monophasic form of the tumour is also controversial.

The usual biphasic synovial sarcoma is readily recognised from its histopathology. Recently, a number of correlated ultrastructural and immunohistochemical studies have been reported (Abenoza et al 1986, Fisher 1986, Krall et al 1981). The epithelial component is composed of cells which appear identical in their fine structure to those of normal ductal structures, with tight junctions, microvilli and a basal lamina. The spindle cells of the stroma are somewhat fibroblastic, but are shorter than fibroblasts, their cytoplasm does not usually branch, and they contain less endoplasmic reticulum. Since this type of cell can predominate within a biphasic tumour, a monophasic spindle-cell variant probably does exist.

Epithelioid sarcoma

Enzinger (1970) pointed out that this tumour can be confused with other neoplasms or granulomatous inflammation. The diagnosis can sometimes be made with confidence by light microscopy, but failure to observe all the histological criteria listed by Enzinger can lead to the inclusion of atypical forms and errors in diagnosis. Most epithelioid sarcomas arise in the distal extremities, and the cells are consistently immunoreactive to cytokeratin antibodies. Some tumours in soft tissues such as the perineal region have close similarities to epithelioid sarcoma but also some histological differences, such as diffuse sheets of cells instead of the characteristic nodules, and they may be more aggressive (Meis et al 1988). Further studies are needed to determine whether these are variants of epithelioid sarcoma.

When a diagnosis of epithelioid sarcoma is in question, electron microscopy can contribute (Mackay et al 1983, Mukai et al 1985). Most of the cells are spherical to ovoid, with irregular surfaces, rare filopodia and desmosome-like junctions at the periphery of the tumour nodules: towards the centre of a nodule, loss of cohesion of the cells is accompanied by a progressive disappearance of the cell junctions. The cells may contain moderate numbers of mitochondria and some lipid droplets but the dominant feature is the occurrence of diffuse zones of intermediate filaments (Mills et al 1981, Fisher 1988), which may occupy much of the cytoplasm, pushing nucleus and organelles to the periphery. The filaments are not always numerous, and they may be confined to scattered cells. In some tumours, denser wavy bundles of cytokeratin filaments are evident. Electron microscopy has not revealed the cell of origin of the epithelioid sarcoma.

Granular cell tumour

A Schwann cell origin for this lesion is supported by its S-100 immunoreactivity, and by the ultrastructural features of the cells which include subdivision into multiple compartments bounded by a unit membrane (Fig. 10.13), microtubules in some compartments, and the many lysosomes (Fig. 10.13) which are seen occasionally in non-neoplastic peripheral nerves. Malignant granular cell tumours are rare, but examples have been studied by electron microscopy (Troncoso et al 1988) and the cells contained the profusion of lysosomes seen in the benign lesions.

Alveolar soft part sarcoma

Much could be written about the ultrastructure of this enigmatic neoplasm. It can be misdiagnosed by light microscopy, especially from a small or distorted biopsy, and electron microscopy is useful for confirmation (Schmidt et al 1981, Unni & Soule 1975, Ordonez et al 1989). The nests of cells are often solid, and the pseudoalveolar appearance results from drop-out of cells. Sustentacular cells are not a consistent component. The smooth cell surfaces are devoid of microvilli and are closely adjacent

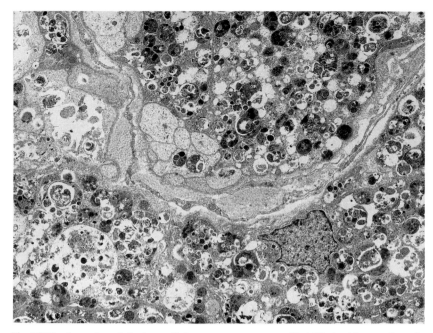

Fig. 10.13   A number of the intracellular compartments are still visible in this granular cell tumour. Others have been obliterated by the numerous lysosomes. × 7500.

within a cell nest. Cell junctions are small and few. Within the abundant cytoplasm, an extensive golgi complex is surrounded by clusters of small dense-core granules (Fig. 10.14). The granules are consistently tiny (around 120 nm) and they are not seen elsewhere in the cytoplasm. The proximity of the granules to the saccules of the golgi complex implies that they are derived from it, and it appears that they coalesce to form larger lysosome-like bodies within which foci of crystallisation appear. The end result is the mature rhomboid crystalloids (Mukai et al 1983) which are occasionally numerous in almost every cell, but are more often confined to scattered cells. In a few tumours, crystalloids can not be found.

Other intriguing appearances in cells of this neoplasm are zones of smooth endoplasmic reticulum, and mitochondria with tubular cristae. Despite these interesting observations, the cell of origin remains obscure.

Conclusions

It has only been possible to survey briefly the extensive field of the soft tissue tumours, but the aim has been to demonstrate that ultrastructural examination of these neoplasms, and sarcomas in particular, is a useful complement to light microscopy, both for diagnosis, and in order to expand our knowledge of the structure of the cells of this fascinating group of neoplasms.

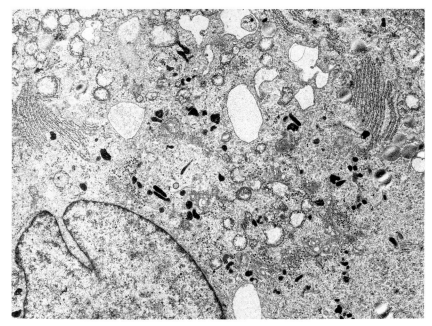

Fig. 10.14 There were only occasional small crystalloids in this alveolar soft part sarcoma, but other distinctive features of the cells are shown in the figure. Many tiny granules surround the golgi complex, and short cisternae of the endoplasmic reticulum are forming stacks. A few lipid droplets and some irregular lysosomes are also present. × 7300.

REFERENCES

Abenoza P, Manivel J C, Swanson P E et al 1986 Synovial sarcoma: ultrastructural study and immunohistochemical analysis by a combined peroxidase-antiperoxidase/avidin-biotin-peroxidase complex procedure. Human Pathology 17: 1107–1115

Benson J D, Kraemer B B, Mackay B 1985 Malignant melanoma of soft parts: An ultrastructural study of four cases. Ultrastructural Pathology 8: 57–70

Bhawan J, Bacchetta C, Joris I et al 1979 A myofibroblastic tumour: infantile digital fibroma (recurrent digital fibrous tumour of childhood). American Journal of Pathology 94: 19–36

Bolen J W, 1987 Tumors of serosal tissue origin. In: Mackay B (ed) Diagnostic electron microscopy of tumors. Clinics in Laboratory Medicine 7/1: 31–50

Bolen J W, Thorning D 1980 Benign lipoblastoma and myxoid liposarcoma: A comparative light and electron microscopic study. American Journal of Surgical Pathology 4: 163–174

Bolen J W, Hammar S P, McNutt M A 1987 Serosal tissue: Reactive tissue as a model for understanding mesotheliomas. Ultrastructural Pathology 11: 251–262

Bruner J M 1987 Tumors of schwann cells and pigmented skin cells. In: Mackay B (ed) Diagnostic electron microscopy of tumors. Clinics in Laboratory Medicine 7/1: 181–198

Chitale A R, Dickersin G R 1983 Electron microscopy in the diagnosis of malignant schwannomas. A report of six cases. Cancer 51: 1448–1461

Chung E B, Enzinger F M 1983 Malignant melanoma of soft parts. A reassessment of clear cell sarcoma. American Journal of Surgical Pathology: 405–413

Churg A M, Kahn L B 1977 Myofibroblasts and related cells in malignant fibrous and fibrohistiocytic tumors. Human Pathology 8: 205–218

Compagno J, Hyams V J 1976 Hemangiopericytoma-like intranasal tumors. A clinicopathologic study of 23 cases. American Journal of Clinical Pathology 66: 672–683

Dardick I 1985 Malignant myoepithelioma of parotid salivary gland. Ultrastructural Pathology 9: 163

DeBlois G, Wang S, Kay S 1986 Microtubular aggregates within rough endoplasmic reticulum: an unusual ultrastructural feature of extra-skeletal myxoid chondrosarcoma. Human Pathology 17: 469–475

Dickersin G R 1987 The electron microscopic spectrum of nerve sheath tumors. Ultrastructural Pathology 11: 103–146

Dickman P S, Triche T J 1986 Extraosseous Ewing's sarcoma versus primitive rhabdomyosarcoma: diagnostic criteria and clinical correlation. Human Pathology 17: 881–893

DiMaio S, Mackay B, Smith J L et al 1982 Neurosarcomatous transformation in malignant melanoma. Cancer 50: 2345–2354

Dupree W B, Langloss J M, Weiss S W 1985 Pigmented dermatofibrosarcoma protuberans (Bednar tumor). A pathologic, ultrastructural and immunohistochemical study. American Journal of Surgical Pathology 9: 630–639

Enzinger F M 1965 Clear-cell sarcoma of tendons and aponeuroses. An analysis of 21 cases. Cancer 18: 1163–1174

Enzinger F M 1970 Epithelioid sarcoma. Cancer 26: 1029–1041

Erlandson R A 1985 Peripheral nerve sheath tumors. Ultrastructural Pathology 9: 113–122

Erlandson R A 1987 The ultrastructural distinction between rhabdomyosarcoma and other undifferentiated sarcomas. Ultrastructural Pathology 11: 83–102

Enzinger F M, Weiss S W 1983 Soft Tissue Tumors. Mosby, St. Louis

Erlandson R A, Woodruff J M 1982 Peripheral nerve sheath tumors: An electron microscopic study of 43 cases. Cancer 49: 273–287

Fisher C 1986 Synovial sarcoma: ultrastructural and immunohistochemical features of epithelial differentiation in monophasic and biphasic tumors. Human Pathology 17: 996–1008

Fisher C 1988 Epithelioid sarcoma: the spectrum of ultrastructural differentiation in seven immunohistochemically defined cases. Human Pathology 19: 265–275

Floyd C, Ro J, Ordonez N G et al 1989 Stromal tumors of the gastrointestinal tract: light microscopic, immunocytochemical and ultrastructural observations on 50 cases. In Digestive Disease Pathology, Vol. 2, Eds. Watanabe S, Wolff M, Sommers S O Field and Wood, pp 165–177

Ghadially F N 1987 Is synovial sarcoma a carcinosarcoma of connective tissue? Ultrastructural Pathology 11: 147–152

Gillespie J J, Roth L M, Wills E R et al 1979 Extraskeletal Ewing's sarcoma: Histologic and ultrastructural observations in three cases. American Journal of Surgical Pathology 3: 99–108

Guarda L A, Silva E G, Ordonez N G et al 1981 Factor VIII in Kaposi's sarcoma. American Journal of Clinical Pathology 76: 197–200

Hammar S P, Bockus D, Remington F et al 1985 Kaposi's sarcoma in a male homosexual. Ultrastructural Pathology 9: 189–194

Hashimoto K et al 1974 Dermatofibrosarcoma protuberans. A tumor with perineural and endoneural cell features. Archives of Dermatology 110: 874–885

Hashimoto H, Daimaru Y, Tsuneyoshi M, Enjoji M 1986 Leiomyosarcoma of the external soft tissues. A clinicopathologic, immunohistochemical and electron microscopic study. Cancer 57: 2077–2088

Hoffman M A, Dickersin G R 1983 Malignant fibrous histiocytoma. An ultrastructural study of eleven cases. Human Pathology 14: 913–922

Kahn H J, Yeger H, Kassim O et al 1983 Immunohistochemical and electron microscopic assessment of childhood rhabdomyosarcoma. Increased frequency of diagnosis over routine histologic methods. Cancer 51: 1897–1903

Krall R A, Kostianovsky M, Patchefsky A S 1981 Synovial sarcoma — a clinical, pathological, and ultrastructural study of 26 cases supporting the recognition of a monophasic variant. American Journal of Surgical Pathology 8: 137–151

Lagace R 1987 The ultrastructural spectrum of malignant fibrous histiocytoma. Ultrastructural Pathology 11: 153–160

Lagace R, Leroy J-P 1987 Comparative electron microscopic study of cutaneous and soft tissue angiosarcomas, post-mastectomy angiosarcoma (Stewart-Treves syndrome) and Kaposi's sarcoma. Ultrastructural Pathology 11: 161–174

Luna M A, Ordonez N G, Mackay B et al 1985 Salivary epithelial-myoepithelial carcinoma of intercalated ducts. A clinical, electron microscopic and immunocytochemical study. Oral Surgery, Oral Medicine, Oral Pathology 59: 482–490

Mackay B, Silva E G 1980 Diagnostic electron microscopy in oncology. Pathology Annual (part 2) 15: 241–270

Mackay B, Rashid R K, Evans H L 1983 Epithelioid sarcoma. Ultrastructural Pathology 5: 329–334

Mackay B, Ordonez N G 1986 The role of the pathologist in the evaluation of poorly differentiated tumors and metastatic tumors of unknown origin. In: Fer M F, Greco F A, Oldham R K (eds) Poorly differentiated neoplasms and tumors of unknown origin. Grune & Stratton, Florida, 3–74

Mackay B, Legha S S, Pickler G H 1981 Coin lesion of the lung in a 19-year-old male. Ultrastructural Pathology 2: 289

Mackay B, Osborne B M, Manning J T 1986 Ultrastructure of lymphomas and leukemias. In: Russo J, Sommers S C (eds) Tumor diagnosis by electron microscopy, vol 1. Field, Rich, New York, p 185–244

Mackay B, Fanning T, Bruner J M et al 1987a Diagnostic electron microscopy using fine needle aspiration biopsies. Ultrastructural Pathology 11: 659–672

Mackay B, Ro J, Floyd C, Ordonez N G 1987b Ultrastructural observations on smooth muscle tumors. Ultrastructural Pathology 11: 593–608.

Meis J M, Mackay B, Ordonez N G 1988 Epithelioid sarcoma: An immunohistochemical and ultrastructural strdy. Surgical Pathology 1: 13–31

Mierau G W 1985 Extraskeletal Ewing's sarcoma (peripheral neuroepithelioma). Ultrastructural Pathology 9: 91–98

Mierau G W, Favara B E 1980 Rhabdomyosarcoma in children: Ultrastructural study of 31 cases. Cancer 46: 2035–2040

Mierau G W, Berry P J, Orsini E N 1985 Small round cell neoplasms: Can electron microscopy and immunohistochemical studies accurately classify them? Ultrastructural Pathology 9: 99–112

Mills S E, Fechner R E, Bruns D E et al 1981 Intermediate filaments in eosinophilic cells of epithelioid sarcoma: A light-microscopic, ultrastructural, and electrophoretic study. American Journal of Surgical Pathology 5: 195–202

Mukai M, Iri H, Nakajima T et al 1983 Alveolar soft part sarcoma. A review on its histogenesis and further studies based on electron microscopy, immunohistochemistry and biochemistry. American Journal of Surgical Pathology 7: 679–689

Mukai M, Torikata C, Iri H et al 1985 Cellular differentiation of epithelioid sarcoma: A light-microscopic, ultrastructural, and electrophoretic study. American Journal of Pathology 119: 44–56

Nunnery E W, Kahn L B, Reddick R L et al 1981 Hemangiopericytoma: A light microscopic and ultrastructural study. Cancer 47: 906–914

Rossouw D J, Cinti S, Dickersin G R 1986 Liposarcoma. An ultrastructural study of 15 cases. American Journal of Clinical Pathology 85: 649–667

Ordonez N G, Ro J Y, Mackay B 1989 Alveolar soft part sarcoma. An ultrastructural and immunocytochemical investigation of its histogenesis. Cancer 63: 1721–1736

Schmidt D, Mackay B 1982 Ultrastructure of human tendon sheath and synovium: Implications for tumor histogenesis. Ultrastructural Pathology 3: 269–278

Schmidt D, Mackay B, Sinkovics J G 1981 Retroperitoneal tumor with vertebral metastasis in a 25-year-old female. Ultrastructural Pathology 2: 383

Schmidt D, Mackay B, Osborne B M et al 1982a Recurring congenital lesion of the cheek. Ultrastructural Pathology 3: 85–90

Schmidt D, Mackay B, Ayala A G 1982b Ewing's sarcoma with neuroblastoma-like features. Ultrastructural Pathology 3: 143–151

Schmidt D, Dickersin Gr, Vawter G F et al (1982) Wilms' tumor: Review of ultrastructure and histogenesis. Pathobiology Annual 12: 281–300

Schmidt D, Harms D, Pilon V A 1987 Small-cell pediatric tumors: histology, immunohistochemistry, and electron microscopy. In: Mackay B (ed) Diagnostic electron microscopy of tumors. Clinics in Laboratory Medicine 7/1: 63

Shimada H, Newton W A, Soule E H. Qualman S J, Aoyama C, Maurer H M 1988 Pathologic features of extraosseous Ewing's sarcoma: a report from the Intergroup Rhabdomyosarcoma Study. Human Pathology 19: 442–453

Suzuki T, Kaneko H, Kojima K, Takatoh M, Hasabe K-I 1988 Extraskeletal myxoid chondrosarcoma characterized by microtubular aggregates in the rough endoplasmic reticulum and tubulin immunoreactivity. Journal of Pathology 156: 51–57

Tetu B, Ordonez N G, Ayala A G et al 1986 Chondrosarcoma with additional mesenchymal component (dedifferentiated chondrosarcoma). II. An immunohistochemical and electron microscopic study. Cancer 58: 287

Troncoso P, Ordonez N G, Raymond A K et al 1988 Malignant granular cell tumor: immunocytochemical and ultrastructural observations. Ultrastructural Pathology 12: 137–144

Tsuneyoshi M, Enjoji M 1982 Glomus tumor. A clinicopathologic and electron microscopic study. Cancer 50: 1601–1607

Tsuneyoshi M, Enjoji M, Shinohara N 1981 Malignant fibrous histiocytoma. An electron microscopic study of 17 cases. Virchow's Archives (Pathological Anatomy) 392: 135–145

Unni K K, Soule E H 1975 Alveolar soft part sarcoma: An electron microscopic study. Mayo Clinic Proceedings 50: 591–598

Wood G S, Beckstead J H, Turner R R et al 1986 Malignant fibrous histiocytoma cells resemble fibroblasts. American Journal of Surgical Pathology 10: 323–335

Wirman J A 1976 Nodular fasciitis: A lesion of myofibroblasts. Cancer 38: 2378–2389

11. The grading and staging of soft tissue sarcomas

J. Costa

INTRODUCTION

Within a given histological type, malignant tumours are not homogeneous. Numerous tumour characteristics, capable of independent progression, combine in a multitude of ways and are responsible for the great diversity of biological behaviour of tumours. Once the diagnosis of a malignant neoplasm is established and confirmed by histopathology, two characteristics of the lesion are determined before deciding therapy: they are the grade and stage of the neoplasm. Whereas grade is attributed on a histological basis, stage results from a combination of an evaluation of the size, local extent and distant spread of the tumour. It can be established clinically or by means of imaging and laboratory techniques. Combined data from both grading and staging are currently the best means of predicting prognosis in soft tissue sarcomas (Mandard et al 1989). Although grading refers to degree of malignancy, thus a biological property, it is common to think of it as histological grade or grade of differentiation. When judging the degree of differentiation, the pathologist compares the tumour tissue to its normal counterpart. It is the degree of architectural and cytological resemblance of the lesion to the tissue it arose from that is translated into a grade. Although, in general, good tissue differentiation correlates with good biological behaviour of tumours, lesions that do not resemble adult or differentiated tissues can exhibit an indolent biological course and thus be at the same time 'undifferentiated' and 'low grade'.

Soft tissue sarcomas (STS) are a heterogeneous group of lesions and this has caused some problems in arriving at a grading system. Grading of large histogenetic groups of neoplasms, like STS, lymphomas or gliomas, carries the danger of ignoring histological typing and classification in favour of a grading system. For soft tissue sarcomas, grading is so intertwined with histological typing that it is hard to conceive that typing could be replaced by grading. The latter is of value because it represents an adjunct for the guidance of therapy and for the stratification of patients entered in prospective randomised studies. It is useful in separating a group of lesions with minimal risk of metastases from lesions with an intermediate risk and a high risk of distant spread. Staging is an approach designed to define the extent of the disease. When this information is derived from the morphological analysis of operative specimens, the stage is qualified as a pathological stage. Staging is crucial at the time of initial diagnosis, but with increasing effectiveness in the rescue of patients with recurrences staging is often repeated at several points in the course of the disease. Diagnosis, grading, staging and treatment of patients with soft tissue tumours are best done in a multidisciplinary centre where close collaboration and exchange exists between surgeons, oncologists, radiotherapists, radiologists and pathologists. The contribution of physical rehabilitation specialists should not be underestimated at the time definitive therapy is planned.

THE GRADING OF SOFT TISSUE SARCOMAS

The clinical presentation and symptomatology of patients with STS is fairly monotonous but histological analysis of the diseased tissue brings considerable diversity to this group of lesions. At least 55 types of malignant tumour are recognised in the most widely accepted classification of STS (Enzinger & Weiss 1983). In 1949, A P Stout clearly stated that the biological behaviour of STS varies with the cell of origin, the location of the lesion and the age of the patient. Since then, numerous studies indicate that each histological type forms a clinicopathological entity but many of the frequent soft tissue tumour types exhibit a wide spectrum of biological aggression and a significant degree of overlap in their clinical evolution or response to therapy. It is thus not surprising that oncologists interested in the multidisciplinary management of STS proposed a classification by histological grade of malignancy. By making histological grade one of the parameters used for staging, the discriminatory prognostic power of staging was enhanced.

Two additional reasons were perhaps also important in establishing the grading of STS. First is the fact that competent pathologists may disagree on the histological classification of a lesion. It is clear that the substantial variation in the reported incidence of the various histological types (Rosenberg et al 1985) reflects differences in pathological opinion rather than true differences in incidence. Second, a significant number of cases defy classification. Between 10% and 20% of STS will be left as unclassified or will be attributed to a category on a highly subjective and arbitrary basis. The majority of unclassified lesions are also biologically aggressive and undifferentiated, but one occasionally encounters a slowly progressing tumour that defies classification. It is clear that, in both these instances, 'grade' constitutes a useful means to convey the malignant potential of a lesion and it thus helps govern therapy and establish prognosis.

The single most important paper giving impulse to grading of STS, already advocated by Broders et al (1939), was the study by Russell et al published in 1977. In the latter paper it is stated that histological grade is the single most important prognostic factor in patients with STS and histological grade is incorporated into the staging system for STS. As Russell had stated earlier

(Suit et al 1975), grading was based in part on subjective evaluation and an assessment of several histological factors. In the last decade a number of multidisciplinary studies have attempted to refine the grading methodology and to remove, at least as far as possible, the subjective facets of this endeavour. Although grading is of undoubted prognostic significance in soft tissue sarcomas, it appears that this practice is not as widely applied as it should be (Henson 1988).

The NCI grading system

The definitions of grades are the following: low grade lesions — grade 1 — are tumours with a tendency to local recurrence if not totally excised, and a minimal risk of metastasis. They differ from benign locally recurring lesions by the fact that they are capable of progression. High grade lesions — grades 2 and 3 — are malignant tumours with an intermediate (grade 2) or a high (grade 3) risk of metastasis from their inception (Fig. 11.1).

The first and most crucial step in arriving at the grade of STS is histological typing or classification. Given its importance it is appropriate to briefly review some general principles of typing. The pathologist must be in possession of the pertinent clinical information (location, size, age, rapidity of growth). When the case is referred to a centre, the histology must be reviewed before therapy is instituted and the gross description of the referring pathologist must accompany the slides. For small lesions up to 3 cm in diameter it is customary to proceed to an excisional biopsy with a carefully planned incision. For larger lesions an incisional biopsy will be preferred. A frozen section on a portion of the incisional biopsy is sometimes useful to ensure that the tissue is adequate for diagnosis and to reserve a small portion for special studies (ultrastructure, biochemical analysis and xenografting). Needle biopsy of large soft tissue masses should be reserved for exceptional occasions and shoud be interpreted with caution by the pathologist. Reactive and benign soft tissue masses can mimic malignancy (Table 11.1) and the overall architectural pattern of the lesion is crucial to arrive at the correct diagnosis. For the same reason, fine-needle aspiration is not an adequate technique to establish the diagnosis of a STS, although it is a useful and efficient technique to document

Table 11.1 Examples of reactive and benign ST lesions containing atypical mesenchymal cells

Reactive conditions	Benign tumours
Myositis ossificans	Degenerating neurofibroma
Proliferative myositis	Ancient schwannoma
Nodular and periosteal fasciitis	Synovial chondromatosis
Radiation changes	Pleomorphic lipoma
Reactive histiocytosis	Giant cell fibroblastoma
Benign vaginal polyps	
Postoperative spindle cell nodules of genitourinary tract	

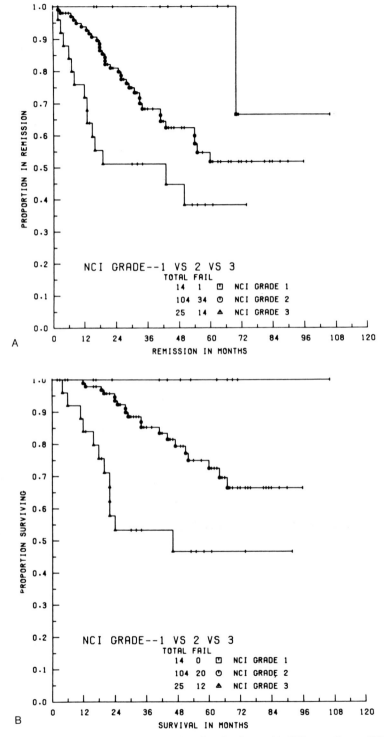

Fig. 11.1   Disease free (**A**) and total survival (**B**) of patients with STS according to NCI grades. (From Costa et al 1984, with permission.)

recurrence (Miralles et al 1986). In practice, 80% to 90% of lesions can be classified on the basis of good haematoxylin-eosin stained sections and conventional special stains, but in some instances electron microscopy and immunohistochemistry will be necessary for histological typing. The latter technique is especially useful, when dealing with undifferentiated tumours, to distinguish between lymphoma, carcinoma, melanoma and sarcoma.

The importance of typing in the grading process resides in the fact that certain histological types, or subtypes, exhibit a narrow spectrum of biological behaviour. They are invariably very aggressive (e.g. alveolar rhabdomyosarcoma) or they will locally recur before metastasising (e.g. lipoma-like liposarcoma). In these cases the histological type directly translates into a histological grade of malignancy. In contrast other types exhibit a wide spectrum of biological aggression. Leiomyosarcomas can vary from a very indolent course to a highly rapid evolution, showing a spectrum from grade 1 to grade 3. Other lesions, such as malignant fibrous histiocytoma and synovial sarcoma, vary between grade 2 and grade 3. What histological criteria can be applied to these neoplasms in order to separate grade 1 lesions from the high-grade group and to distinguish those with an intermediate risk of metastasis from the very aggressive STS?

For tumours with a wide spectrum of biological behaviour, grade 1 lesions can be identified by their well-differentiated character and the mitotic count (Table 11.2). In many instances the grade 1 lesions are those in which their benign versus malignant nature is seriously pondered by the pathologist and can be thus regarded as 'borderline lesions'. Conditions that can morphologically mimic malignancy but that never metastasise, such as desmoid fibromatosis, should not be included with the grade 1 tumours. The crucial difference between a locally recurring benign lesion and a grade 1 sarcoma is the capacity for progression of the latter. Table 11.1 provides a non-exhaustive list of the lesions that can mimic malignancy but that, lacking the potential for progression, should be separated from grade 1 sarcomas.

For the histological types of variable behaviour in which cytological differentiation is sometimes difficult to judge, it is architecture and mitoses that compel the pathologist to classify a lesion as a grade 1 sarcoma. Perhaps one of the most difficult situations is the focal malignant transformation of neurofibromas in patients with von Recklinghausen's disease. I have found foci of hypercellularity containing mitotic figures one of the most reliable signs indicating malignant conversion, and when focal and contained within the mass, I classify the lesion as a grade 1 neurofibrosarcoma (Fig. 11.2).

What histological features distinguish grade 2 from grade 3 lesions ? Studies conducted at the US National Cancer Institute (Costa et al 1984) strongly suggest that a single histological criterion is a powerful discriminator between two groups of metastasising lesions, one of intermediate aggressiveness and a highly malignant one. This criterion was found to be the extent of necrosis present in the primary tumour. Other histological criteria such as pleomorphism, matrix, cellularity and histological type were not as predictively useful as necrosis. In our study, necrosis was approximately quantified in four

Table 11.2 The grading of soft tissue sarcomas

Grade	Morphological criteria used for grading	Common histological types
G1	Histological type or subtype	Lipoma-like liposarcoma
		Myxoid liposarcoma
		Epith. haemangioendothelioma
		Spindle cell haemangioendothelioma
		Infantile fibrosarcoma
	Histological type and location	Deep-seated dermatofibrosarcoma protuberans
		Subcutaneous myxoid MFH
	Histological type, mitoses and differentiation	Well-differentiated malignant haemangiopericytoma
		Well-differentiated leiomyosarcoma
		Well-differentiated neurofibrosarcoma
		Well-differentiated fibrosarcoma
		Myxoid chondrosarcoma
G2/3	Histotype and necrosis	Pleomorphic liposarcoma
	$N < 15\%m = G2$	Round cell liposarcoma
	$N < 15\%m = G3$	Fibrosarcoma
		MFH
		Malignant haemangiopericytoma
		Synovial sarcoma
		Epithelioid sarcoma
		Neurofibrosarcoma
		Leiomyosarcoma
		Angiosarcoma
		Unclassified sarcoma
G3	Histological type	Alveolar rhabdomyosarcoma
		Extraskeletal Ewing's sarcoma
		Mesenchymal chondrosarcoma

groups: absent 0, up to 15% minimal, 15% to 30% moderate and over 30% marked. The difference in behaviour was found to be most significant between the groups 'absent and minimal' versus 'moderate and marked'. This is why 15% necrosis was given as the threshold for separating grade 2 from grade 3 lesions. Although 15% represents an estimate, it is important that it be based on adequate gross and histological sampling and grade can be only regarded as accurately established when it is arrived at after examination of the whole tumour specimen. Next to necrosis, mitotic rate (more or less than 5 per 10 high power fields) showed discriminatory power to distinguish between grade 2 and grade 3 but it failed to reach statistical significance. Other studies have confirmed the prognostic significance of necrosis for STS, and it is of interest that it appears also to carry prognostic implications in Ewing's sarcoma of bone (Llombart-Bosch et al 1986). The NCI study strongly suggests that necrosis did not depend on the histological type of STS and it was found to have prognostic value even among 'unclassified sarcomas'.

Clearly, necrosis could be in direct relation to tumour size, large lesions often having necrotic area. In order to test if necrosis was independent of size, the predictive value of necrosis was tested for lesions less than 100 cm^3 in volume. Although necrosis was more prevalent among large lesions, it retained its predictive power among the 'small size' group. The NCI grading

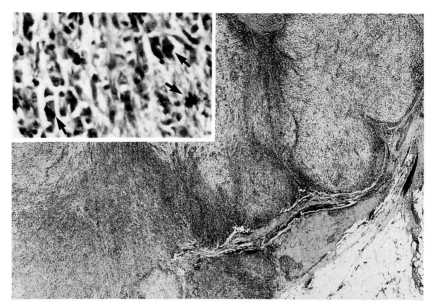

Fig. 11.2 Focal malignant change within a plexiform neurofibroma in a patient with neurofibromatosis. Inset shows dense cellularity with abundant mitotic figures. H + E × 8, inset 330–330.

strategy has been applied to patients treated with surgery alone or with combined modality therapies. In both cases it correlates with disease-free survival and total survival suggesting that it is mostly dependent on a tumour characteristic(s), rather than being strongly influenced by the form of therapy. An interesting result was seen in patients with grade 2 and 3 STS when patient survival was analysed according to the grade of the primary lesion after the first recurrence had taken place. It was found that patients with grade 2 primaries were more often salvaged than patients with grade 3 primaries, even when surgery rendered both grade 2 and 3 patients disease free.

Should local recurrences be graded? For grade 1 STS, grading of local recurrences is essential to govern therapy. Grade 1 lesions that retain their grade when they recur can be treated with a conservative surgical approach and no adjuvant therapy has proven of benefit. However, it is possible for the recurrence of a grade 1 lesion to show histological signs of 'upgrading' (Fig. 11.3). When the round cell component of a recurrent myxoid liposarcoma goes beyond 20% of the lesion, the grade should be changed to grade 2 or 3 depending on necrosis.

For grade 2 and 3 lesions the most common site of initial recurrence is the lung. It has been my experience that a change in grade is seldom observed in local recurrences or in the metastases. Increase in necrosis is not often seen, and other histological features of the local recurrence (mitoses, pleomorphism, cell to matrix ratio) vary in what appears to be a random fashion (Table 11.3) (Restrepo & Costa, unpublished results).

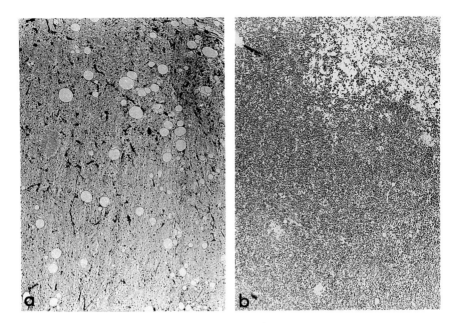

Fig. 11.3 Upgrading of recurrent liposarcoma: **a** primary myxoid liposarcoma. H + E ×
33. **b** 1st recurrence of the tumour depicted in **a** shows conversion to a round cell
liposarcoma H + E × 33.

Table 11.3   Evolution of histological variables with recurrence in five cases of malignant
fibrous histiocytoma

	Recurrence	Histological criteria		
		Mit.	Pleo.	Cellul.
Case 1	1st R	↓	↓	—
	2 R	↑	—	—
Case 2	1 R	↓	↑	↓
	2 R	↑	↑	↓
Case 3	1 R	—	↓	—
	2 R	—	↑	—
Case 4	1 R	↓	—	↓
	2 R	—	—	—
Case 5	1 R	↓	↑	—
	2 R	↓	↓	—
	3 R	↑	—	—

Five cases of NCI grade 2 MFH with two or more local recurrences were quantitatively
analysed in terms of number of mitoses, number of pleomorphic cells and cell to matrix ratio
(cellularity). For 1 R (first recurrence), the comparison is with the primary tissue and the
previous recurrence for each subsequent sample analysed. Analysis of 128 samples belonging
to 33 other patients with other types of sarcoma failed to show any consistent patterns.
[↑ = increase, ↓ = decrease, – = no change.]

Other grading systems

Data from published series in which a 3 or 4 grade scale is used are consistent in indicating a correlation of survival with histological grade. Given the variation observed between grade 2 and 3 or 3 and 4 in four-point systems, it is my feeling that a two-grade system, as proposed by Enneking et al (1980) or by Hajdu (1979), is not discriminative enough and that at least a three-grade system should be used.

Many grading systems are based on cellular pleomorphism, mitotic figures and cellularity (Markhede et al 1982), sometimes modified depending on the histological group of lesions analysed (Rydholm et al 1984). A system derived in France at the Fondation Bergonié and Institut Gustave Roussy (Trojani et al 1984, Coindre et al 1986) is based on a score generated by evaluating three histological criteria: tumour differentiation, mitotic rate and necrosis. Such a grade correlates with disease-free and total survival, and appears to be the most significant prognostic factor in the patient population studied by these authors (Trojani et al 1984). The difference between the Bergonié-Roussy system of grading and the NCI method may be more dependent on terminology than objective criteria. Since differentiation can only be judged by arriving at a histological type and the two other criteria (necrosis and mitosis) are used in both systems, one would predict that if the same patient population is graded by both systems there will be a major overlap.

A study by Rydholm et al (1984), using a four-grade system, found a good correlation with survival (100% grade 1; 91% grade 2; 69% grade 3 and 38% grade 4) and none of the grade 1 lesions metastasised. In addition, Rydholm et al found interesting correlations between grade, depth and size, grade 4 tumours being more often deeper and of larger size that the other grades. This type of correlation should be more often attempted in studies of STS. A recent study (Tsujimoto et al 1988) has, in fact, concluded that the depth of a lesion and its mitotic rate are the best prognostic factors.

THE STAGING OF STS

Staging allows the classification of a neoplasm according to a system which uses size, presence or absence of nodal metastases and presence or absence of distant metastases. The purpose of a staging system is to evaluate the extent of the disease, in order to guide the primary therapeutic modality and the use of adjunctive therapies. Attributing a patient to a stage carries not only therapeutic and prognostic implications, but it is also very useful in order to stratify prospective randomised clinical studies and to be able to compare the resuts of studies conducted in different treatment centres. As emphasised by Suit et al (1985), staging systems are, by design, simplistic and not suited for serious and detailed analysis of clinical results. Some authors regard staging as being unable to provide any more prognostic information than grading alone (Rooser 1987). Staging systems require revision as knowledge expands and therapies become more effective. Detailed clinical and pathological information of each case should be recorded, be available for analysis and compared with the staging system used, in order for the latter to be refined or remodelled if new parameters are proven to be more relevant to establish prognosis and guide therapy.

The different systems of STS staging make use of size, local spread, metastases and histological grade. The inclusion of grade was proposed by Russell et al (1977) and carries the implication that there will be as many different staging systems as grading methodologies. This situation is well illustrated in the paper of Lindberg et al (1985), in which the stage of patients was significantly altered (60% of the sarcomas classified as stage 2 became stage 3) because a change in grading method intervened at a certain moment in time.

The staging systems in use for STS are summarised in Table 11.4. Rather than arguing the merits and problems of each system, usually shown to be useful by its proponents, I will discuss some of the information that should be

Table 11.4 Staging systems for STS

AJC staging for soft tissue sarcomas (Russell et al 1977)

T	Primary tumour
	T_1 Tumour less than 5 cm
	T_2 Tumour 5 cm or greater
	T_3 that grossly invades bone, major vessel or major nerve
N	Regional lymph nodes
	N_0 No histologically verified metastases to regional lymph nodes
	N_1 Histologically verified regional lymph node metastasis
M	Distant metastasis
	M_0 No distant metastasis
	M_1 Distant metastasis
G	Histological grade of malignancy
	G_1 Low
	G_2 Moderate
	G_3 High

Stage I		
Ia	$G_1T_1N_0M_0$	Grade 1 tumour less than 5 cm in diameter with no regional lymph nodes or distant metastases
Ib	$G_1T_2 N_0M_0$	Grade 1 tumour 5 cm or greater in diameter with no regional lymph nodes or distant metastases
Stage II		
IIa	$G_2T_1 N_0M_0$	Grade 2 tumour less than 5 cm in diameter with no regional lymph nodes or distant metastases
IIb	$G_2T_2 N_0M_0$	Grade 2 tumour 5 cm or greater in diameter with no regional lymph nodes or distant metastases
Stage III		
IIIa	$G_3T_1 N_0M_0$	Grade 3 tumour less than 5 cm in diameter with no regional lymph nodes or distant metastases
IIIc	Any $GT_{1-2} N_1M_0$	Tumour of any grade or size (no invasion) with regional lymph nodes but no distant metastases
Stage IV		
IVa	Any $GT_3 N_{0-1}M_0$	Tumour of any grade grossly invades bone, major vessel, or major nerve with or without regional lymph node metastases but without distant metastases
IVb	Any $GTNM_1$	Tumour with distant metastases

recorded to gain knowledge about the natural history of STS. The *size* of the tumour should be recorded in three dimensions and the *extent* of the tumour should mapped and a cartography of spread constructed (Figs 11.4 and 11.5). The main body of the lesion is easily measured but satellite nodules should be taken into account and should be separately measured. Infiltration of adjacent structures should be documented histologically, even if it is well established that malignant soft tissue tumours grow by expansion and tend to respect preformed barriers (Stener 1984). It is well known that a 'shell out' procedure gives a 90% chance of local recurrence because of the persistence of residual disease. The risk of local recurrence when wide local excision is used as the sole therapy varies widely, but is superior to 50% (Rosenberg et al 1985).

The importance of the anatomical setting (intra-versus extra-compartmental) with respect to local spread has been emphasised by Enneking et al (1981). Tumours that arise in intercompartmental planes will

Table 11.4   Staging systems for STS (*Continued*)

Musculoskeletal Society staging system (Enneking et al 1980)

Stage I-A	Low-grade intracompartmental lesion without metastases
Stage I-B	Low-grade extracompartmental lesion without metastases
Stage II-A	High-grade intracompartmental lesion without metastases
Stage II-B	High-grade extracompartmental lesion without metastases
Stage III	Any grade with metastases

Memorial Sloan Kettering Hospital staging system (Hajdu 1979)

Stage O		< 5 cm	Superficial	Low grade
Stage	Ia	< 5 cm	Superficial	High grade
	Ib	< 5 cm	Deep	Low grade
	Ic	> 5 cm	Superficial	Low grade
Stage	IIa	< 5 cm	Deep	High grade
	IIb	> 5 cm	Superficial	High grade
	IIc	> 5 cm	Deep	Low grade
Stage III		> 5 cm	Deep	High grade

MGH proposed staging for the T category (Suit et al 1985)

	Size of primary tumour (cm)	Compartment	Invasion of adjacent structures
T1a	≤ 5	Intracompartmental	No
T1b	≤ 5	Extracompartmental	No
T1c	≤ 5	Extracompartmental	Yes
T2a	5.1–15	Intracompartmental	No
T2b	5.1–15	Extracompartmental	No
T2c	5.1–15	Extracompartmental	Yes
T3a	> 15	Intracompartmental	No
T3b	> 15	Extracompartmental	No
T3c	> 15	Extracompartmental	Yes

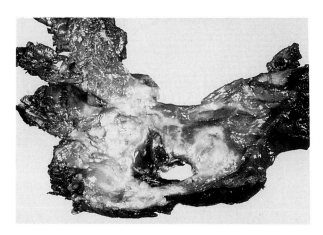

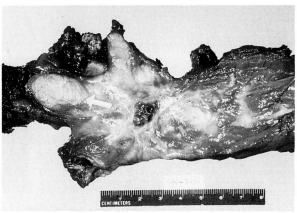

Fig. 11.4 **A** and **B** Serial gross sections through a resection specimen for liposarcoma show the cavity where the primary mass had been excised and satellite intracompartmental nodule (arrow) (**B**).

more easily and rapidly extend longitudinally, as is also the case for intracompartmental lesions that have extended outside their compartment of origin. Bleeding (haematoma) and oedema may encourage tumour cell implants at considerable distances and are a risk of biopsy procedures. It is therefore worthwhile to sample biopsy tracts (Fig. 11.6) and potentially contaminated loose areolar tissue (iron-laden macrophages are a good marker) in order to ascertain the local spread of sarcomas.

If specimens are carefully sectioned it is possible to define the extent of spread. After gross and microscopic study, sarcomas can be classified into three groups:

1. Those with a single mass and no grossly visible satellite nodules
2. Those with satellite nodules no further than 3 cm from the margin of the main mass
3. Those with nodules at a greater distance from the margin of the main mass.

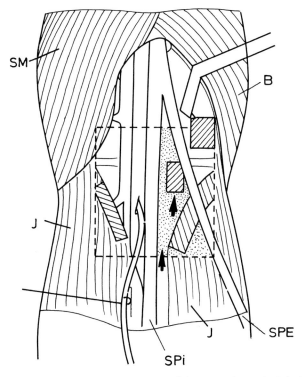

Fig. 11.5 Schema illustrating the exact provenance of tissue samples excised during conservative surgical treatment of an extracompartmental synovial sarcoma of the popliteal space. A single microscopic focus of tumour was found in the specimen marked with an arrow. (Prepared by Dr Reinberg, Division of Paediatric Surgery, University of Lausanne.)

In my experience, satellites within the 3 cm range are found in about half the cases of grade 2 and 3 STS whereas 'distant spread' is less frequent (Table 11.5).

Surgical margins

Surgical margins of resection specimens require a very careful macroscopic study with histological sampling of all suspicious areas. The distance of the margin to gross and microscopic tumour should be measured and recorded in the pathology protocol. Tumour can be at the margin (intralesional) or at a measurable distance. Information on the margin status in 66 patients treated at the NCI (Table 11.6) with conservative surgery, radiation therapy and chemotherapy in 40 cases shows that 6 out of 8 local recurrences took place in patients who had tumour at, or close (within 1 cm) to the surgical margin. The fact that most recurrences are seen in the trunk, head and neck category underscores the difficulties in treating those patients. It is remarkable that a significant number of patients with intralesional excision margins (Table 11.6) did not suffer local recurrence, reflecting the effectiveness of radiotherapy and perhaps systemic chemotherapy in controlling microscopic local disease.

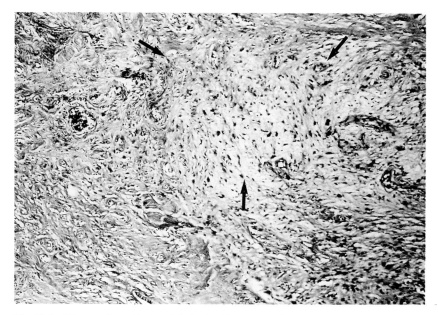

Fig. 11.6 Microscopic residual nodule in the biopsy tract of a subcutaneous myxoid malignant fibrous histiocytoma. Re-excision was performed 2 weeks after the initial excisional biopsy. H + E × 85.

Extension of STS of lymph nodes

Extension of STS to lymph nodes is unusual (5.8% of all STS) except in specific types such as alveolar rhabdomyosarcoma, synovial sarcoma and epithelioid sarcoma. Because the evidence that clear cell sarcoma represents a malignant melanoma arising in soft tissues is strong, I am not including this type among the 'sarcomas metastasising to lymph nodes'. In any event, lymph node metastasis per se has been shown to correlate with a very poor prognosis (Ruka et al 1988).

Table 11.5 Distribution of types of 'local spread' in 60 cases of STS (G2 and G3) and correlation with local recurrence

	Extrem (Loc R)	HN-T (Loc R)	All loc (Loc R)
Local mass	17 (0)	6 (1)	23 (1)
Close nodules	21 (1)	8 (1)	29 (2)
Distant nodules	6 (3)	2 (1)	8 (4)
Total	44 (4)	16 (3)	60 (7)
Local mass:	no gross or microscopic evidence of disease beyond the main tumour mass		
Close nodules:	all gross and microscopic disease within 3 cm of the margin of the main tumour mass		
Distant nodules:	gross and microscopic disease beyond 3 cm of the margin of the main tumour mass		

Loc R (local recurrence) : number of patients that showed a local recurrence. Median follow up: 1539 days.
HN-T: head, neck and trunk.

Table 11.6 Distribution of surgical margin categories in 66 patients and correlation with local recurrence

	Extrem (Loc R)	HN-T (Loc R)	All loc (Loc R)
T at M	12 (1)	14 (4)	26 (5)
M within 1 cm of T	10 (1)	5 (0)	15 (1)
M beyond 1 cm of T	12 (0)	13 (2)	25 (2)
Total	34 (2)	32 (6)	66 (8)
T at M	Margin intralesional gross or microscopic		
T within 1 cm	Gross or microscopic disease within 1 cm of the margin		
M beyond 1 cm	More than 1 cm of tissue free of microscopic disease		

Loc-R: local recurrence; HN-T: head, neck and trunk.
Median follow up: 1539 days.

Lung metastases

The histological diagnosis of lung metastases seldom causes problems to the pathologist. On occasion a solitary metastasis will mimic a pulmonary primary sarcoma. An occult, usually retroperitoneal, primary will be detected later. I have seen synovial sarcoma in the retroperioneum metastasise and mimic a primary pulmonary malignant haemangiopericytoma, one year before the retroperitoneal primary mass became symptomatic.

When examining lung metastases of unclassified sarcomas, the pathologist should be careful not to interpret entrapped reactive terminal bronchioles or alveolar epithelium as tumour glands and reclassify the case as a synovial sarcoma. Regression of pulmonary metastasis after intensive chemotherapy can be histologically proven, with total necrosis of the neoplastic tissue and subsequent fibrosis.

SPECIAL PROBLEMS IN THE GRADING AND STAGING OF SARCOMAS

There are three situations which deserve a brief special comment. The first one is the problem of *sarcomas of childhood* (Miser & Pizzo 1985). Soft tissue sarcomas account for approximately 6% of all malignant neoplasms under the age of 15. Five per cent of all solid tumours are rhabdomyosarcomas of embryonal or alveolar subtype, with a survival, when treated with combined therapy, of approximately 70%. Although, in terms of their natural history, they are aggressive lesions that disseminate (grade 3), two 'histologies', one 'favourable' (89% 2-year survival) and one 'unfavourable' (72% 2-year survival), have been proposed by the Intergroup Rhabdomyosarcoma Study (IRS) (Miser & Pizzo 1985). These histologies are defined by cytological characteristics, rather than tissue pattern. The two unfavourable cytological categories are 'anaplastic', characteristised by the focal or diffuse presence of enlarged, bizarre, mitotic figures and diffuse nuclear pleomorphism and hyperchromatism, and the 'monomorphic round cell', characterised by round cells of uniform size and constant cytological features. It remains to be confirmed if such a distinction allows the selection of patients who are at increased risk of recurrence and who may profit from more intensive therapy. The IRS has used a 'clinical grouping system' instead of stages for childhood rhabdomysarcomas, and the stages are defined in Table 11.7.

Fibrosarcoma of childhood accounts for up to 11% of non-myogenous neoplasms in children. When seen under the age of 5, this neoplasm practically never metastasises and it should be therefore classified as a grade 1 lesion (Table 11.2). In children older than 10 years of age, the lesion behaves in a similar fashion as in adults.

The second area that will require attention in the future is the pathological *staging and grading of tumours treated preoperatively.* Radiation therapy has been advocated as a preoperative modality by Suit et al (1985) on the basis that one can restrict treatment volume, increase resectability, and decrease the chance of autotransplantation from exfoliation. Regional preoperative chemotherapy has also been used as a limb salvage strategy in patients with extremity sarcomas by Eilber et al (1985), as well as by Honnegger et al (1986). Clearly, preoperative radiation and chemotherapy will modify the degree of 'spontaneous' tumour necrosis, which is one of the grading criteria used in many systems. It is also likely that it will make typing difficult when the diagnosis is not unequivocally established in the biopsy.

It has been claimed that the pathological estimation of the degree of regression is the main objective after preoperative chemotherapy (Azzarelli et al 1986) but the following difficulties must be acknowledged :

1. Areas of induced necrosis are indistinguishable from spontaneous necrosis

2. It is difficult to evaluate irreversible cytological damage that does not give an image of massive necrosis

3. Sampling of the tissue is likely to be crucial.

Beside necrosis, extensive hyaline sclerosis surrounding small rests of morphologically intact tumour cells has been observed after preoperative chemotherapy.

Table 11.7 The clinical grouping system of the Intergroup rhabdomyosarcoma studies

Group 1	Localised disease, completely resected Regional nodes not involved Confined to muscle or organ of origin Contiguous involvement-infiltration outside the muscle or organ of origin, as through fascial planes
Group 2	Regional disease Grossly resected tumor with microscopic residual disease. No evidence of gross residual disease. No clinical or microscopic evidence of regional node involvement Regional disease, completely resected (regional nodes involved and completely resected with no microscopic residual) Regional disease with involved nodes, grossly resected, but with evidence of microscopic residual
Group 3	Incomplete resection or biopsy with gross residual disease
Group 4	Metastatic disease present at onset

Finally the question is asked: can the knowledge gained about mesenchymal tumours in the soft tissue be applied to *visceral lesions* ? For sarcomas arising in the mammary gland there is a suggestion that certain morphological parameters, such as tissue type, can be useful in predicting prognosis (Austin & Dupree 1986). Other visceral locations, such as uterine sarcomas, should be studied from this point of view. Although I use the NCI grading system for visceral lesions, I do not believe that therapeutic decisions for visceral lesions should be based heavily on the histological grade of malignancy until the pertinent studies are carried out.

REFERENCES

Austin R M, Dupree W B 1986 Liposarcoma of the breast: a clinicopathologic study of 20 cases. Human Pathology 17: 906–913

Azzarelli A, Gennari L, Vaglini M et al 1986 Intra-arterial infusion and perfusion chemotherapy for soft tissue sarcomas of the extremities. In: Pinedo H M, Verweij J (eds) Clinical management of soft tissue sarcomas. Martinus Nijhoff, Boston, p 103

Broders A C, Hargrave R, Meyerding H W 1939 Pathologic features of soft tissue fibrosarcoma. Surgery, Gynecology and Obstetrics 69: 267–272

Coindre J M, Trojani M, Contesso G et al 1986 Reproducibility of a histopathological grading system for adult soft tissue sarcoma. Cancer 58: 306–309

Costa J, Wesley R A, Glatstein E et al 1984 The grading of soft tissue sarcomas. Results of a clinicopathologic correlation in a series of 163 cases. Cancer 53: 530–541

Eilber F R, Guiliano A E, Husk J et al 1985 Limb salvage for high grade soft tissue sarcomas of the extremity: Experience at University of California, Los Angeles. Cancer Treatment Symposia 3: 49–57

Enneking W F, Spanier S S, Goodman M A 1980 A system for the surgical staging of musculo-skeletal sarcoma. Clinical Orthopaedics and Related Research 153: 106–120

Enneking W F, Spanier S S, Malawer M M 1981 The effect of the anatomic setting on the results of surgical procedures for soft parts sarcoma of the thigh. Cancer 47: 1005–1022

Enzinger F M, Weiss S W 1983 In: Soft tissue tumors. Mosby C V, St Louis

Hajdu S I 1979 Pathology of soft tissue tumors. Lea and Febiger, Philadelphia

Henson D E 1988 The histological grading of neoplasms. Archives of Pathology and Laboratory Medicine 112: 1091–1096

Honegger H P, Cserhati M, von Hochstetter A R et al 1986 A pilot study of chemotherapy containing Adriamycin by continuous infusion, Cytoxan and DTIC in patients with soft tissue sarcoma, applied preoperatively and in metastatic disease. In: Neoadjuvant chemotherapy. Colloque INSERM. John Libbey Eurotext 137: 599–605

Lindberg R 1985 Treatment of localized soft tissue sarcomas in adults at MD Anderson Hospital and Tumor Institute. Cancer Treatment Symposia 3: 59–65

Llombart-Bosch A, Contesso G, Henry-Amar M et al 1986 Histopathological predictive factors in Ewing's sarcoma of bone and clinicopathological correlations. A retrospective study of 261 cases. Virchows Archiv A 409: 627–640

Mandard A M, Petiot J F, Marnay J et al 1989 Prognostic factors in soft tissue sarcoma. A multivariate analysis of 109 cases. Cancer 63: 1437–1451

Markhede G, Angervall L, Stener B 1982 A multivariate analysis of the prognosis after surgical treatment of soft tissue tumors. Cancer 49: 1721–1733

Miralles T G, Gosalbez F, Menendez P et al 1986 Fine needle aspiration cytology of soft tissue lesions. Acta Cytologica (Baltimore) 30: 671–678

Miser J S, Pizzo P A 1985 Soft tissue sarcomas in childhood. Pediatric Clinics of North America 32: 779–800

Rooser B 1987 Prognosis in soft tissue sarcoma. Acta Orthopaedica Scandinavica 58 Supplement 225: 1–54

Rosenberg S A, Suit H D, Baker L H 1985 Sarcomas of the soft tissues. In DeVita, Hellman,

Rosenberg (eds) Cancer principles and practice of oncology, 2nd edn. Lippincott J B, Philadelphia, p 1249

Ruka W, Emrich L J, Driscoll D L, Karakousis C P 1988 Prognostic significance of lymph node metastasis and bone, major vessel or nerve involvement in adults with high-grade soft tissue sarcomas. Cancer 62: 999–1006

Russell W O, Cohen J, Enzinger F M et al 1977 A clinical and pathological staging system for soft tissue sarcomas. Cancer 40: 1562–1570

Rydholm A, Berg N O, Gullberg B et al 1984 Epidemiology of soft tissue sarcomas in the locomotor system. A retrospective population based study of the inter-relationships between clinical and morphological variables. Acta Pathologica, Microbiologica et Immunologica Scandinavica Section A Pathology 92: 363–374

Stener B 1984 Musculo-skeletal tumor surgery in Goeteborg. Clinical Orthopaedics and Related Research 191: 8–20

Suit H D, Russell W O, Martin R G 1975 Management of patients with sarcoma of soft tissue in an extremity. Cancer 35: 1478–1483

Suit H D, Mankin H J, Shiller A et al 1985 Staging systems for sarcoma of soft tissue and sarcoma of bone. Cancer Treatment Symposia 3: 29–36

Suit H D, Mankin H J, Wood W C et al 1985 Preoperative, intraoperative and postoperative radiation in the treatment of primary soft tissue sarcoma. Cancer 55: 2659–2667

Trojani M, Contesso G, Oindre J M et al 1984 Soft tissue sarcomas of adults: Study of pathological and prognostic variables and definition of a grading system. International Journal of Cancer 33: 37–42

Tsujimoto M, Aozasa K, Ueda T, Morimura Y, Komatsubara Y, Doi T 1988 Multivariate analysis for histologic prognostic factors in soft tissue sarcomas. Cancer 62: 994–998

12. Progress in benign soft tissue tumours

C. D. M. Fletcher   P. H. McKee

While advances are occasionally made in determining the histogenesis or aetiology of a given lesion, arguably the most important step forward is the recognition or accurate clinicopathological delineation of new entities, particularly of those tumours which had frequently been misclassified as sarcomas. Such progress has a profound effect on clinical management and, of course, makes a great difference to the patient. Despite such a dogmatic statement, the significant contribution of work which has increased our understanding of tumour biology, without any apparent clinical effect as yet, should not be underestimated.

Most of the benign tumours which had formerly often been mislabelled as malignant, such as pleomorphic lipoma or fibrosseous pseudotumour of the digits, are covered in Chapter 13. This group accounts for the majority of newly described benign soft tissue neoplasms. However, it is also important that *histologically* benign lesions be accurately classified for two principal reasons. Firstly, this facilitates accurate prediction of the clinical course (particularly with regard to the possibilities of local recurrence, spontaneous regression or the development of multicentric lesions). Infantile myofibromatosis (Chung & Enzinger 1981, Fletcher et al 1987) illustrates this point well: correct diagnosis allows the assurance that most cases regress spontaneously (hence overenthusiastic surgery may be avoided in a small child) and multicentricity may be anticipated in 25% of patients, preventing misinterpretation as metastatic spread. Secondly, appropriate histological categorisation is the only means by which our insight into the biological nature of a given lesion is ever increased. In most cases, it is simply not acceptable on the basis of a confidently benign diagnosis to avoid or ignore further classification where this might have been possible. Furthermore, such shoddy practices will inevitably lead to dangerous errors, since in no other group of tumours is there such a propensity for benign lesions to appear cytologically malignant and vice versa.

In this chapter, some of the recently recognised benign tumours, which should not be confused with sarcomas, are described and new data about some of the better known entities are briefly discussed.

NEW ENTITIES

Giant cell fibroblastoma

This tumour was first described by Shmookler and Enzinger in 1982. To date their own findings have only been published in Abstract form,[*] although the AFIP material (25 cases) has been described in rather more detail in an extensive review of infantile and childhood soft tissue tumours by Chung (1985). Three further cases were described by Abdul-Karim et al (1985) and, most recently, seven cases have been reported and comprehensively illustrated by Dymock et al (1987).

Combining these data with our own experience of this lesion (Fletcher 1988), giant cell fibroblastoma arises most often before the age of 5 years, although occasional cases present in adolescence or adulthood. Approximately 70% of patients are male. The trunk is the single commonest site, although almost any location may be affected. The tumour, which is solitary, arises in superficial soft tissue, is slowly growing and painless and seems always to measure less than 6 cm in diameter.

Histologically, there are two principal components — solid and 'angiectoid' (Dymock et al 1987, Fletcher 1988). The solid areas (Fig. 12.1) are composed of variably cellular fibrous tissue, ranging from a fascicular, rather neural-looking pattern of spindle cells with wavy collagen fibres and a myxoid stroma

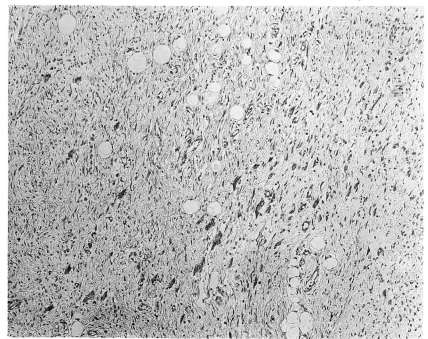

Fig. 12.1   Giant cell fibroblastoma. The solid areas have a rather neural appearance, with admixed multinucleate giant cells. × 100.

[*] The AFIP series has very recently appeared in Cancer 64, 2154–2161 1989.

to densely sclerotic, hyalinised foci. Scattered bizarre giant cells with apparently multiple nuclei are present in the solid component, as are occasional adipocytes. The 'angiectoid' areas (Fig. 12.2) are the most striking feature of this tumour and consist principally of irregular, branching and often dilated spaces with an incomplete lining of bizarre giant cells and hyperchromatic mononuclear cells. These spaces do not seem to have an endothelial lining and contain palely staining acid mucopolysaccharides. Electron microscopy has suggested that the spindle cells and bizarre giant cells are of fibroblastic origin and that the latter cells, in fact, contain only one very large multilobated nucleus. Cells lining the lymphatic-like spaces show no ultrastructural or immunohistochemical evidence of endothelial differentiation (Fletcher 1988, Chou et al 1989).

Follow up reveals a local recurrence rate of about 50%, but, despite this high figure, these tumours do not seem to be locally destructive in the manner of desmoid fibromatoses. The very distinctive histological appearances do not allow any differential diagnosis.

Aggressive angiomyxoma

This tumour was originally reported by Steeper and Rosai (1983) and, at that time, was thought to be confined to females. Subsequently identical lesions

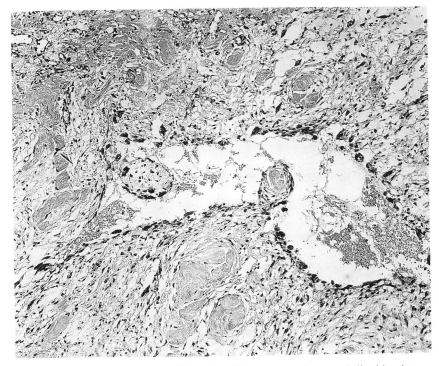

Fig. 12.2 Giant cell fibroblastoma. The angiectoid spaces are at least partly lined by giant cells and often contain small amounts of mucin. × 100.

have been described in males (Begin et al 1985). All published cases to date have arisen in the pelvic region, most notably the vulva and perineum. The overwhelming majority present in adult life, particularly in the third and fourth decades, as a large, ill-defined mass which is often thought clinically to be cystic. Macroscopically, these lesions are typically greater than 10 cm in diameter, are only partially encapsulated and have a soft, gelatinous cut surface.

Histologically, aggressive angiomyxoma has infiltrative margins and is composed of small, stellate, or spindle-shaped cells set in a copious, pale myxoid matrix (Fig. 12.3). The distinctive feature is the presence of large numbers of variably sized blood vessels, showing characteristically marked thickening or hyalinisation of their walls (Fig. 12.4). Extravasated red cells are common. These vessels do not have the arborising pattern of myxoid liposarcoma, nor are lipoblasts identifiable. While the stroma of primary tumours is relatively hypocellular, local recurrence may be associated with a marked increase in cellularity, but mitoses are generally not seen. Ultrastructurally, the stromal cells have the features of myofibroblasts and recent work has suggested that they express desmin, actin and vimentin (Manivel et al 1987). The myxoid matrix appears, non-specifically, to be composed mainly of hyaluronic acid.

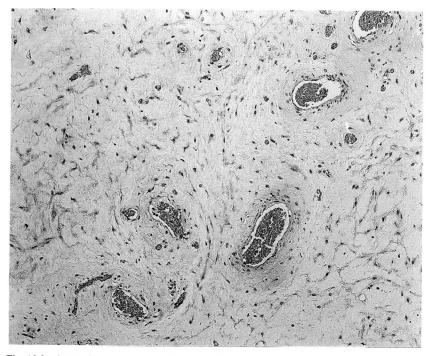

Fig. 12.3 Aggressive angiomyxoma. Rather stellate cells are set in an aboundant myxoid matrix containing prominent vessels. × 100.

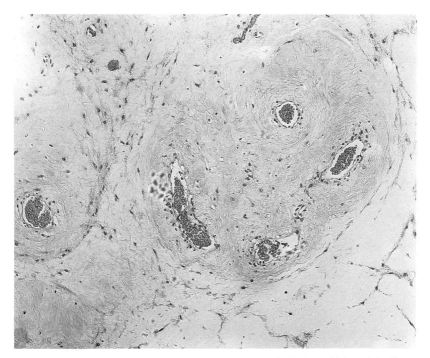

Fig. 12.4 Aggressive angiomyxoma. The blood vessels typically have thickened, hyaline walls. × 100.

The designation 'aggressive' is well earned, since at least 70% of cases recur locally, often after a long period and the recurrences are often very large. Wide excision of the primary lesion seems advisable if later, more destructive surgery is to be avoided. However, the typically infiltrative nature of this unusual tumour often makes this impossible.

Differential diagnosis is usually straightforward. Myxoid neurofibroma is excluded by the prominent vascular pattern and the absence of ultrastructural or immunohistochemical evidence of Schwann cell differentiation. Intramuscular myxoma is almost totally devoid of blood vessels and is rare in the pelvis. Myxoid malignant fibrous histiocytoma shows obvious pleomorphism with multinucleate giant cells and almost always has extremely cellular foci. Embryonal rhabdomyosarcoma is uncommon at this age and either contains identifiable rhabdomyoblasts or shows evidence of myogenic differentiation by more specialised techniques. As mentioned above, myxoid liposarcoma is excluded by the absence of either a plexiform vascular pattern or lipoblasts.

Interestingly, one of us (CDMF) has seen a small number of histologically similar tumours arising in superficial soft tissue outside the pelvis. Such lesions occur in either sex, seem to be smaller and appear less likely to recur. A fairly substantial series of such cases has recently been published under the name 'superficial angiomyxoma' (Allen et al 1988).

Fibrolipomatous hamartoma of nerve

This is a very rare and clinicopathologically unusual entity which, despite scattered case reports (e.g. Patel et al 1979) dating back over 30 years, was not properly delineated until the AFIP series of 26 cases was published by Silverman and Enzinger in 1985.

Fibrolipomatous hamartoma of nerve presents most often in adolescence or early adulthood as a slowly expanding mass, most often located in the wrist or hand. About 25% of patients have diffuse enlargement of an associated digit, affecting both soft tissues and bone, and in this group females seem to be most often affected. In the absence of macrodactyly, the sex incidence is approximately equal. In many patients the mass seems to have been noticed since birth or early childhood and a proportion develop neurological symptoms, often indicative of a compression neuropathy.

At operation, the mass is found to represent fusiform expansion of a nerve by fibrofatty tissue. Most often the median nerve or one of its branches is affected.

By light microscopy, it may be hard to appreciate that the lesion is intraneural since there is gross expansion of the epineurium by mature fibrofatty tissue, which widely separates the individual nerve bundles (Fig. 12.5). The nerve bundles themselves often show striking perineural and endoneural fibrosis (Fig. 12.6). Perivascular fibrosis may also be prominent.

Silverman and Enzinger (1985) regarded this lesion as hamartomatous since it seemed to represent disorderly overgrowth of normal fat and fibrous tissue within the epineurium from an early age. Such a suggestion is impossible to refute, although it remains unclear why some cases have associated macrodactyly.

Since excision of the lesion inevitably leads to a severe neurological deficit, it seems most approriate, if possible, to make the diagnosis on a small biopsy and then to treat any neurological symptoms separately, e.g. by carpal tunnel decompression.

Cellular schwannoma

This tumour is included in the 'benign' rather than 'pseudosarcomatous' chapter, since in real terms it is only likely to be labelled malignant if its neural origin is not appreciated. It is most often mistaken, nowadays, for a smooth muscle tumour of deep soft tissue, in which case the presence of mitotic activity might precipitate a diagnosis of leiomyosarcoma.

Cellular schwannoma was first defined as a clinicopathological entity by Woodruff et al in 1981. For some time, doubt was cast on the existence of this entity, since some reputable authors felt that Woodruff's cases were low-grade malignant nerve sheath tumours which had been inadequately followed up (Ducatman et al 1986), and a recent authoritative review article classified cellular schwannoma as a 'soft tissue tumour of uncertain malignancy' (Angervall et al 1986). However, a recently published series has confirmed Woodruff and

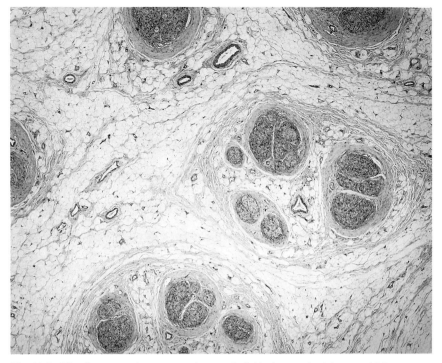

Fig. 12.5 Fibrolipomatous hamartoma of nerve. Individual nerve fascicles are widely separated by fibroadipose tissue. (Case courtesy of Dr J. Van der Walt, The London Hospital Medical College.) × 25.

colleagues' findings and, by obtaining a median follow-up of 12 years, has proved the truly benign nature of this neoplasm (Fletcher et al 1987).

Cellular schwannoma accounts for rather less than 10% of all schwannomas (neurilemmomas), has an equal sex incidence and presents most often in the 4th to 6th decades. It frequently arises in the mediastinum or retroperitoneum, often in a paravertebral location, where it may attain a considerable size. Up to 20% of cases are asymptomatic and are found incidentally on routine radiological examination. Intraoperatively, demonstrable origin from a major nerve is common and occasional cases may be associated with neurofibromatosis.

Macroscopically, these lesions are well-circumscribed, often encapsulated and may show degenerative myxoid or cystic change. Necrosis is not a feature, although haemorrhage may sometimes be evident.

Histologically, cellular schwannoma is predominantly composed of interlacing fascicles or whorls of eosinophilic spindle cells, which, although superficially resembling smooth muscle cells, have slender, wavy nuclei of neural type (Fig. 12.7). Nuclear palisading is uncommon and Verocay bodies are almost always absent. In the spindle cell areas, the stroma is sometimes hyalinised or myxoid. Elsewhere, foci of Antoni B type tissue may be evident, and typical thick-walled vessels with hyalinised walls are common. A dense

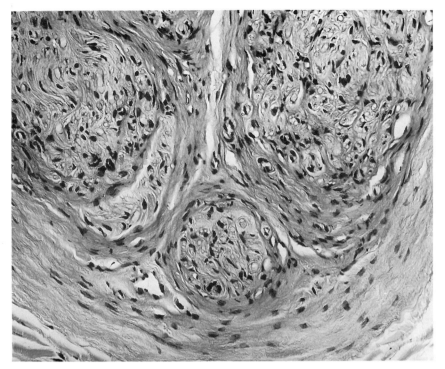

Fig. 12.6 Fibrolipomatous hamartoma of nerve. Note the marked perineurial and endoneurial fibrosis (Case courtesy of Dr J. Van der Walt, The London Hospital Medical College.) × 250.

peripheral lymphocytic infiltrate is frequently present and about 30% of cases contain striking collections of large, foamy histiocytes. In about half the cases, scattered mitoses are identified in the spindle cell element, but these are always of normal configuration and never exceed 5 per 20 high power fields in number. Nuclear pleomorphism and hyperchromasia may be evident adjacent to degenerate cystic or hyalinised foci, but in these areas mitoses are not seen.

Differential diagnosis from a smooth muscle tumour is best achieved by the invariable S-100 positivity in cellular schwannoma, combined with the frequent history of origin from a nerve. Smooth muscle tumours are also distinguished by their blunt, cigar-shaped nuclei and longitudinal myofibrils on a trichome or PTAH stain. Malignant nerve sheath tumours are more mitotically active, show greater pleomorphism and frequently show foci of necrosis. Perivascular whorling and invasion of vessel walls are common features and heterologous differentiation is quite often present.

Plexiform schwannoma

Although this tumour was described in Abstract form by Harkin et al in 1978 and two short reports followed (Woodruff et al 1983, Barbosa & Hansen

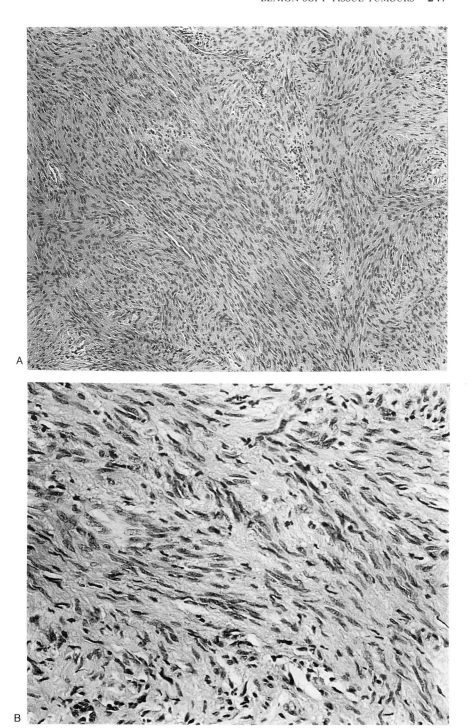

Fig. 12.7 Cellular schwannoma. At lower power, note the resemblance to a smooth muscle tumour (**A**), although at higher magnification the nuclei have a neural quality (**B**). (**A**) × 100 (**B**) × 400.

1984), it was not formally delineated as a clinicopathological entity until quite recently (Fletcher & Davies 1986).

Plexiform (multinodular) schwannoma accounts for between 4% and 5% of all schwannomas (neurilemmomas) and presents most often before the age of 40 years, frequently having been noticed as a slowly growing nodule since early childhood. The sex incidence is equal. It typically arises in the head and neck region or trunk (in contrast to conventional schwanno-mas) and was not thought to be associated with von Recklinghausen's neurofibromatosis. However, one case has been associated with what the authors describe as 'schwannomatosis' (Qureshi et al 1986) and two very recently published examples were apparently found in patients with von Recklinghausen's disease (Iwashita & Enjoji 1987). Even so, it would appear that only about 7% of cases have shown such an association, in stark distinction to plexiform neurofibroma which is *always* indicative of neurofibromatosis.

Macroscopically, most lesions are situated in the dermis or subcutis and the majority measure less than 5 cm in diameter. Multinodularity is not always evident to the naked eye.

Histologically, plexiform schwannoma is composed of multiple (usually 10 to 20), discrete encapsulated nodules, predominantly composed of Antoni A type cellular tissue showing frequent nuclear palisading (Fig. 12.8). As in ordinary schwannomas, Verocay bodies are by no means always identified. Areas of hypercellularity and nuclear pleomorphism are quite common, but mitotic activity is only evident in occasional cases (Woodruff et al 1983, Iwashita & Enjoji 1987). Electron microscopy confirms that the lesion is composed of hyperplastic schwann cells (Harkin et al 1978).

Follow-up reveals that only occasional cases recur locally and, in contrast to plexiform neurofibroma, malignant transformation has never been docu-mented. For this reason, distinction from plexiform neurofibroma, although fairly easy, is vital. This distinction is also important because pleomorphism and mitotic activity in a plexiform neurofibroma could be construed as evidence of malignancy.

Intravenous pyogenic granuloma

This rare lesion was first described by Cooper et al in 1979. Since then only occasional cases have been reported (Ulbright & Santa Cruz 1980).

Intravenous pyogenic granuloma presents most often as a solitary nodule in the neck or upper limb of an adult, typically in the 3rd or 4th decades, with an equal sex incidence. Most examples have been present for less than 2 months. Clinically, there are no features to suggest the tumour's vascular nature but, at operation, the nodule is usually recognised to be situated within a vein and typically measures less than 2 cm in diameter.

By light microscopy, the lesion consists of a pedunculated intravascular mass composed of lobulated collections of small, often uncanalised capillaries

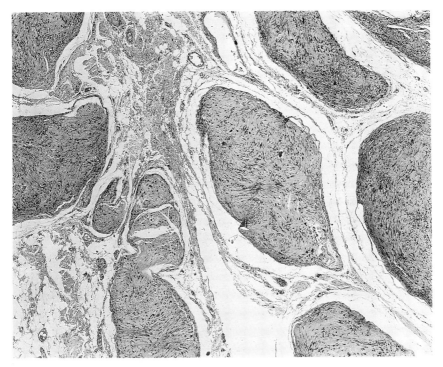

Fig. 12.8 Plexiform schwannoma. Multiple discrete nodules of schwannomatous tissue, predominantly Antoni A in type, are evident. × 40.

set in a fibrous stroma (Fig. 12.9). The capillary endothelial cells are frequently rather plump and mitotically active and the stroma contains moderate numbers of mixed inflammatory cells, However, unlike cutaneous pyogenic granuloma, surface ulceration and a prominent polymorph infiltrate are not seen. These lesions always seem to extend into the vein wall, at which site they are associated with a small feeding artery, branches of which extend into the tumour's stroma.

Differential diagnosis is usually not a problem, since there is no other comparable intravascular neoplasm. Perhaps the only lesion which may look similar is the intravascular variant of epithelioid haemangioma (angiolymphoid hyperplasia with eosinophilia) (Rosai & Ackerman 1974), which, however, shows the characteristic endothelial appearances (see below) and typically has an adjacent extravascular component in the dermis or subcutis.

Plexiform fibrohistiocytic tumour

This is a very recently described but distinctive neoplasm (Enzinger & Zhang 1988), which typically arises as a solitary nodule in the deep dermis and subcutis of children and young adults. There is an apparent predominance of females and the upper limb is by far the commonest site.

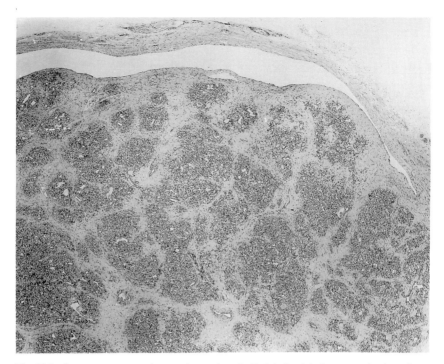

Fig. 12.9   Intravenous pyogenic granuloma. A typically lobulated lesion protrudes into the lumen of this large vein. × 25.

Histologically there are two principal components, the relative proportions of which are very variable (Fig. 12.10). The first and much the most distinctive is composed of nodules of plump, eosinophilic histiocyte-like cells, often associated with osteoclast-like multinucleate giant cells and peripheral hyalinisation. The second element consists of an ill-defined, plexiform array of monomorphic fibroblasts arranged in fascicles, closely resembling those seen in a desmoid fibromatosis. Mitoses are scarce and cytological pleomorphism or necrosis are not present. Occasional cases may show intravascular spread by the tumour.

Clinically, around a third of these lesions recur locally (although not in a destructive fashion). Two of the 65 cases reported by Enzinger and Zhang metastasised to lymph nodes, but widespread dissemination is not known to occur and there have been no fatalities. Wide excision seems the most appropriate treatment. Interestingly, the only published case to have been examined cytogenetically showed complex chromosomal abnormalities (Smith et al 1990).

Intranodal myofibroblastoma

This is a fascinating tumour which was accurately delineated for the first time by both Weiss et al and Suster and Rosai in two separate papers published in May 1989. It presents most often with enlargement of a single lymph node in

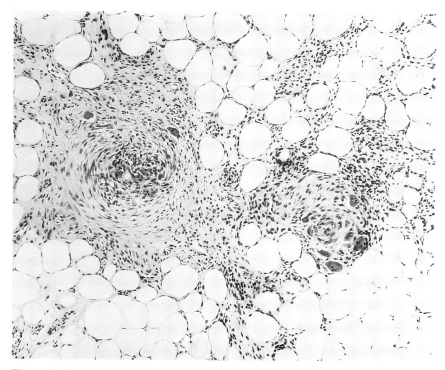

Fig. 12.10 Plexiform fibrohistiocytic tumour. Part of a typically ill-defined lesion showing an admixture of fibroblasts, histiocyte-like cells and osteoclast-type giant cells. × 100.

the groin, although occasionally other sites may be affected (Fletcher & Stirling 1990), and appears to be confined to adults of either sex.

Histologically, most of the lymph node is replaced by a well-circum-scribed mass of bland eosinophilic spindle cells, which is separated from the compressed cortex by a dense fibrous pseudocapsule (Fig. 12.11). The spindle cells quite closely resemble smooth muscle cells, are arranged in short intersecting fascicles and frequently show a degree of nuclear pali-sading (hence the previous mistaken name of lymph node schwannoma). Extravasation of red blood cells may be prominent, leading to confusion with Kaposi's sarcoma, and another striking, but not invariable, feature is the presence of nodular or band-like hyalinisation with a rather frayed or stellate outline, known as 'amianthoid fibres'. Tumour cells are desmin negative but actin positive and ultrastructurally appear to be myofibro-blasts. Whether that is truly the case or whether they represent specialised myoid cells (normally found in lymph nodes) is uncertain. The clinical course is entirely benign and, to date, no case has even recurred locally.

OTHER RECENT DEVELOPMENTS

In this section, a wide variety of new developments applicable to a disparate group of benign soft tissue tumours are discussed. These are not arranged in

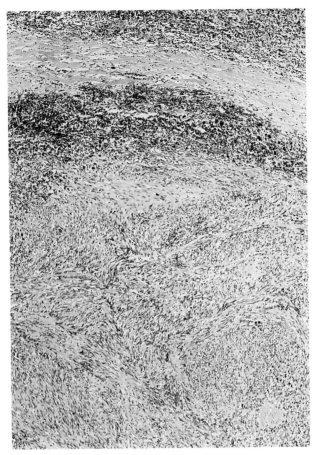

Fig. 12.11 Intranodal myofibroblastoma. Note the hyaline subcortical capsule (top) and the prominent extravasation of red blood cells. (Case courtesy of Dr Juan Rosai, Yale University School of Medicine.) × 63.

any particular order, since it is impossible to rank them in terms of significance.

Angiolymphoid hyperplasia with eosinophilia (epithelioid haemangioma) and Kimura's disease

Despite long-standing aetiological hypotheses and its beautifully descriptive name, angiolymphoid hyperplasia with eosinophilia (ALHE) is now regarded by many authorities as a neoplasm (Rosai 1982, Enzinger & Weiss 1983). The principal reasons for this are that these lesions show little if any tendency spontaneously to involute, not infrequently recur after local excision and may arise at deeply located sites, including skeletal muscle (Buchanan et al 1980), lymph nodes (Suster 1987) and a major arterial wall (Reed & Terazakis 1972, Morton et al 1987). Furthermore, a single case with lymph node micrometastasis has been recorded (Reed & Terazakis 1972). All these features argue against a cutaneous reactive phenomenon as originally proposed (Wells & Whimster 1969, Wilson Jones & Bleehen 1969). Furthermore, those reactive conditions said to be similar or allied to ALHE, such as persistent insect bite reactions or responses to aluminium-containing immunisations, totally lack the characteristic epithelioid endothelial cells (see below), which are the diagnostic *sine qua non* of this condition.

The alternative names of 'histiocytoid' (Rosai et al 1979, Rosai 1982) and 'epithelioid' (Enzinger & Weiss 1983) haemangioma have been suggested, principally because of the strikingly plump, eosinophilic endothelial cells which characterise this entity (Fig. 12.12) and which contain histiocytic-type enzymes (Castro & Winkelmann 1974, Rosai et al 1979). Descriptively there is nothing to choose between these names, but we would favour Enzinger and Weiss's designation 'epithelioid' for two reasons. Firstly, Rosai et al (1979) have lumped together a spectrum of clinically different tumours under the term histiocytoid haemangioma, including epithelioid haemangioendothelioma which is histologically and behaviourly different (Weiss et al 1986), which could therefore lead to clinical confusion. Secondly, the term epithelioid underlines the basic cytological similarity to the other epithelioid endothelial neoplasms, such as the borderline-malignant epithelioid

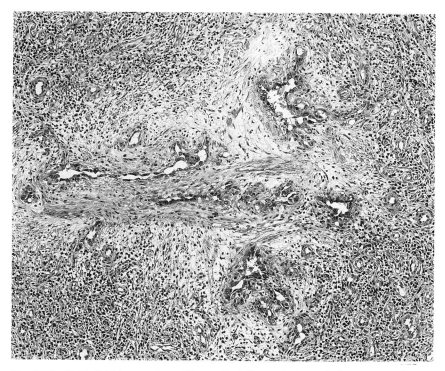

Fig. 12.12 Epithelioid haemangioma. The cardinal diagnostic feature is the presence of very plump endothelial cells with copious esoinophilic cytoplasm. × 100.

haemangioendothelioma (see Ch.13) and the frankly malignant epithelioid angiosarcoma. This then helps create a generic group of tumours with a spectrum of biological behaviour (Weiss et al 1986), notwithstanding that this grouping may be artificial and simply convenient.

Probably more significant, however, than these problems of nomenclature, is the perennial question regarding the relationship, if any, between epithelioid haemangioma and Kimura's disease, the latter having been described 20 years earlier in Orientals (Kimura et al 1948). In our view these two entities are probably different and not even related. Our reasons are based on nothing more sophisticated than the manifest clinical and histological differences.

Epithelioid haemangioma, which has predominantly been reported in Caucasians, characteristically arises in the head and neck region of either sex (mainly females) in the 3rd to 5th decades, although almost any site may be occasionally affected. Patients only occasionally have a circulating eosinophilia or an associated lymphadenopathy. In contrast, Kimura's disease (Kawada et al 1966, Kung et al 1984, Kuo et al 1988), while topographically similar, is largely confined to patients of Oriental extraction, shows a very marked predilection for males and typically presents in adolescence or early adulthood. The majority of cases have an associated lymphadenopathy and circulating eosinophilia. The characteristic histological features of lymph node involvement in Kimura's disease have recently been described (Hui et al 1989). Salivary gland involvement is common.

Histologically there are also striking differences (Rosai et al 1979, Kung et al 1984, Urabe et al 1987), the most notable of which is the lack of plump, epithelioid endothelial cells in the proliferating vessels of Kimura's disease. In fact, the vascular component is altogether less prominent in Kimura's disease than in epithelioid haemangioma, while the lymphocytic infiltrate is more profuse (Fig. 12.13) and lymphoid follicle formation is much more marked. Personally, however, we do not accept Kung and colleagues' suggestion that fibrosis is much greater in Kimura's disease, since long-standing cases of epithelioid haemangioma may sometimes have a very 'burnt-out' fibrotic stroma.

Overall, then, there are good reasons for regarding haemangioma and Kimura's disease as separate entities, at least until such time as racially-predetermined differences in response to an identical initiating stimulus can be demonstrated. This view now appears to have wide support (Weiss et al 1986, Urabe et al 1987, Kuo et al 1988). Recent evidence suggests that Kimura's disease is, in fact, an immunologically-mediated reactive phenomenon characterised by IgE deposition in germinal centres and elevated circulating levels of IgE (Hui et al 1989, Kuo et al 1988).

Irrespective of this contentious terminological discussion, other interesting features of epithelioid haemangioma have emerged in recent years, most notable of which is the demonstration of arteriovenous shunts in the deeper aspect of up to 42% of cases (Olsen & Helwig 1985). The origin of these

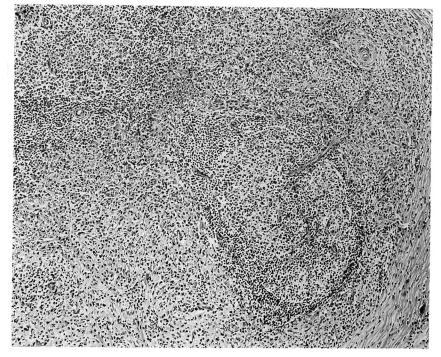

Fig. 12.13   Kimura's disease. This condition is characterised by a more prominent lymphoid infiltrate, often with follicle formation, stromal fibrosis and fairly banal thin-walled vessels. × 100.

shunts is uncertain, but the latter authors have postulated that they may be derived from the vasa vasorum of the large thick-walled vessels around which epithelioid haemangioma often seems to be orientated. Olsen and Helwig also suggested that these shunts represent a neovascularisation process, perhaps resulting directly from whatever the inciting stimulus to these lesions is, and that, if the shunts persist following surgical excision, then they may be responsible for the significant local recurrence rate.

Another much more extraordinary finding has been the demonstration of renin within perivascular stromal cells in seven out of nine cases of epithelioid haemangioma (Fernandez et al 1986). These authors also noted that hypertension in their index patient remitted after removal of two typical subcutaneous lesions. They postulated that the renin-containing cells, by releasing renin in response to ischaemia (perhaps due to the shunts described above), may play a role in tumour angiogenesis within epithelioid haemangioma. Quite what one makes of these thought-provoking results is hard to say, but until they have been substantiated by other authors they should probably be regarded with caution. Fernandez et al provided no data as to the source of their renin antiserum, nor how it was raised. The use of antirenin antibodies of dubious specificity in the past led DeSchryver-Kecskemeti et al

(1982) to suggest that alveolar soft part sarcoma was in fact a malignant angioreninoma, a hypothesis which has subsequently been disproved (Mukai et al 1983).

Infantile digital fibromatosis

Since the original description of this lesion (Reye 1965), the nature of the characteristic, brightly eosinophilic intracytoplasmic inclusions has been a source of both interest and controversy. No convincing evidence has been found to support early proposals of a viral aetiology (Reye 1965, Burry et al 1970) and the possibilities of an altered cellular constituent or abnormal metabolic product have long been favoured (Grunnet et al 1973, Mehregan et al 1972, Stiller & Katenkamp 1975). That this constituent represented an accumulation of contractile filaments became apparent from more recent ultrastructural studies (Faraggiana et al 1981, Mortimer & Gibson 1982) and, latterly, Iwasaki et al (1983) have demonstrated that these filaments appear to be actin by their characteristic binding pattern with heavy meromyosin in tissue culture studies. These authors have suggested, therefore, that the inclusions represent abnormally contracted actin filament bundles within the myofibroblastic tumour cells. To date this seems much the most plausible hypothesis, although the aetiological defect responsible for this phenomenon remains unknown and a subsequent study was unable to confirm the presence of actin (Yun 1988).

New clinicopathological features of this unusual, but readily recognised, tumour have also come to light, which may in due course necessitate a change in this lesion's name.

Firstly, histologically identical tumours have now been recognised in adulthood (Sarma & Hoffman 1980, Viale et al 1988, Fletcher—personal observations). This occurrence may not be as rare as it seems, since the entrenched belief that these lesions only arise in infancy means that bland dermal fibrous proliferations in adulthood may often not be examined closely for characteristic inclusions. Such a proposition would be worthy of careful study in the future.

Secondly, there are now several reports of microscopically classical examples arising outside the digit (Sarma & Hoffman 1980, Purdy & Colby 1984). This would appear to be of no great significance, other than the fact that at other sites this diagnosis might be missed and hence the significant risk of local recurrence may be overlooked. Certainly it is very hard to come up with a good anatomical or biological reason why these neoplasms should be confined to the fingers.

Infantile myofibromatosis

Interest has centred recently on the extent to which these rare lesions are inherited and by what mode. Familial cases have been recorded for many years (Bartlett et al 1961), but their significance was not easily appreciated, since there was much confusion over nomenclature until the seminal paper of Chung and Enzinger (1981). Within the 61 cases recorded by the latter authors were two pairs of siblings and, up to that time, all the evidence culled from the literature pointed to an autosomal recessive mode of inheritance.

However, Jennings et al (1984) recorded the development of identical tumours in both a female infant and her father and then mentioned a second family also afflicted over two successive generations in a short addendum to their paper. In reviewing all the familial cases reported up to that time, they concluded that infantile myofibromatosis was an autosomal dominant condition with incomplete penetrance and that some gene carriers may go unnoticed owing to spontaneous regression of small lesions soon after birth.

The situation has been further confused by a recent report of another set of affected siblings in the absence of parental lesions (Venencie et al 1987), which, like most of the previous familial cases, supports an autosomal recessive disease.

Since infantile myofibromatosis is so rare, it is unlikely that very large numbers of familial cases will be collected in such a way that this question can be resolved. It is possible, however, that the gene responsible may be identified and hence carriers might be identified, perhaps by DNA hybridisation techniques. This would be a potentially very valuable advance, since multicentric visceral involvement is frequently fatal and therefore worth preventing if possible. Furthermore, a fact which published reports of familial cases have not laid emphasis on is that all inherited cases to date have been of the multicentric (although not necessarily visceral) type. Multicentric involvement, which is seen in 26% of all cases of infantile myofibromatosis (Chung & Enzinger 1981), is clearly the disease form most in need of prevention. In addition, if only the multicentric type appears to be inherited, this would fit better with Jennings and colleagues' hypothesis of a generalised, genetically-influenced abnormality of myofibroblastic proliferation.

Benign neural tumours showing Pacinian differentiation

This seemingly banal topic is included since there seems to be much confusion over such lesions, particularly with regard to nomenclature. All manner of tumours seem to be labelled 'Pacinian neurofibroma', often without much justification.

Pacinian differentiation in neural tumours of whatever type is very rare, in contrast to Meissnerian differentiation which is quite common, particularly in diffuse neurofibromata. This is especially true if one retains strict criteria for the recognition of each type of tactile corpuscle. Under normal circumstances, Pacinian corpuscles are large, rounded structures, composed of thin flattened cells arranged in up to 60 closely-packed concentric lamellae, hence the onion-skin appearance. Meissnerian corpuscles, on the other hand, are much smaller ovoid structures with a rather hyalinised, collagenous core containing small numbers of transversely orientated cells.

There appear to be three principal types of benign neural tumour which show Pacinian differentiation, all of which are sufficiently uncommon that hard clinicopathological data are generally lacking. Firstly, there are histologically atypical neurofibromata (Prichard & Custer 1952), which may be of the plexiform type (Schochet & Barrett 1974) within which rather poorly formed, often rather cellular Pacinian corpuscles may be seen (Fig. 12.14). Such lesions seem to be associated with von Recklinghausen's neurofibromatosis. Secondly, there are tumours which would conventionally be classified as schwannomas (neurilemmomas), with typical Antoni A and B areas, which also contain rudimentary Pacinian corpuscles (Fig. 12.15). These cases do not seem to be associated with neurofibromatosis. Thirdly, and perhaps most commonly, there are lesions composed solely of an ill-defined mass of relatively mature Pacinian corpuscles (Fig. 12.16) (Prose et al 1957, Bennin et al 1976, Fletcher & Theaker 1989), which seem to present most often as a painful nodule in the hand or foot (frequently in a digit). These also are not associated with neurofibromatosis and it is tempting to suggest that they usually represent post-traumatic hyperplasia of a structure which is normally pre-eminent at those sites. Whatever their origin, digital Pacinian neuroma would seem the most appropriate name for such tumours.

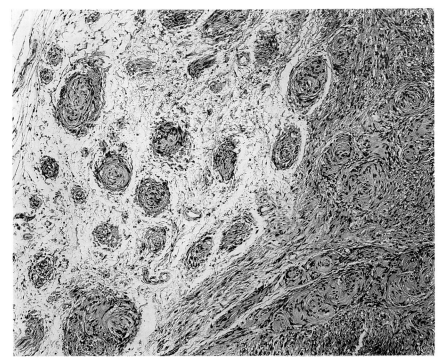

Fig. 12.14 Pacinian neurofibroma. An unusual lesion containing whorled structures resembling Pacinian corpuscles, as well as areas suggestive of Meissnerian differentiation. × 100.

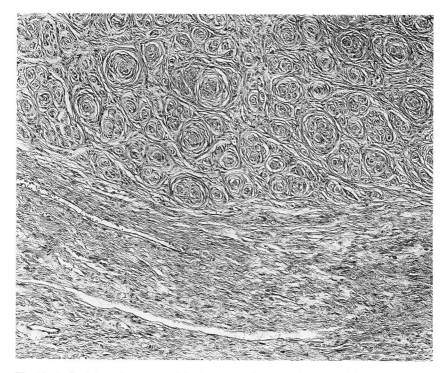

Fig. 12.15 Pacinian schwannoma. A benign encapsulated neoplasm containing numerous whorled structures. × 100.

In addition, Bale (1980) has described two similar cases, composed of innumerable Pacinian corpuscles, overlying the sacrococcygeal region in infants with spina bifida. She regarded these lesions as congenital malformation.

Finally, MacDonald and Wilson Jones (1977) described four cases of a tumour which they labelled Pacinian neurofibroma, but which, in fact, probably represented the first reported series of what is now called dermal nerve sheath myxoma or neurothekeoma (Gallager & Helwig 1980, Fletcher et al 1986). It is interesting to note that all neural tumours showing convincing Pacinian differentiation which have been described to date have been benign.

APPLICATIONS OF MODERN TECHNIQUES

Much of the information covering the use of modern techniques in benign soft tissue tumours has been covered in preceding chapters, particularly Chapter 8 on immunohistochemistry. Soft tissue neoplasms, particularly those that are non-aggressive, have generally been neglected during the molecular biology boom of the last 5–10 years, although this may to some extent reflect the comparative rarity of the more interesting lesions and the general difficulties in obtaining suitably prepared material.

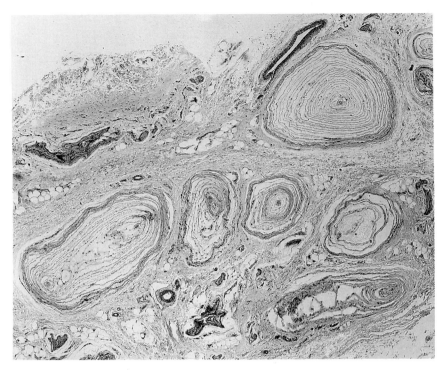

Fig. 12.16   Digital Pacinian neuroma. An example of this rather more common lesion, which is probably hyperplastic in nature. × 40.

Cytogenetic studies have so far revealed a strikingly consistent chromosomal alteration in an admittedly small number of lipomas, perhaps the most mundane but readily available soft tissue tumour. These tumours seem to manifest a non-random translocation between chromosome 3 and the breakpoint q14 on chromosome 12 (Sandberg & Turc-Carel 1987). This finding has, as yet no known significance and, in particular, is not related to sarcomatous change in a lipoma, which appears for all practical purposes not to occur. This point is of some importance since particular chromosomal changes in various non-mesenchymal 'benign' tumours have been associated with a significant risk of malignant transformation. More recent data has now suggested that lipomata may be divisible into several cytogenetic subgroups, some of which show ring chromosomes and some show abnormalities of chromosome 6 (Sait et al 1989). Chromosomal abnormalities have now also been identified in angioleiomyomata (Nilbert et al 1989).

With regard to the analysis of DNA content and proliferative activity of benign soft tissue neoplasms, there is similarly very little published work. In 1980, Eeckhaut et al demonstrated that benign cutaneous fibrous histiocytomas were diploid, using Feulgen-DNA analysis on a microdensitometer. Since then Kreicbergs et al (1987) have shown, by standard flow cytometry, that all of a rather undetailed selection of 23 benign lesion were diploid with a low proportion of cells in S-phase. Those authors, however, had not concerned themselves with examining pseudosarcomatous tumours, in which analysis of DNA content might have proved to be diagnostically useful. However, Angervall et al (1986) quote as yet unpublished work in which nodular fasciitis proved to be consistently diploid. How useful this technique is going to be in the context of soft tissue neoplasia is hard to predict. However, personal preliminary studies (Fletcher & Camplejohn 1987), using flow cytometry, failed to distinguish benign from malignant haemangiopericytomas. In fact this particular question, which is not infrequently a problem, was more reliably solved by simple mitosis counting.

REFERENCES

Abdul-Karim F W, Evans H L, Silva E G 1985 Giant cell fibroblastoma: a report of three cases. American Journal of Clinical Pathology 83: 165–170

Allen P W, Dymock R B, MacCormac L B 1988 Superficial angiomyxomas with and without epithelial components. Report of 30 tumors in 28 patients. American Journal of Surgical Pathology 12: 519–530

Angervall L, Kindblom L-G, Rydholm A, Stener B 1986 The diagnosis and prognosis of soft tissue tumors. Seminars in Diagnostic Pathology 3: 240–258

Bale P M 1980 Sacrococcygeal Pacinioma. Pathology 12: 231–235

Barbosa J, Hansen L S 1984 Solitary multilobular schwannoma of the oral cavity. Journal of Oral Medicine 39: 232–235

Bartlett R C, Otis R D, Laakso A O 1961 Multiple congenital neoplasms of soft tissues. Report of 4 cases in 1 family. Cancer 14: 913–920

Begin L R, Clement P B, Kirk M F, Jothy S, McGauhey W T E, Ferenczy A 1985 Aggressive angiomyxoma of pelvic soft parts: a clinicopathologic study of nine cases. Human Pathology 16: 621–628

Bennin B, Barsky S, Salgia K 1976 Pacinian neurofibroma. Archives of Dermatology 112: 1558

Buchanan R, Sworn M J, Monsley J M 1980 Angiolymphoid hyperplasia with eosinophilia involving skeletal muscle. Histopathology 4: 197–204

Burry A F, Kerr J F R, Pope J H 1970 Recurring digital fibrous tumour of childhood: an electron microscope and virological study. Pathology 2: 287–291

Castro C, Winkelmann R K 1974 Angiolymphoid hyperplasia with eosinophilia. Cancer 34: 1696–1705

Chou P, Gonzalez-Crussi F, Mangkornkanok M 1989 Giant cell fibroblastoma. Cancer 63: 756–762

Chung E B 1985 Pitfalls in diagnosing benign soft tissue tumors in infancy and childhood. In: Sommers S C, Rosen P P, Fechner R E (eds) Pathology Annual, vol 20. Appleton-Century-Crofts, Connecticut, p 323–386

Chung E B, Enzinger F M 1981 Infantile myofibromatosis. Cancer 48: 1807–1818

Cooper P H, McAllister H A, Helwig E B 1979 Intravenous pyogenic granuloma. A study of 18 cases. American Journal of Surgical Pathology 3: 221–228

Deschryver-Kecskemeti K, Kraus F T, Engleman B A 1982 Alveolar soft part sarcoma — a malignant angioreninoma. Histochemical, immunocytochemical and electron microscopic study of four cases. American Journal of Surgical Pathology 6: 5–18

Ducatman B S, Scheithauer B W, Piepgras D G, Reiman H M, Ilstrup D M 1986 Malignant peripheral nerve sheath tumors. A clinicopathologic study of 120 cases. Cancer 57: 2006–2021

Dymock R B, Allen P W, Stirling J W, Gilbert E F, Thornbery J M 1987 Giant cell fibroblastoma. A distinctive, recurrent tumour of childhood. American Journal of Surgical Pathology 11: 263–271

Eeckhaut W, Roels H, MacKenzie D H 1980 Cytophotometric investigation of the Feulgen-DNA content of cell nuclei of fibrous histiocytomas. Histopathology 4: 45–52

Enzinger F M, Weiss S W 1983 Soft tissue tumors. C V Mosby, St Louis
Enzinger F M, Zhang R 1988 Plexiform fibrohistiocytic tumor presenting in children and young adults. An analysis of 65 cases. American Journal of Surgical Pathology 12: 818–826
Faraggiana T, Churg J, Strauss L, Voglino A 1981 Ultrastructural histochemistry of infantile digital fibromatosis. Ultrastructural Pathology 2: 241–247
Fernandez L A, Olsen T G, Barwick K W, Sanders M, Kaliszewski C, Inagami T 1986 Renin in angiolymphoid hyperplasia with eosinophilia. Its possible effect on vascular proliferation. Archives of Pathology and Laboratory Medicine 110: 1131–1135
Fletcher C D M 1988 Giant cell fibroblastoma of soft tissue: a clinicopathological and immunohistochemical study. Histopathology 13: 499–508
Fletcher C D M, Camplejohn R S 1987 DNA flow cytometry in haemangiopericytomas is of no prognostic value. Journal of Pathology 151: 31A (Abstract)
Fletcher C D M, Davies S E 1986 Benign plexiform (multinodular) schwannoma: a rare tumour unassociated with neurofibromatosis. Histopathology 10: 971–980
Fletcher C D M, Davies S E, McKee P H 1987 Cellular schwannoma: a distinct pseudosarcomatous entity. Histopathology 11: 21–35
Fletcher C D M, Stirling R W 1990 Intranodal myofibroblastoma presenting in the submandibular region: evidence of a broader clinical and histological spectrum. Histopathology, 16: 287–294
Fletcher C D M, Theaker J M, 1989 Digital Pacinian neuroma: a distinctive hyperplastic lesion. Histopathology 15: 249–256
Fletcher C D M, Chan J K-C, McKee P H 1986 Dermal nerve sheath myxoma: a study of three cases. Histopathology 10: 135–145
Fletcher C D M, Achu P, van Noorden S, McKee P H 1987 Infantile myofibromatosis: a light microscopic, histochemical and immunohistochemical study suggesting true smooth muscle differentiation. Histopathology 11: 245–258
Gallager R L, Helwig E B 1980 Neurothekeoma — a benign cutaneous tumor of neural origin. American Journal of Clinical Pathology 74: 759–764
Grunnet N, Genner J, Mogensen B, Myhre-Jensen O 1973 Recurring digital fibrous tumour of childhood. Case report and survey. Acta Pathologica Microbiologica Scandinavia Section A 81: 167–173
Harkin J C, Arrington J H, Reed R J 1978 Benign plexiform schwannoma, a lesion distinct from plexiform neurofibroma. Journal Neuropathology and Experimental Neurology 37: 622 (Abstract)
Hui P K, Chan J K C, N G C S, Kung I T M, Gwi E 1989 Lymphadenopathy of Kimura's disease. American Journal of Surgical Pathology 13: 177–186
Iwasaki H, Kikuchi M, Ohtsuki I, Enjoji M, Suenaga N, Mori R 1983 Infantile digital fibromatosis. Identification of actin filaments in cytoplasmic inclusions by heavy meromyosin binding. Cancer 52: 1653–1661
Iwashita T, Enjoji M 1987 Plexiform neurilemoma: a clinicopathological and immunohistochemical analysis of 23 tumours from 20 patients. Virchows Archiv A Pathological Anatomy and Histology 411: 305–310
Jennings T A, Duray P H, Collins F S, Sabetta J, Enzinger F M 1984 Infantile myofibromatosis. Evidence for an autosomal dominant disorder. American Journal of Surgical Pathology 8: 529–538
Kawada A, Takahashi H, Anzai T 1966 Eosinophilic lymph-folliculosis of the skin (Kimura's disease). Japanese Journal of Dermatology (Series B) 76: 61–72
Kimura T, Yoshimura S, Ishikawa E 1948 On the unusual granulation combined with hyperplastic changes of lymphatic tissues. Transactiones Societatis Pathologicae Japonicae 37: 179–180
Kreicbergs A, Tribukait B, Willems J, Bauer H C F 1987 DNA flow analysis of soft tissue tumors. Cancer 59: 128–133
Kung ITM, Gibson J B, Bannatyne P M 1984 Kimura's disease: a clinicopathological study of 21 cases and its distinction from angiolymphoid hyperplasia with eosinophilia. Pathology 16: 39–44
Kuo T, Shih L-Y, Chan H-L 1988 Kimura's disease. Involvement of regional lymph nodes and distinction from angiolymphoid hyperplasia with eosinophilia. American Journal of Surgical Pathology 12: 843–854
MacDonald D M, Wilson Jones E 1977 Pacinian neurofibroma. Histopathology 1: 247–255
Manivel C, Steeper T, Swanson P, Wick M 1987 Aggressive angiomyxoma of the pelvis: an

immunoperoxidase study. Laboratory Investigation 56: 46A (Abstract)

Mehregan A H, Nabai H, Matthews J E 1972 Recurring digital fibrous tumor of childhood. Archives of Dermatology 106: 375–378

Mortimer G, Gibson A A M 1982 Recurring digital fibroma. Journal of Clinical Pathology 35: 849–854

Morton K, Robertson A J, Hadden W 1987 Angiolymphoid hyperplasia with eosinophilia: report of a case arising from the radial artery. Histopathology 11: 963–969

Mukai M, Iri H, Nakajima T et al 1983 Alveolar soft part sarcoma. A review on its histogenesis and further studies based on electron microscopy, immunohistochemistry and biochemistry. American Journal of Surgical Pathology 7: 679–689

Nilbert M, Mandahl N, Heim S et al 1989 Cytogenetic abnormalities in an angioleiomyoma. Cancer Genetics and Cytogenetics 37: 61–64

Olsen T G, Helwig E B 1985 Angiolymphoid hyperplasia with eosinophilia. A clinicopathologic study of 116 patients. Journal of the American Academy of Dermatology 12: 781–796

Patel M E, Silver J W, Lipton D E, Pearman H S 1979 Lipofibroma of the median nerve in the palm and digits of the hand. Journal of Bone and Joint Surgery 61A: 393–397

Prichard R W, Custer R P 1952 Pacinian neurofibroma. Cancer 5: 297–301

Prose P H, Gherardi G J, Coblenz A 1957 Pacinian neurofibroma. Archives of Dermatology 76: 65–69

Purdy L J, Colby T V 1984 Infantile digital fibromatosis occurring outside the digit. American Journal of Surgical Pathology 8: 787–790

Qureshi F, Hozakewich H, Perez-Atayde A 1986 Plexiform schwannoma in children. Laboratory Investigation 54: 7p (Abstract)

Reed R J, Terazakis N 1972 Subcutaneous angioblastic lymphoid hyperplasia with eosinophilia (Kimura's disease) Cancer 29: 289–497

Reye R D K 1965 Recurring digital fibrous tumors of childhood. Archives of Pathology 80: 228–231

Rosai J 1982 Angiolymphoid hyperplasia with eosinophilia of the skin: Its nosological position in the spectrum of histiocytoid hemangioma. American Journal of Dermatopathology 4: 175–184

Rosai J, Ackerman L R 1974 Intravenous atypical vascular proliferation: a cutaneous lesion simulating a malignant blood vessel tumor. Archives of Dermatology 109: 714–717.

Rosai J, Gold J, Landy R 1979 The histiocytoid hemangiomas. A unifying concept embracing several previously described entities of skin, soft tissue, large vessels, bone and heart. Human Pathology 10:707–730

Sait S N J, Dal Cin P, Sandberg A A et al 1989 Involvement of 6p in benign lipomas. A new cytogenetic entity. Cancer Genetics and Cytogenetics 37: 281–283

Sandberg A A, Turc-Carel C 1987 The cytogenetics of solid tumors. Relation to diagnosis, classification and pathology. Cancer 59: 387–395

Sarma D P, Hoffmann E O 1980 Infantile digital fibroma-like tumor in an adult. Archives of Dermatology 116: 578–579

Schochet S S, Barrett D A 1974 Neurofibroma with aberrant tactile corpuscles. Acta Neuropathologica 28: 161–165

Shmookler B M, Enzinger F M 1982 Giant cell fibroblastoma; a peculiar childhood tumor. Laboratory Investigation 46: 76A (Abstract)

Silverman T A, Enzinger F M 1985 Fibrolipomatous hamartoma of nerve. A clinicopathologic analysis of 26 cases. American Journal of Surgical Pathology 9: 7–14

Smith S, Fletcher C D M, Smith M A, Gusterson B A 1990 Cytogenetic analysis of a plexiform fibrohistiocytic tumour. Cancer Genetics and Cytogenetics, in press

Steeper T A, Rosai J 1983 Aggressive angiomyxoma of the female pelvis and perineum. Report of nine cases of a distinctive type of gynecologic soft tissue neoplasm. American Journal of Surgical Pathology 7: 463–475

Stiller D, Katenkamp D 1975 Morphogenesis of intracytoplasmic dense (inclusion) bodies in a recurring digital fibrous tumour of childhood. Light- and electron-microscopic investigations. Virchows Archiv A Pathological Anatomy and Histology 367: 73–81

Suster S 1987 Nodal angiolymphoid hyperplasia with eosinophilia. American Journal of Clinical Pathology 88: 236–239

Suster S, Rosai J 1989 Intranodal hemorrhagic spindle cell tumor with amianthoid fibers. Report of six cases of a distinctive mesenchymal neoplasm of the inguinal region that simulates Kaposi's sarcoma. American Journal of Surgical Pathology 13: 347–357

Ulbright T M, Santa Cruz D J 1980 Intravenous pyogenic granuloma. Case report with ultrastructural findings. Cancer 45: 1646–1652

Urabe A, Tsuneyoshi M, Enjoji M 1987 Epithelioid haemangioma versus Kimura's disease. A comparative clinicopathologic study. American Journal of Surgical Pathology 11: 758–766

Venencie P Y, Bigel P, Desgruelles C, Lortat-Jacob S, Dufier J L, Saurat J H 1987 Infantile myofibromatosis. Report of two cases in one family. British Journal of Dermatology 117: 255–259

Viale G, Doglioni C, Iuzzolina P et al 1988 Infantile digital fibromatosis-like tumour (inclusion body fibromatosis) of adulthood: report of two cases with ultrastructural and immunocytochemical findings. Histopathology 12: 415–424

Weiss S W, Gnepp D R, Bratthauer G L 1989 Palisaded myofibroblastoma. A benign mesenchymal tumor of lymph node. American Journal of Surgical Pathology 13: 347–357

Weiss S W, Ishak K G, Dail D H, Sweet D E, Enzinger F M 1986 Epithelioid hemangioendothelioma and related lesions. Seminars in Diagnostic Pathology 3: 259–287

Wells G C, Whimster I W 1969 Subcutaneous angiolymphoid hyperplasia with eosinophilia. British Journal of Dermatology 81; 1–15

Wilson Jones E, Bleehen S S 1969 Inflammatory angiomatous nodules with abnormal blood vessels occurring about the ears and scalp (pseudo-or atypical pyogenic granuloma). British Journal of Dermatology 81; 804–816

Woodruff J M, Godwin T A, Erlandson R A, Susin M, Martini N 1981 Cellular schwannoma. A variety of schwannoma sometimes mistaken for a malignant tumor. American Journal of Surgical Pathology 5: 733–744

Woodruff J M, Marshall M L, Godwin T A, Funkhouser J W, Thompson N J, Erlandson R A 1983 Plexiform (multinodular) schwannoma. A tumor simulating the plexiform neurofibroma. American Journal of Surgical Pathology 7: 691–697

Yun K 1988 Infantile digital fibromatosis. Immunohistochemical and ultrastructural observation of cytoplasmic inclusions. Cancer 61: 500–507

13. Progress in pseudosarcomatous and borderline soft tissue tumours

W. B. Dupree

If you can look into the seeds of time and say which will grow and which will not, speak then to me ...

(Macbeth, Act I, Scene III)

Collective experience is the keystone in the understanding of pseudosarcomatous and borderline soft tissue lesions. Numerous clinicopathological studies have dispelled some of the uncertainties surrounding these entities. Once posing diagnostic and therapeutic dilemmas, lesions such as nodular fasciitis are now most often diagnosed and treated with unassuming facility. Through continuing efforts in description and correlation, new pseudosarcomatous and borderline lesions are being recognised. More recently described entities will be reviewed in this chapter.

Pseudosarcomas display morphological hallmarks often associated with clinical aggressiveness, yet invariably behave in a benign fashion. Borderline lesions may follow either a benign or malignant course unheralded by their morphology. This discordance between morphology and biological potential underscores the inconsistency of our present ability to predict 'which will grow and which will not'. The tools of modern molecular biology are refining our diagnostic ability to 'look into the seeds of time'. As a consequence, diagnoses with greater predictive value are being made. Diagnostic applications of modern molecular biology techniques will be explored in regard to soft tissue lesions.

PSEUDOSARCOMAS

Benign fibroblastic proliferations

Introduction

A proliferation of terms often surrounds a lesion in the early stages of understanding. Over time, numerous variations are described, and the merits of classification systems are debated. With experience, grand unification sometimes occurs. The study of proliferative fibroblastic lesions may be approaching a unification phase. As early as 1979, Meister et al suggested that nodular fasciitis, proliferative fasciitis and myositis ossificans represent a

Table.13.1   Pseudosarcomatous (proliferative) fibroblastic lesions (Soule et al 1986)

Nodular fasciitis
Subcutaneous pseudosarcomatous fasciitis
Proliferative fasciitis
Infiltrative fasciitis
Pseudosarcomatous fasciitis
Fasciitis ossificans
Parosteal fasciitis
Intravasular fasciitis
Cranial fasciitis
Proliferative myositis
Myositis ossificans, florid phase
Pseudomalignant myositis ossificans

spectrum of tissue responses which are variants of one disease process. This concept is central to Soule's classification of proliferative fibroblastic lesions (Table 13.1). While total agreement concerning classification is lacking, Soule's grouping emphasises common clinical and morphological themes (Soule et al 1986, Enzinger & Weiss 1983a, WHO International 1969).

Although a clinicomorphological spectrum has become apparent which links these benign pseudosarcomatous fibroblastic proliferations, knowledge of their aetiology and pathogenesis remains incomplete. An aberrant inflammatory response has long been considered a likely mechanism (Enzinger & Weiss 1983b). Variable numbers of lymphocytes admixed with proliferative fibroblasts are a common feature of pseudosarcomatous fibroblastic tumours. In vivo and in vitro observations indicate that lymphocytes and monocytes participate in the regulation of fibroblast growth and function (Leibovich & Ross 1975, Spielvogel et al 1977, Fleischmajer et al 1977). Recent studies suggest that T lymphocytes and monocytes/macrophages can effectively modulate several fibroblast functions through the production and release of soluble macromolecular factors collectively categorised as lymphokines (LK) and monokines (MK). LK and MK preparations have been found to stimulate and inhibit fibroblast movement (Postlethwaite et al 1976, Tsukamato et al 1981, Rola-Pleszczynski et al 1982), proliferation (Wahl & Gately 1982, Schmidt et al 1982, Korotzer et al 1982, Korn et al 1980, Duncan et al 1984), and collagen production (Postlethwaite et al 1984). How these fibroblast regulatory factors figure in the pathogenesis of benign fibroblastic proliferations remains an unanswered question in soft tissue pathology. The answer may further unify our thinking in regard to benign fibroblastic proliferations.

Fasciitis

Variants of fasciitis occurring in unusual clinical settings may cause diagnostic problems. Three uncommon clinicopathological presentations of fasciitis have been better described in recent years:

1. Intravascular fasciitis

2. Cranial fasciitis
3. Fibroosseous pseudotumour of digits.

1. Intravascular fasciitis. Rarely nodular fasciitis may involve small- to medium-sized arteries or veins in a luminal, mural or extramural distribution. The participation of these vessels suggests vascular invasion, raising the question of malignancy. Patchefsky and Enzinger clarified the clinicopathological features of this potentially confusing variant of nodular fasciitis in their report of 17 cases (Patchefsky & Enzinger 1981).

Intravascular fasciitis [IVF] presents as a slow growing mass most commonly in individuals under 30 years of age. Predilection for sex or a specific anatomic site have not been identified in the limited number of cases studied. Although some lesions may range up to 4–5 cm in length, most are small with a mean diameter of 1.5 cm. Intimate association with vessels along their course gives intravascular fasciitis a characteristic multinodular or rope-like gross configuration. In many lesions the bulk of the proliferation is distributed in a linear perivascular fashion. Often elastin and Masson Trichome stains are required to demonstrate luminal or mural involvement. Multiple noncontiguous foci may be identified within a vessel some distance from the major growth centre. This, in conjunction with multiple vessel involvement, suggests a pathogenesis which centres around a field effect. Microscopically, IVF is distinguished from more classic forms of nodular fasciitis by its intimate association with blood vessels (Fig. 13.1) and the

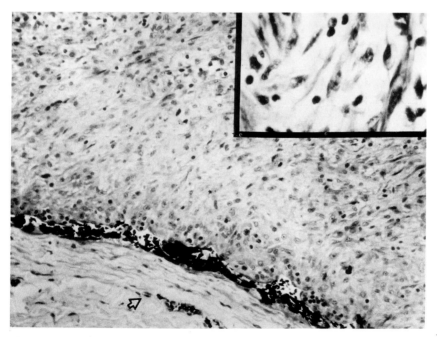

Fig. 13.1 Intravascular fascitis. Low power showing growth within dilated vein (arrow, vein wall). Inset, characteristic matrix separation of tissue culture-like fibroblasts.

sporadic presence of benign, non-ganglion-type giant cells. Awareness of IVF and recognition of the rope-like or multinodular gross presentation in conjunction with the classical matrix-separated arrangement of fibroblasts (Fig. 13.1 inset) help to avert a diagnosis of sarcoma. Luminal obstruction by IVF significant enough to cause infarction has not been reported.

2. Cranial fasciitis. In 1980, Lauer and Enzinger described a variant of nodular fasciitis occurring exclusively in the cranial region of infants and small children. The lesion was termed 'cranial fasciitis of childhood' to focus attention on the characteristic age incidence of fasciitis arising at this anatomic location.

Cranial fasciitis presents as a rapidly growing soft tissue mass, located deep in the scalp, which is obvious and disconcerting to the child's parents. Spontaneous growth stabilisation after a phase of rapid enlargement, as seen in classic nodular fasciitis, may also be encountered in cranial fasciitis. The lesion occurs congenitally, and has been reported in children from 3 weeks to 7 years of age (Lauer & Enzinger 1980, Patterson et al 1988). While fasciitis in the head and neck region is rare in adults, the cranium is the most common single site in infants and children. However, one possible case of cranial fasciitis has recently been reported in a 40-year-old (Oliver et al 1987). Fibroblastic lesions often show male predominance, a fact reflected in cranial fasciitis, which has a 2:1 male to female incidence (Enzinger 1965). Radiographs usually display a saucer-like erosion of the outer table of the calvarium, which sometimes exhibits a sclerotic margin. Rarely the lesion may extend to involve or penetrate the inner table of the skull. Involvement of the bone plate probably constitutes a secondary erosion, which lacks new bone-forming characteristics. The propensity of these lesions to involve underlying bone may be, in part, due to the incomplete ossification of the membranous bones of the skull in infants. Cranial fasciitis averages 2–5 cm in greatest dimension, with the largest examples in the range of 9.0 cm. Gross and microscopic features parallel those of more typical nodular fasciitis. Conservative surgical excision is usually the treatment of choice. In some instances, curettage of the affected underlying bone may be indicated.

3. Fibro-osseous pseudotumour of digits. The zonal pattern of myositis ossificans is well described and recognised as a key diagnostic clue in distinguishing myositis ossificans from sarcomatous bone-forming lesions (Ackerman 1958). Unlike classic myositis ossificans, benign fibroblastic lesions with foci of mature osseous differentiation occurring in the digits often lack the characteristic peripheral zone of mature bone. This fact coupled with the presence of a dense population of immature fibroblasts (Fig. 13.2) may lead to an erroneous diagnosis of sarcoma with resultant needless digital amputation. Spjut and Dorfman (1981) studied a small series of these lesions under the heading of 'florid reactive perostitis of tubular bones of the hands and feet'. More recently, Dupree and Enzinger (1986) reported a series of 21 cases which they termed 'fibro-osseous pseudotumor of digit'. Attention was focused on the lesion's close relationship to myositis ossificans with emphasis

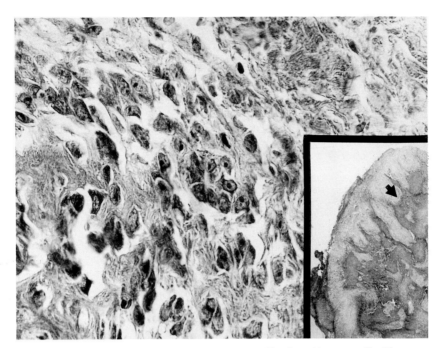

Fig. 13.2   Fibro-osseous pseudotumour of digits. A proliferation of immature fibroblasts coupled with haphazardly arranged trabeculae of bone (lower inset, arrow) may lead to an erroneous diagnosis of sarcoma.

on diagnostic criteria. In keeping with Soule's grouping of myositis ossificans and its variants with other forms of fasciitis, fibro-osseous pseudotumour of digits is discussed here.

Fibro-osseous pseudotumour of digits presents most commonly in young adults as a fusiform swelling, often of sudden onset which is sometimes accompanied by pain and erythema. The lesion does not demonstrate racial or sexual predilection. Roentgenograms display an ill-defined soft tissue mass which may or may not exhibit calcification. When present, the calcification is unevenly distributed without X-ray evidence of geographical distribution or zoning of the calcified material. Periosteal thickening adjacent to the lesion and cortical erosion are sporadic associated findings. Macroscopically, the lesion consists of a circumscribed firm or rubbery grey-white nodule, ranging from 1 to 3 cm in greatest diameter. Microscopically, the lesion is characterised by four morphological features:

1. Localisation in the subcutaneous tissue without muscular involvement.

2. A disorderly multinodular growth pattern with indistinct borders.

3. A fibroblastic proliferation showing varying degrees of cellular atypia (Fig. 13.2).

4. Haphazardly arranged osseous trabeculae without the zoning phenomenon of myositis ossificans (Fig. 13.2 lower inset).

The above clinicomorphological features, in conjunction with the virtual absence of atypia in the osteoblasts lining the osseous trabeculae and the absence of atypical mitotic figures, point to the diagnosis of fibroosseous pseudotumour of digits rather than sarcoma. A substantiated explanation for the haphazard arrangement of the cellular elements and osseous trabeculae is lacking. Conceivably, the small and narrow tissue compartments in the digits may preclude an orderly expansion of the lesion which contributes to the haphazard array. Fibro-osseous pseudotumour of digits behaves in a non-aggressive fashion and is curable by complete local excision.

Pseudosarcomatous lesions of adipose tissue

Introduction

Benign tumours of adipose tissue are some of the most frequently encountered neoplasms in surgical pathology. While ordinary lipomas seldom cause diagnostic problems, certain variants of lipoma have posed dilemmas which have only been resolved through meticulous descriptive clinicopathological studies. Lipomas containing heterogeneous mesenchymal elements (angiolipoma — Enjoji et al 1976, Belcher et al 1974; myelolipoma — Tulcinsky 1970; angiomyolipoma — Hajdu & Foote 1969; chondrolipoma — Murphy 1974; and hibernoma — Mori & Yumoto 1975) are now easily recognised. Fatty lesions distinguished by their clincal presentation or anatomic location (fibrolipomatous hamartoma of nerve — Silverman & Enzinger 1985; lumbrosacral lipoma — Rickwood et al 1979; and lipoma of tendon sheath — Sullivan et al 1956) are now well described. Despite invasive or destructive growth patterns, the inability of diffuse lipomatous lesions (intermuscular lipoma — Kindblom et al 1974; intramuscular lipoma — Dionne & Seemayer 1974 Fletcher & Martin Bates 1988; cervical symmetrical lipomatosis—Schuler et al 1976; pelvic lipomatosis — Cook et al 1973; and diffuse lipomatosis — McCarthy et al 1969) to metastasise is commonly acknowledged. Less familiar variants of lipoma continue to challenge the diagnostician. Spindle cell lipomas are characterised by a dense cellularity which may mask their relationship to adipocytes (Enzinger & Harvey 1975, Angervall et al 1976, Bolen & Thorning 1981). The unusual degree of cellular atypia encountered in pleomorphic lipomas can lead to a mistaken diagnosis of liposarcoma (Shmookler & Enzinger 1983, Azzopardi et al 1979). Parameters which distinguish atypical lipomas from well-differentiated lipoma-like liposarcomas remain one of the 'unresolved issues' of soft tissue pathology (Azumi et al 1987). These potentially problematic variants of lipoma are reviewed in this section.

Spindle cell lipoma

Enzinger and Harvey (1975) reported a series of 114 superficial tumours characterised by a proliferation of fibroblast-like spindle cells and variable numbers of mature adipocytes. The label spindle cell lipoma was chosen to reflect the uncertain histogenesis of the spindle cell element and the overall cellular composition of the neoplasm. Attention was focused on the morphological features distinguishing spindle cell lipoma from spindle cell variants of liposarcoma. Subsequent reports have confirmed the benign nature of this neoplasm (Angervall & Kindblom 1976, Fletcher & Martin-Bates 1987).

Spindle cell lipomas occur almost exclusively in the shoulder and neck regions of males older than 50 years. The lesion presents as a slow-growing, painless nodule centred in the dermis or subcutis. Grossly, the neoplasm consists of a circumscribed nodule of fat, ranging from 1.0 cm to 13.0 cm in greatest dimension. Microscopically uniform spindle cells (Fig. 13.3) are admixed with variable numbers of mature adipocytes set in a background of mucinous material traversed by ropey collagen fibers. A bipolar cytoplasmic membrane encloses the spindle cells' single elongated nucleus. While well circumscribed, the lesion is seldom encapsulated. Variables such as cellularity, collagen content and the ratio of spindle cells to mature adipocytes create a broad morphological spectrum. On occasion, the spindle cells are oriented along bundles of collagen to form fascicles of cells. When the nuclei happen to be in register, nuclear 'palisading' may be present. This appearance can simulate a leiomyoma or neurilemmoma. These entities are usually easily excluded by the intimate relationship of non-grouped spindle cells with mature adipocytes elsewhere in the lesion. Mast cells are numerous in nearly

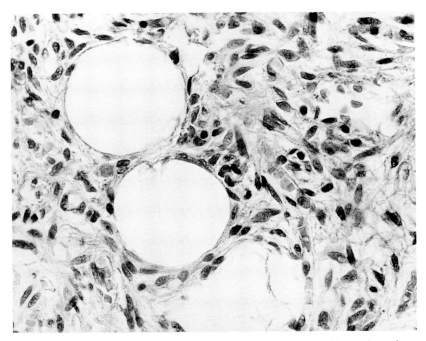

Fig. 13.3 Spindle cell lipoma. Uniform spindle cells admixed with variable numbers of mature adipocytes.

all cases of spindle cell lipoma. Less commonly, prominent endothelium-lined sinusoidal channels divide the tumour into small irregular lobules. While the precise histogenesis of the spindle cell remains uncertain, ultrastructural studies in four cases favour a common lineage with fibroblasts or cells closely related to fibroblasts, perhaps arising from a pluripotential cloud of mesenchyme surrounding blood vessels. Primitive mesenchymal origin is also favoured by immunohistochemical analysis (Beham et al 1989). Follow-up has proven spindle cell lipomas incapable of distant metastasis and rarely locally aggressive. Conservative simple excision is the apparent treatment of choice. The absence of: 1. diagnostic lipoblasts, 2. marked cellular atypia and 3. atypical mitotic figures, in conjunction with the clinical setting and histological pattern described above, exclude the diagnosis of spindle cell variant of liposarcoma.

Pleomorphic lipoma

Pleomorphic lipoma ia a benign lesion of the dermis and subcutaneous tissue which is often microscopically mistaken for liposarcoma (Shmookler & Enzinger 1981, Azzopardi et al 1979). The lesion is characterised by a population of bizzare multinucleated giant cells (Fig. 13.4) containing moderate amounts of eosinophilic cytoplasm. Some of these pleomorphic

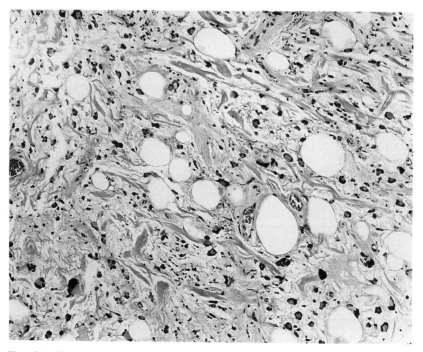

Fig. 13.4 Pleomorphic lipoma. Showing characteristic floret-like giant cells and bizarre giant cells.

multinucleated cells exhibit a distinctive, circular, marginal distribution of overlapping nuclei (Fig. 13.4), which is configurationally reminiscent of a small flower. In view of this morphology, Shmookler and Enzinger designated these cells 'floret-like' multinucleated giant cells. Despite bizarre cellular features and the presence of occasional lipoblasts (Fig. 13.5) pleomorphic lipomas always behave in a benign fashion.

Pleomorphic lipoma and spindle cell lipoma share many clinical and morphological features. Like spindle cell lipoma, the great majority of pleomorphic lipomas affect the neck and shoulder region of men in their fifth to seventh decades. These lesions present as a superficial, slow-growing mass which grossly resembles an encapsulated or partially circumscribed typical lipoma. As with spindle cell lipoma, pleomorphic lipomas encompass a wide morphological spectrum, brought about in part by the marked heterogeneity of cellular elements. These neoplasms contain varying combinations of bizarre multinucleate giant cells, floret-like giant cells, and irregular atypical adipocytes. Up to 50% of cases display lipoblasts and approximately 25% contain areas histologically indistinguishable from spindle cell lipoma. Like spindle cell lipoma, the background is often mucinous, containing thick bundles of birefringent collagen and foci of myxoid change. An inflammatory infiltrate composed of lymphocytes, plasma cells, mast cells and occasional histiocytes may be seen in a diffuse stromal or perivasular distribution.

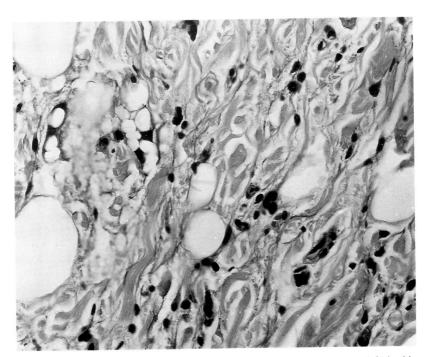

Fig. 13.5 Plemorphic lipoma. Showing two multivacuolated lipoblasts (upper left) in this clinically typical case.

Occasional normal mitotic figures may be present. Commonly, the lesion is completely or partially circumscribed. Less often, the tumour can appear as a sharply demarcated nodule within an otherwise typical lipoma. No single parameter excludes liposarcoma and points without qualification to a diagnosis of pleomorphic lipoma. Only a multivariate approach consistently leads to a correct diagnosis. Attention must be focused on: 1. age and sex of the patient, 2. regional anatomic location, 3. size, 4. epicentre of growth (deep or superficial), 5. degree of local invasion and 6. the presence or absence of floret-like giant cells, thick birefringent collagen fibres, and mast cells. Lipoblasts and atypical irregular adipocytes may be seen in both liposarcoma and pleomorphic lipoma. Numerous atypical mitoic figures and/or abundant necrosis would be unusual features in pleomorphic lipoma. As with spindle cell lipoma, the precise histogenesis of pleomorphic lipoma remains to be determined. In view of the clinical and morphological overlap with spindle cell lipoma, Shmookler and Enzinger (1981) suggested that pleomorphic lipoma might represent 'the end stage in a progression of cellular changes, possibly degenerative, occurring in a previously existing spindle cell lipoma'. This sequence would be analogous to the findings in the so-called 'ancient schwannoma' (Dahl 1977). Follow-up reveals an invariably benign course, with the real danger arising from an erroneous morphological diagnosis of liposarcoma.

Atypical lipoma—the need for a multivariate diagnostic approach

Stout called liposarcoma the malignant tumour of lipoblasts in 1944, and the diagnosis of liposarcoma still rests in part on the identification of these cells in the appropriate histological background and clinical setting. Newer pseudosarcomatous adipose lesions highlight the importance of clinical parameters in the diagnosis of adipose neoplasms (Enzinger & Harvey 1975, Shmookler & Enzinger 1981, Azumi et al 1987).

Perhaps only the quest for classic Reed-Sternberg cells in cases of Hodgkin's lymphoma has caused as much frustation as the microscopic search for diagnostic lipoblasts. During differentiation, normal lipocytes go through a sequence of morphological changes en route to maturity (Napolitano 1963). Diagnostic malignant lipoblasts may recapitulate any stage in this sequence creating a broad spectrum of potential cellular changes. The common denominator of recognisable lipoblasts is the presence of well-demarcated intracytoplasmic lipid, which often peripherally displaces one or more irregular nuclei (Enterline et al 1960). In most instances the nucleus conforms to the contour of the lipid droplets, causing an apparent delicate scalloping of the nuclear membrane. Hyperchromasia and irregularity from lipoblast to lipoblast helps to support a malignant diagnosis. However, the distinction between lipoblast and 'atypical lipocyte' can at times be subjective, especially in the more well-differentiatied variants of liposarcoma. The diagnostic pitfalls of lesions containing vacuolated cells mimicking malignant lipoblasts (fat necrosis—Schrier et al 1965; myxoid fatty change, lipogranu-loma—Smetana & Bernhard 1950; lymphoma with signet ring changes—Kim et al 1978; and carcinoma) can often be avoided by obtaining an adequate clinical history. Lesions such as pleomorphic lipoma or lipoblastoma illustrate that even unequivocal lipoblasts do not always portend a malignant pathobi-ology. As with most surgical pathology problems, the assessment of adipose neoplasms requires careful clinical morphological correlation in order to arrive at a diagnosis with the greatest clinical predictive value.

The infantile counterparts of lipoma, lipoblastoma and lipoblastomatosis, clearly illustrate the importance of age in the evaluation of an adipose tumour (Chaudhuri et al 1980, Chung & Enzinger 1973, Vellios et al 1958). These lesions display numerous lipoblasts set in a prominent myxoid stroma containing a delicate capillary proliferation. When taken out of clinical context, such features can easily lead to a mistaken diagnosis of myxoid liposarcoma. The age of the patient, overall lobular nature of the fat, and regularity of the lipoblasts point to the proper diagnosis. While occasional liposarcomas do arise in children between 10 and 15 years old, they are extremely rare in individuals younger than 10 years (Shmookler & Enzinger 1983).

Anatomical location is playing an increasingly significant role in the evaluation of adipose neoplasms. Recent reports have suggested that the clinical outcome of well-differentiated lipoma-like liposarcomas can best be predicted on the basis of anatomical location (Azumi et al 1987). These studies indicate that well-differentiatied liposarcomas in superficial soft tissue are invariably benign, since they never metastasise. In contrast, morpholog-ically indistinguishable retroperitoneal well-differentiated liposarcomas were found to behave in an aggressive fashion. Several new terminologies— atypical lipoma (Evans et al 1979, Kindblom et al 1982), differentiated fatty neoplasms of somatic soft tissues (DFT-S) (Azumi et al 1987)—have been proposed to distinguish the site-dependent pathobiology of these histologically indistin-guishable adipose neoplasms. The natural history and proper diagnostic label for well-differentiated lipoma-like liposarcomas arising in somatic soft tissue remains controversial. However, this controversy focuses attention on the diagnostic significance of clinical parameters in predicting the pathobiology of adipose neoplasms. Only a multivariate approach which carefully considers the patient's age and sex, the basic location, epicentre of growth (deep or superficial), as well as morphology, will lead to an adequate assessment of an adipose neoplasm's potential clinical outcome (see Ch. 14).

BORDERLINE SOFT TISSUE LESIONS

Introduction

With the development of the flexible enteroscope (Zavala 1975), more sensitive clinical imaging techniques (Webb 1986) and fine-needle aspiration

(Woolner 1981), pathologists are now commonly called upon to evaluate the earliest stages of malignancy. This new demand has focused diagnostic attention on the morphology which occurs at the border between stages of premalignant and malignant transformation. Prior knowledge of the pathobiology and histology at this interface stems largely from tissue systems which are readily observed over time through serial screenings. The uterine cervix has been the classic model (Jenson 1986).

In the cervix, constellations of light microscopic changes are often found in association with malignancy (Jenson 1986). These changes commonly form a morphological continuum (Jenson 1986). Clinicopathological studies indicate that lesions in this continuum, with similar light microscopic phenotypes, may exhibit entirely different clinical outcomes (Jenson 1986). Because of the apparent discordance between morphology and pathobiological potential, in many instances, 'those that will grow' (progress to metastatic malignancy) cannot be distinguished at the light microscopic level from those that will remain dormant or regress. Similar ambiguous situations exist in many tissue systems (Henson & Albores-Saavedra 1986). Because of this uncertainty, such lesions are often considered, as a group, potential precursors of invasive malignancy. A host of terms including intermediate lesion, minimal cancer, tumourlet, grade ½ carcinoma and borderline lesion have been used to describe these entities which reside at the morphological interface between premalignant and malignant transformation (Henson & Albores-Saavedra 1986).

Because soft tissue sarcomas often clinically declare their presence relatively late in their development, and frequently occur at inaccessible anatomic sites, very little is known about the earliest phases in their development. Unlike a sarcoma arising in bone, whose early course is sometimes captured by serial X-rays, there is no sensitive means of demonstrating sequential change over time for lesions based in soft tissue. With the exception of the neurofibroma—malignant schwannoma transformation seen in cases of von Recklinghausen's disease—the antecedent lesions of soft tissue sarcomas remain ill defined. Malignant transformation of most benign soft tissue tumours is presently thought to be an extremely rare event (Enzinger & Weiss 1983c). However, in most classification systems, many histogenetic categories are divided into a benign and malignant group (Table 13.2). From a purely diagnostic standpoint, the parameters which separate the low-grade malignant mesenchymal neoplasm from its benign counterpart are often difficult to apply. The recent appearance of a borderline or intermediate category in classification schemes reflects the realisation that certain soft tissue neoplasms cannot be accurately classified on histological grounds as to their ultimate biological behaviour (Enzinger & Weiss 1983d). Epithelioid haemangioendothelioma, spindle cell haemangioendothelioma, dermatofibrosarcoma protuberans and pigmented dermatofibrosarcoma protuberans are among the first soft tissue neoplasms tentatively placed into this category.

Table 13.2   Borderline diagnostic problems in soft tissue pathology

Benign (atypical)	Diagnostic parameters favouring malignancy	Low 'grade' malignant
Lipoma	Age, anatomic location, lipoblasts	Well differentiated, lipoma-like liposarcoma
Leiomyoma	Anatomic location, necrosis Mitotic figures: 1–4/10 HPF 'potentially malignant' (cellular atypia of limited value)	Leiomyosarcoma (non-uterine)
Haemangiopericytoma	4 or more mitotic figures/10 HPF, hypercellularity, cellular pleomorphism, haemorrhage, necrosis	Malignant haemangiopericytoma
Fibrous histiocytoma	Anatomic location Presence of both pleomorphism and mitotic activity Necrosis	Malignant fibrous histiocytoma
Myxoma	Hypercellularity Cellular pleomorphism 'Elevated' mitotic activity	Myxoid variant of malignant fibrous histiocytoma
Giant Cell Tumour	Decreased numbers of giant cells. Large mononuclear cells with prominent nucleoli. Atypical & typical mitotic figures present in a diffuse distribution Haemorrhage, necrosis	Malignant giant cell tumour (giant cell variant of malignant fibrous histiocytoma)
Von Recklinghausen's disease (neurofibromatosis)	Clinical setting: Disease present 10 years or longer. Rapid painful enlargement. Elevated mitotic rate Necrosis — harmorrhage (nuclear atypia of limited value)	Malignant schwannoma
Granular cell tumour	(May be virtually devoid of malignant features) 2 or more mitoses/10 HPF or tumour greater than 5 cm diameter raises index of suspicion Hypercellularity small elongated cells (cellular variability or cellular pleomorphism alone not reliable)	Malignant granular cell tumours
Haemangioma	Clinical setting, anatomic location Irregular vascular channels permeating between collagen bundles Anastamosing network of vessels Endothelial hyperchromasia	Angiosarcoma
Chondroma	Cellular pleomorphism Hypercellularity Loose 'soupy' matrix	Chondrosarcoma
Fibro-osseous pseudotumour	Absence of zonation Infiltrative growth pattern Absence of bone trabeculae with ossification front and osteoblast rim Elevated mitotic rate Cellular pleomorphism	Extraskeletal osteosarcoma

Recent progress in borderline soft tissue lesions

Epithelioid haemangioendothelioma

Epithelioid haemangioendothelioma sometimes masks its potential for a malignant clinical course with a deceptively non-malignant morphological appearance. This lesion was first described by Dail and Liebow (1975) under the term intravascular bronchiolo-alveolar tumour (IVBAT). It was initially thought to be epithelial in origin until Corrin et al (1979) recognised its endothelial features by electron microscopy; this was confirmed later by immunohistochemical studies for factor VIII-related antigen (Weldon-Linne et al 1981). Subsequently, the lesion was reported at other anatomical locations under a wide variety of names obscuring the common clinicomorphological features (Weiss et al 1986). In 1979, Rosai et al used the term histiocytoid haemangioma for this entity and emphasised a unifying histological spectrum embracing several previously described lesions of bone, soft tissue, skin, large vessels and heart. A study of 41 cases of the soft tissue counterpart of IVBAT was reported by Weiss and Enzinger in 1982. The term epithelioid haemangioendothelioma was suggested because of the tumour cells' focal resemblence to epithelium and a clinical course intermediate between those of haemangioma and angiosarcoma.

Epithelioid haemangioendothelioma may affect all age groups, but usually excludes the very young. These neoplasms can arise in deep or superficial soft tissue and are associated with medium to large veins in approximately two-thirds of cases. Epithelioid haemangioendothelioma presents grossly as a white circumscribed mass which seldom displays haemorrhage.

Microscopically, the lesion is characterised by plump polygonal or slightly spindled epithelioid cells containing abundant eosinophilic cytoplasm and ovoid nucleoli (Fig. 13.6). These cells often lie within a myxoid or hyalinised matrix. Intracytoplasmic spaces containing erythrocytes are commonly observed (Fig. 13.7 B and C). Four distinct growth patterns of the neoplastic epithelioid cells are encountered: 1. solid areas with a vague nested pattern (Fig. 13.6 upper inset), 2. cords, 3. vascular tubes, and 4. isolated individual cells often of a signet-ring shape. These distinct growth patterns are linked by zones of transition. Cellular variation is limited and, in most cases, few mitoses are identified.

At the electron microscopic level, packets and cords of polygonal cells are surrounded by an incomplete basement membrane of variable thickness. Individual cells demonstrate prominent oval nuclei with smooth nuclear membranes, diffuse chromatin, and rare nucleoli. An abundance of parallel, wavy, intermediate (100 Å), cytoplasmic filaments (Fig. 13.8A) accounts for the copious eosinophilic cytoplasm. These cells are equipped with various cytoplasmic organelles, including short, straight segments of smooth endoplasmic reticulum, free ribosomes and small round mitochondria. Numerous pinocytotic vesicles occur along plasma membranes (Fig. 13.8B). In addition, many cells demonstrate a distinctive endothelial-type contact with neighbour-

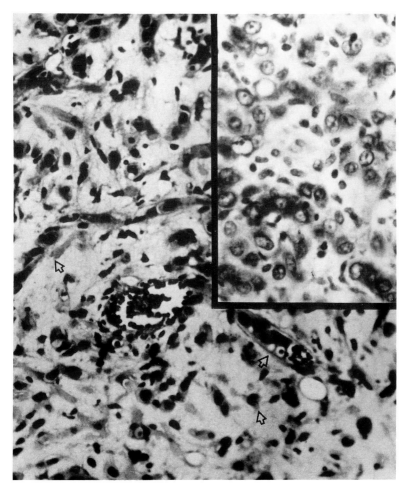

Fig. 13.6 Epithelioid haemangioendothelioma. Four distinct growth patterns are encountered: 1. solid areas with a vague nested pattern (upper inset, factor VIII stain), 2. cords, 3. vascular tubes, 4. isolated individual cells. (Courtesy Dr Bruce Ragsdale.)

ing cells characterised by specialised junction of interlocking flaps of membrane-bound cytoplasm ('mortice junctions') (Fig. 13.8C). The presence of Weibel Palade bodies is variable. Factor VIII-associated antigen, when identified (Fig. 13.7D), is useful in distinguishing the nested pattern from metastatic carcinoma.

Epithelioid haemangioendothelioma must be distinguished from metastatic carcinoma and chondrosarcoma on the basis of the above clinicomorphological features. The differential between epithelioid haemangioma and epithelioid haemangioendothelioma is sometimes impossible at the light microscopic level (Cooper 1988) with some clearly morphologically benign 'epithelioid haemangiomas' metastasising after a very long latency period. In general, epithelioid haemangiomas present with microscopic lobulation

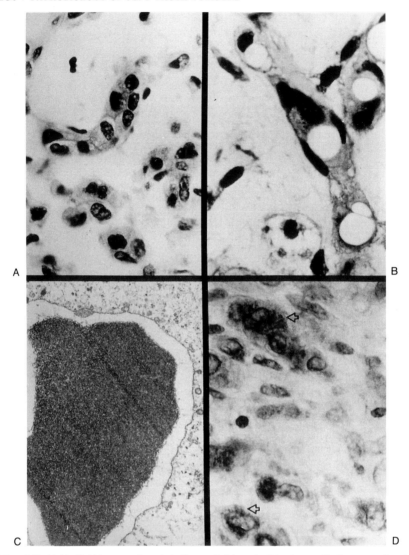

Fig. 13.7 Epithelioid haemangioendothelioma. Solid cords (**A**) whose cells form cytoplasmic vacuoles may link to form a common vascular channel containing red blood cells (EM **C**). Those epithelioid cells are factor-VIII-related antigen positive (**D**). (Courtesy Dr Bruce Ragsdale.)

consisting of small vessels grouped around a larger parent 'feeder' vessel. A brisk inflammatory infiltrate is a common element in epithelioid hae-mangioma, which is ordinarily minimal or absent in epithelioid haeman-gioendothelioma.

Numerous mitotic figures, (greater than 1/10 HPF), abundant necrosis or extreme cellular pleomorphism all suggest epithelioid angiosarcoma. Weiss and Enzinger report that approximately 50% of patients undergoing surgical therapy for epithelioid haemangioendothelioma usually have no further

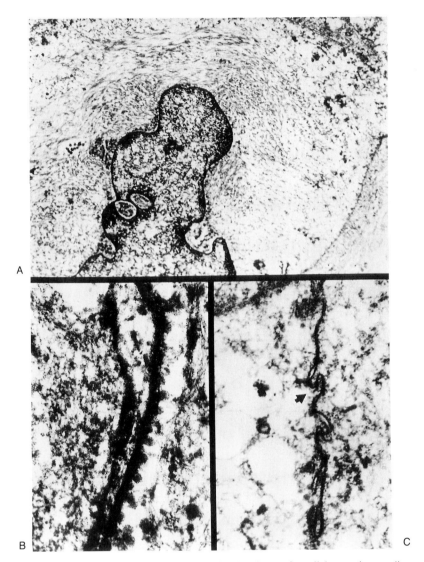

Fig. 13.8   Epithelioid haemangioendothelioma. An abundance of parallel, wavy intermediate filaments (**A**) accounts for the copious eosinophilic cytoplasm. Numerous pinocyctotic vesicles occur along the plasma membrane (**B**). Mortice junction characteristic of endothelial cell contacts (**C**). (Courtesy Dr. Bruce Ragsdale.)

disease. In their experience about 15% suffer a local recurrence with 30% developing distant metastasis.

Following the general theme of borderline lesions, epithelioid haemangioendotheliomas represent a group of biologically heterogenous lesions which display a common morphological phenotype at some point in their course. As indicated by the development of solid cords whose cells form cytoplasmic vacuoles which may link to form a common vascular channel, some epithelioid haemangioendotheliomas closely recapitulate normal angio-genesis. The orchestration of the sequential steps in normal capillary growth no doubt requires many chemical mediators. The discovery of tumour angiogenesis factors initiated the hot pursuit of the chemical factors in tumours that stimulate the growth of blood vessels (Folkman 1983). Basic science research has most recently led to the resolution, purification and amino acid sequencing of a hormone dubbed 'angiogenin' (Strydom et al 1985). This capillary growth hormone, unlike Folkman's hormones, does not bind heparin or stimulate endothelial cells. Instead, it appears to generate and extend preformed capillaries within tissue. Angiogenin then may initiate normal angiogenesis. In view of epithelioid haemangioendothelioma's pro-pensity to closely recapitulate normal angiogenesis and its common associa-tion with more normal medium and large veins, the role of angiogenin, if any, in the pathogenesis of some benign-acting variants of epithelioid haeman-gioendothelioma remains an intriguing question.

Spindle cell haemangioendothelioma

Spindle cell haemangioendothelioma (SCH) is a recently recognised vascular neoplasm which combines histological and clinical features of both cavernous haemangioma and Kaposi's sarcoma (Weiss et al 1986). While the latter author's experience with spindle cell haemangioendothelioma was limited (26 reported cases, 14 cases with followup), the disease appears to potentially follow a locally aggressive course with numerous recurrences, sometimes separated by long latency periods. This has since been borne out by Scott and Rosai (1988). Although the apparent multifocal nature of the disease makes it difficult to exclude local metastasis, unequivocal distant metastasis has been reported in only one case. This patient experienced 19 recurrences over a 40-year period and received local irradiation before developing a regional lymph node metastasis.

SCH may occur in any age or sex, but exhibits a predilection for males less than 25 years of age. The tumour most often presents as a dermal or subcutaneous nodule in a distal extremity. Spindle cell haemangioendothe-lioma has a tendency to grow locally or develop multifocally in a generalized area over a long period of time. Macroscopically, these neoplasms present as small reddish tumours sometimes containing phleboliths. Microscopically the lesion is composed of gaping, thin-walled vascular channels (Fig. 13.9) separated by a proliferation of relatively bland-appearing spindle cells. Within the spindle cell component, occasional epithelioid or vacuolated endothelial cells are identified which help to distinguish SCH from Kaposi's sarcoma. The cells lining the dilated, well-formed, gaping vascular channels possess many ultrastructural features of normal endothelial cells including basal lamina, elaborate cell–cell interdigitations, numerous pinocytotic vesicles, abundant intermediate filaments, and occasional Weibel-Palade bodies. Epi-theloid endothelial cells not lining vascular channels show less specific

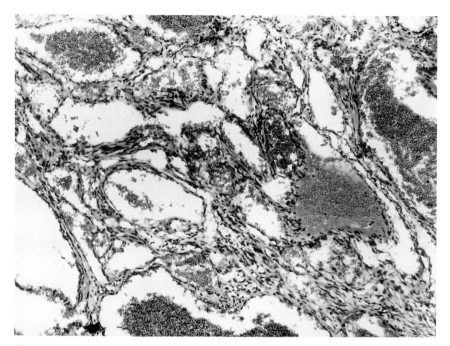

Fig. 13.9 Spindle cell haemangioendothelioma. Gaping, thin-walled vascular channels separated by a proliferation of bland appearing spindle cells. Vacuolated epithelioid endothelial cells are found admixed with spindle cell elements.

ultrastructural features, but suggest partial endothelial differentiation through intimate association with one another in small cohesive groups. Both cells lining the vascular channels and epithelioid endothelial cells within the spindle cell areas stain positively for immunoreactive factor VIII-associated protein. Spindle cells staining unequivocally for factor VIII-related protein are rarely, if ever, present. Curiously, one case of SCH has been reported in association with adjacent epithelioid haemangioendothelium, raising the possibility that rare transitional forms may exist. As with epithelioid haemangioendothelioma, spindle cell haemangioendothelioma is tentatively regarded as a borderline tumour, recognising that experience with greater numbers of cases and extended followup information may require its reclassification as an angiosarcoma.

Non-pigmented dermatofibrosarcoma protuberans

Dermatofibrosaroma protuberans (DFSP) and its pigmented counterpart (Bednar tumor) are classified by some experts as borderline lesions (Enzinger & Weiss 1983e). Non-pigmented DFSP grows in an infiltrative fashion, possesses a great propensity for aggressive local recurrence, and in some cases metastasises (Adams & Salzstein 1963). The true metastatic incidence of non-pigmented DFSP is difficult to glean from the literature; however, in 400 reported cases, fewer than 1% have documented metastasis (Brenner et al 1975, Fletcher et al 1985). As with most other soft tissue sarcomas, haematogenous spread to the lungs is the most common avenue of metastasis, when it does occur. Regional lymph nodes are involved in approximately one quarter of metastatic cases. To predict morphologically which cases of non-pigmented DFSP 'will grow' (metastasise) and 'which will not' is difficult. Those cases which show fibrosarcomatous change in subsequent recurrences are at increased risk of metastasis (Enzinger & Weiss 1983f, Ding et al 1989), although this is disputed (Wrotnowski et al 1988). Those cases which do not show fibrosarcomatous change over time give little morphological indication of their metastatic potential. From a clinical perspective, however, metastasising lesions are almost always recurrent lesions, and there is usually a period of several years between diagnosis and metastasis (Enzinger & Weiss 1983f).

Pigmented dermatofibrosarcoma protuberans (Bednar tumour)

First described by Bednar in 1957 as a variant of neurofibroma (storiform neurofibroma), pigmented dermatofibrosarcoma is a rare neoplasm accounting for approximately 1% to 5% of all cases of dermatofibrosarcoma protuberans (DFSP). Stout, who initially regarded the lesion to be a variant of fibrosarcoma, subsequently reported a similar lesion as a 'neoplasm of uncertain histogenesis' and finally entertained the possible diagnosis of melanosarcoma (Stout 1948, 1953). Dupree and Weiss reported 20 cases in 1985 emphasising clinical, morphological, electron microscopic and immuno-histochemical evidence supporting this tumour's close relationship to non-pigmented DFSP (Dupree et al 1985). While pigmented DFSP may be locally aggressive, cases with distant metastasis have not been documented (Dupree et al 1985). This may, in part, reflect the limited number of cases studied to date (follow-up in 9 out of 20 cases).

Pigmented DFSP commonly presents as an exophytic multinodular neoplasm in the dermis or subcutaneous tissue. The lesion occurs predominantly in blacks and shows no sex predilection. The trunk is the most common anatomic site, with the remaining cases almost equally distributed in the upper and lower extremities and the head and neck. At the light microscopic level, spindled cells are focally arranged in a tight storiform pattern (Fig. 13.10) and in areas infiltrate fat forming a honeycomb-like pattern. Melanin-containing dendritic cells admixed with the spindle cell element distinguishes this lesion from nonpigmented DFSP (Fig. 13.10). Ultrastructurally, three cell populations are usually identified. Most cells display electron microscopic features of fibroblasts. The next most prominent cell population displays long, slender processes, partially or completely invested with basal lamina (Fig. 13.11 lower left inset). The most quantitatively limited cell population is also invested by basal lamina but, in addition, contains both melanosomes and premelanosomes (Fig. 13.11 lower right

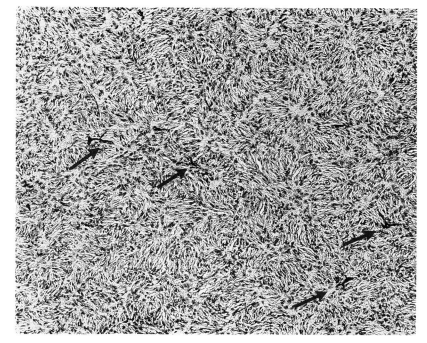

Fig. 13.10   Pigmented dermatofibrosarcoma protuberans (Bednar tumour). Delicate spindle cells admixed with melanin containing cells (arrows) arranged in a tight storiform pattern.

inset). While the histogenesis of this neoplasm remains controversial, ultrastructural studies and the presence of melanosomes in variable stages of maturation, suggest a neuroectodermal origin or possible perineural cell lineage, although this has recently been questioned (Fletcher et al 1988) and the possibility of melanocyte colonisation from the epidermis has been suggested. The Bednar tumor is tentatively classified as a borderline lesion in view of its close relationship to classic non-pigmented DFSP.

New diagnostic methods: probes and DNA analysis

Introduction

Over the years a number of ancillary techniques (including special stains, histochemical reactions, electron microscopy, immunofluorescence, and immunohistochemistry) have been devised to supplement the haematoxylin and eosin microscopic impression. While all of these tools have proved useful in specific diagnostic settings, none has significantly improved our ability to predict which borderline lesion 'will grow' (metastasise) and 'which will not'. The uncertainty reflected in a borderline diagnosis remains unsettling to the clinical oncologist attempting to tailor the optimal therapeutic intervention.

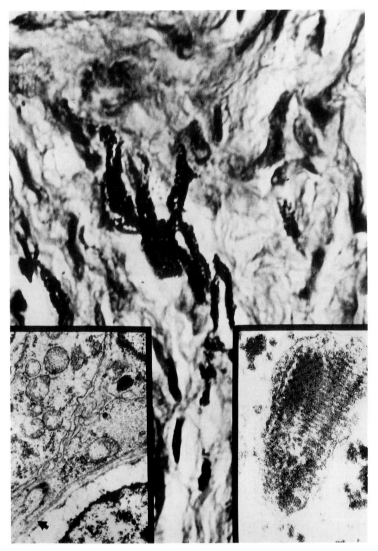

Fig. 13.11 Pigmented dermatofibrosarcoma protuberans (Bednar tumour). Melanin containing dentritic cell (top) displaying melanosomes (lower right inset) in various stages of maturation. Both pigmented cells and cells displaying slender cytoplasmic processes may be partially or completely invested with basal lamina (lower left inset, arrow).

Recent advances in molecular biology promise diagnostic avenues which may dispel ambiguity in these cases and lead to more confident therapy.

Diagnostic probes which penetrate the molecular confines of a cell's nucleic acid machinery have been made possible through enormous advances in recombinant DNA technology (Sklar 1985). Nucleic acid probes consist of suitably labelled single strands of DNA, engineered to bind through hydrogen bonds to specific complementary DNA or RNA sequences which may be present in the material under examination (Sklar 1985). These probes have permitted in depth study of genes, gene organisation, gene products, and the genetic basis for morphological changes in cells. Initially, hybridisation reactions were performed on target DNA that had been bound and immobilised on nitrocellulose or other filter membranes (Southern 1975). The probes were radioactively labelled and detected by autoradiography. While in vitro procedures remain the standard, the development of in situ hybridisation of DNA probes to endogenous nucleic acid sequences in tissue sections and cytological smears is well under way (Grody et al 1987).

From these advances, DNA rearrangement analysis has emerged as a diagnostic tool which complements conventional tissue studies. Information regarding clonality (Arnold et al 1983), lineage (Waldmann et al 1985), and specific chromosomal translocations (Furlet et al 1986) is now being applied to resolve issues in classification, differential diagnosis, histogenesis and, most relevant to the present discussion, the detection of early morphologically occult malignant transformation (Cossman et al 1986). While these probes have been predominantly applied in the evaluation of haematopoietic and lymphoid malignancies (Raffeld et al 1987), recent insights into the pathobiology of neuroblastoma suggest an impending significant impact on the diagnosis and management of solid tumours (Israel 1986).

Neuroblastoma—a biologically heterogenous group of morphologically similar lesions

Several lines of evidence suggest that neuroblastoma as presently defined clinically and morphologically is a biologically heterogenous group of morphologically similar lesions.

Neuroblastoma is a unique neoplasm which often undergoes spontaneous regression and in vivo morphologic maturation (Evans et al 1976). Incidental microscopic nodules of primitive neuroblasts (occasionally invading blood vessels), which are clinically and morphologically indistinguishable from neuroblastoma, are found in a comparatively high percentage of fetuses between 17 to 20 weeks gestation (Beckwith & Perin 1963, Evans et al 1976). While neuroblastoma is the most common extracranial solid tumour in children, there are only about 500 new cases diagnosed each year in the USA (Young & Miller 1975). Extrapolations from the above fetal autopsy studies would predict 25 000 new cases each year if these incidental lesions became clinically significant or failed to regress.

Prognosis is intimately related to the patient's age at presentation (Breslow & McCann 1971). Children who are diagnosed at less than 1 year of age have a much better prognosis than children who are older than 1 year at the time of diagnosis, regardless of the primary site or extent of disease (Green & Hayes 1984). Aggressive therapeutic intervention has not improved prognosis in older children, while limited intervention, including partial surgical resection, has resulted in extended survival in young infants (Finklestein et al

1979). These observations have spawned speculation that some 'neuroblastomas' are outgrowths of a cell which is truly neoplastic, while other lesions may represent a simple physiological expansion of cells behaving in a manner appropriate to their stage of maturation or specific milieu of growth-regulating factors. Our ability to distinguish those that 'will grow' (true metastatic neoplasms) from those that will regress (physiologic proliferations) based on conventional modalities is presently limited.

DNA rearrangement analysis: (11;22) (q24; q12) translocation

Neuroepithelioma (peripheral neuroectodermal tumour) is a variant of neuroblastoma for which genetic characterisation has provided diagnostically relevant information (Israel 1986). In most cases, neuroepithelioma is histopathologically indistinguishable from other childhood neuroblastomas (Bolen & Thorning 1980).

Neuroepithelioma is defined by its clinical presentation as an extremity mass in an adolescent or young adult. In the past, the diagnosis of neuroepithelioma was made only when no tumour could be identified in the common sites of neuroblastoma, i.e. the adrenal medulla or sympathetic ganglia (Seemayer et al 1975). When the clinical presentation of neuroepithelioma occurred in a young child, the lesion was considered by many to be a neuroblastoma in which the primary tumour had regressed. Traditionally, neuroepithelioma was treated with the standard neuroblastoma regimens with almost universally poor results (Lopez et al 1980).

Exciting preliminary studies in gene analysis indicate that the presence of a reciprocal (11;22) (q24;q12) translocation separates neuroepithelioma from other neuroblastomas (Israel 1986). This genetic marker has also been identified in four tumour specimens and six tumour cell lines from patients with the malignant round cell tumour of the chest wall described by Askin et al in 1979 (Israel 1986). In a similar fashion another morphologically similar neoplasm, Ewing's sarcoma, seems invariably to carry a reciprocal (11;22) (q24;12) translocation indistinguishable from neuroepithelioma (Israel 1986). While cytogenetic characterisation of a translocation breakpoint serves only as an estimate, there are presently very few examples of different tumour types bearing indistinguishable cytogenetic alterations. Are these break points in fact functionally identical? Is the small round cell tumour described by Askin identical to neuroepithelioma? Does Ewing's sarcoma arise in cells of neuroectodermal origin rather than from mesoderm? Will neuroepithelioma better respond to multimodality therapeutic regimens known to be effective in Ewing's sarcoma (Israel 1986)? While the new technology provides the means to explore these issues, the answers await the test of clinicopathological experience. This topic is further discussed in Chapter 14.

Oncogene amplification

Neuroblastomas display a wide variety of cytogenetic abnormalities including homogeneously staining regions and double minute chromosomes (Balaban-

Malerbaum & Gilbert 1977). Both of these features are manifestations of gene amplification (Cowell 1982). Biochemical characterisation of this amplified DNA in neuroblastoma has identified a base sequence, N-myc, which is homologous to the cellular oncogene c-myc (Schwab et al 1983, Salmon et al 1986). The availability of probes corresponding to the N-myc region could lead to diagnostic applications which may help to predict which neuroblastoma 'will grow and which will not'.

Recent research has been aimed at understanding genetic sequences which may be responsible for the induction or maintenance of malignancy (oncogenes) (Bishop 1983, Salmon et al 1984). The molecular characterisation of the genome of the rapidly transforming retrovirus first led to the identification of oncogenic sequences. Curiously the paradigm of these viruses is the Rous sarcoma virus. When specific viral oncogenes were used as probes, homologues to all oncogenic sequences were found in normal vertebrate DNA including that of humans. This observation led to the now generally accepted hypothesis that viral oncogenes arose from a group of normal cellular genes (proto-oncogenes) during transit of the retrovirus through the host cell. While it is difficult to conceive of a selective advantage conferred by genes capable of aiding malignancy, these DNA sequences span a broad range of vertebrate and invertebrate evolution. Current theories about the role of proto-oncogenes suggest that they play a part in normal cellular proliferation and differentiation. At least 3 of 20 identified oncogenes are related to known growth factors or growth factor receptors.

There is a close correlation between N-myc amplification in neuroblastoma and Evans stage III–IV lesions (Israel 1986). Approximately 50% of these aggressive variants of neuroblastoma are found to have multiple copies of detectable N-myc DNA (Schwab et al 1984). Most localised tumours have not been found to have amplified N-myc sequences. When Evans stage II lesions contained amplified N-myc sequences, they behaved in a manner unlike non-N-myc positive cases, progressed rapidly, did not respond to therapy well, and carried a poor clinical prognosis (Seeger et al 1985). With refinement, the identification of N-myc amplification may provide a more sensitive index of potential biological behaviour than the present clinical staging system. Recent evidence suggests that immunohistochemical demonstration of the N-myc gene product in paraffin-embedded neuroblastomas may provide such prognostic information by relatively simple and widely available means (Hashimoto et al 1989).

CONCLUSION

Over the past century, pathologists have become expert in recognising neoplastic disease by visual examination of suitably prepared tissue and cells. During recent years, it has become increasingly apparent that tumours are composed of behaviourally heterogenous subpopulations of cells. Borderline soft tissue lesions represent a group of biologically diverse entities which display a common morphological phenotype at some point in their course.

Despite often similar presentations, their true potential clinical character at a given time is defined at the molecular level. Diagnosticians must be ready to go beyond the limits of vision to distinguish outgrowths of cells which are truly neoplastic from those that may represent a simple physiological expansion of cells behaving in a manner appropriate to their stage of maturation or specific milieu. The tools of modern molecular biology, coupled with computer-assisted image analysis, promise to play a major role in future attempts to look into the seeds of time and predict which will grow and which will not.

REFERENCES

Ackerman L V 1958 Extraosseous localized nonneoplastic bone and cartilage formation (so-called myositis ossificans). Journal of Bone and Joint Surgery 40A (2): 279–298

Adams J T, Salzstein S L 1963 Metastasizing dermatofibrosarcoma protuberans metastatic to a regional lymph node. American Journal of Surgery 29: 879–886

Angervall L, Dahl I, Kindblom L G et al 1976 Spindle cell lipoma: a clinical light and electron microscopic study. Acta Pathologica Microbiologica Scandinavia 84: 477–487

Arnold A, Cossman J, Bakhshi A 1983 Immunoglobulin-gene rearrangements as unique clonal markers in human lymphoid neoplasms. New England Journal of Medicine 313: 776

Askin F B, Rosai J, Sibley R K et al 1979 Malignant small cell tumor of the thoracopulmonary region in childhood. Cancer 43: 2438–2451

Azumi N, Curtis J, Kempson R L, Hendrickson M R 1987 Atypical and malignant neoplasms showing lipomatous differentiation: a study of 111 cases. American Journal of Surgical Pathology 11(3): 161–183

Azzopardi J G, Iocco J, Salm R 1979 Pleomorphic lipoma: a tumour simulating liposarcoma. Histopathology 7: 511-523

Balaban–Malenbaum G, Gilbert F 1977 Double minute chromosomes and the homogeneously staining regions in chromosomes of a human neuroblastoma cell line. Science 198: 739–741

Beckwith J B, Perrin E V 1963 In situ neuroblastoma: a contribution to the natural history of neural crest tumors. American Journal of Pathology 43: 1089–1104

Bednar B 1957 Storiform neurofibromas of the skin, pigmented and nonpigmented. Cancer 10: 368–376

Beham A, Schmid C, Hodl S, Fletcher C D M 1989 Spindle cell and pleomorphic lipoma: an immunohistochemical study and histogenetic analysis. Journal of Pathology 158: 219–222

Belcher R W, Czarnetzki B M, Carney J F et al 1974 Multiple (subcutaneous) angiolipomas, clinical, pathologic and pharmacologic studies. Archives of Dermatology 110: 583

Bishop J M 1983 Cellular oncogenes and retroviruses. Annual Review Biochemistry 52: 301–354

Bolen J W, Thorning D 1980 Peripheral neuroepithelioma: a light and electron microscopic study. Cancer 46: 2456–2462

Bolen J W, Thorning D 1981 Spindle cell lipoma: a clinical light and electron microscopic study. American Journal of Surgical Pathology 5: 435–441

Brenner W, Schaefler K, Chabra H et al 1975 Dermatofibrosarcoma protuberans metastatic to a regional lymph node. Cancer 36: 1897–1902

Breslow N, McCann B 1971 Statistical estimation of prognosis for children with neuroblastoma. Cancer Research 31: 2098–2103

Chaudhuri B, Ronan S, Ghosh L 1980 Benign lipoblastoma: report of a case. Cancer 46: 611–614

Chung E B, Enzinger F M 1973 Benign lipoblastomatosis: an analysis of 35 cases. Cancer 32: 482–492

Cook S A, Hayaskik, Lalli A F 1973 Pelvic lipomatosis. Cleveland Clinic Quarterly 40: 35

Cooper P H 1988 Is histiocytoid hemangioma a specific pathologic entity? American Journal of Surgical Pathology 12: 815–817

Corrin B, Manners B, Millard M et al 1979 Histogenesis of the so-called 'Intravascular bronchioloalveolar tumour'. Journal of Pathology 128: 163

Cossman J, Bakhshi A, Korsmeyer S 1986 Gene rearrangements applied to diagnostic pathology. In: Rose N R, Friedman H, Fabely J L (eds) Manual of clinical laboratory immunology. American Society of Microbiology, Washington DC p 168–173

Cowell J K 1982 Double minutes and homogeneously staining regions: gene amplification in mammalian cells. Annual Review of Genetics 16: 21–59

Dahl I 1977 Ancient neurilemoma (schwannoma). Acta Pathologica Microbilogica Scandinavica (A) 85: 812–818

Dail D H, Liebow A A 1975 Intravascular bronchioalveolar tumor. American Journal Of Pathology 78: 61a

Ding J, Hashimoto H, Enjoji M 1989 Dermatofibrosarcoma protuberans with fibrosarcomatous areas. A clinicopathologic study of nine cases and a comparison with allied tumours. Cancer 64: 721–729

Dionne G P, Seemayer T A 1974 Infiltrating lipomas and angiolipomas revisited. Cancer 33: 732–738

Duncan M R, Perlish J S, Fleischmajer 1984 Lymphokine/monokine inhibition of fibroblast proliferation and collagen production: role in progressive systemic sclerosis (PSS). Journal of Investigative Dermatology 83: 377

Dupree W B, Enzinger F M 1986 Fibroosseous pseudotumor of the digits. Cancer 58: 2103–2109

Dupree W B, Langloss J M, Weiss S W 1985 Pigmented dermatofibrosarcoma protuberans (Bednar tumor): a pathologic, ultrastructural and immunohistochemical study. American Journal of Surgical Pathology 9: 630–639

Enjoji M, Tsuneyoshi M, Hashimoto, H 1976 Subcutaneous angiolipoma, a clinicopathologic observation. Fukuoka Acta Medica 67: 82–89

Enterline H T, Culberson J D, Rochlin D B et al 1960 Liposarcoma: A clinical and pathologic study of 53 cases. Cancer 13: 932–950

Enzinger F M 1965 Fibrous tumors of infancy. In: Tumors of bone and soft tissue (a collection of papers presented at the Eighth Annual Clinical Conference on Cancer, 1963 at the University of Texas M. D. Anderson Hospital and Tumor Institute, Houston, Texas). Year Book Medical Publishers, Chicago

Enzinger F M, Harvey D A 1975 Spindle cell lipoma. Cancer 36: 1852–1859

Enzinger F M, Weiss S W 1983a Benign tumors and tumorlike lesions of fibrous tissue. In: Soft tissue tumors. CV Mosby, St Louis, p 14–44

Enzinger F M, Weiss S W 1983b Benign tumors and tumorlike lesions of fibrous tissue. In: Soft tissue tumors. CV Mosby, St Louis, p 22

Enzinger F M, Weiss S W 1983c Soft tissue tumors, general considerations. In: Soft tissue tumors. CV Mosby, St Louis, p 8

Enzinger F M, Weiss S W 1983d Soft tissue tumors, general considerations. In: Soft Tissue tumors. CV Mosby, St Louis p 6–7

Enzinger F M, Weiss S W 1983e Fibrohistiocytic tumors of intermediate malignancy. In: Soft tissue tumors. CV Mosby, St Louis, p 154–165

Enzinger F M, Weiss S Z 1983f Fibrohistiocytic tumors of intermediate malignancy. In: Soft tissue tumors. CV Mosby, St Louis, p 161

Evans A E, Gerson J, Schnaufer L 1976 Spontaneous recession of neuroblastoma. National Cancer Institute Monogram 44: 49–54

Evans H L 1979 Liposarcoma, a study of 55 cases with a reassessment of its classification. American Journal of Surgical Pathology 3: 507–523

Finklestein J Z, Klemperer M R, Evans A E et al 1979 Chemotherapy for metastatic neuroblastoma. Med Pediatric Oncology 6: 179–188

Fleischmajer R, Perlish J S, West W P 1977 Ultrastructure of cutaneous cellular infiltrates in scleroderma. Archives of Dermatology 113: 1661

Fletcher C D M, Evans B J, Macartney J C, Smith N, Wilson Jones E, McKee P H 1985 Dermatofibrosarcoma protuberans : a clinicopathological and immunohistochemical study with a review of the literature. Histopathology 9: 921–938

Fletcher C D M, Martin-Bates E 1987 Spindle cell lipoma: a clinicopathological study with some original observations. Histopathology 11: 803–817

Fletcher C D M, Martin-Bates E 1988 Intramuscular and intermuscular lipoma: neglected diagnoses. Histopathology 12: 275–287

Fletcher C D M, Theaker J M, Flanagan A, Krausz T 1988 Pigmented dermatofibrosarcoma protuberans (Bednar tumour): melanocytic colonisation or neuroectodermal differentiation?

A clinicopathological and immunohistochemical study. Histopathology 13: 631–643

Folkman J 1983 Angiogeneisis: initiation and modulation. Symposium Fundamental Cancer Research 36: 201–208

Furley A J, Mizutani S, Weilbaecher K et al 1986 Developmentally regulated rearrangement and expression of genes encoding the T-cell receptor T3 complex. Cell 46: 75

Green A A, Hayes F A 1984 Neuroblastoma presenting in the first year of life —surgical staging and therapy. American Society of Clinical Oncology 3: 84

Grody W W, Cheng L, Lewin K J 1987 In situ viral DNA hybridization in diagnostic surgical pathology. Human Pathology 18(6): 535–543

Hajdu S I, Foote F W Jr 1969 Angiomyolipoma of the kidney, report of 27 cases and review of the literature. Urology 102: 396

Hashimoto H, Daimaru Y, Enjoji M, Nakagawara A 1989 N-myc gene product expression in neuroblastoma. Journal of Clinical Pathology 42: 52–55

Henson D E, Albores–Saavedra J (eds) 1986 The pathology of incipient neoplasia. W B Saunders, Philadelphia PA

Israel M 1986 The evolution of clinical molecular genetics. American Journal of Pediatric Hematology/Oncology 8(2): 163–172

Jenson A B, Lancaster W D, Kurnan R J 1986 Uterine cervix. In: Henson E Albores–Saavedra J (eds) The pathology of incipient neoplasia. W B Saunders, Philadelphia PA

Kim H, Dorfman R, Rappaport H 1978 Signet ring cell lymphoma. American Journal of Surgical Pathology 2: 119–132

Kindblom L G, Angervall L, Fassina A S 1982 Atypical lipoma. Acta Pathologica Microbiologica Immunologica Scandinavia (A) 90: 27-36

Kindblom L G, Angervall L, Stener B et al 1974 Intermuscular lipomas and intramuscular lipomas and hibernoma, a clinical, roentgenologic, histologic and prognostic study of 46 cases. Cancer 33: 754-762

Korotzer T I, Page R C, Granger G A, Rabinovitch P S 1982 Regulation of growth of human diploid fibroblasts by factors elaborated by activated lymphoid cells. Journal of Cell Physiology 111: 247

Korn J H, Halushka P V, LeRoy E C 1980 Mononuclear cell modulation of connective tissue function. Journal of Clinical Investigation 65: 543

Lauer D, Enzinger F M 1980 Cranial fasciitis. Cancer 45: 401–406

Leibovich S J, Ross R 1975 The role of the macrophage in wound repair: a study with hydrocortisone and antimacrophage serum. American Journal of Pathology 78: 71

Lopez R, Karakausis C, Rao U 1980 Treatment of adult neuroblastoma. Cancer 45: 840–844

McArthur W, Derr M, Dixon S, Jimenez A, Rosenbloom J 1982 Immune modulation of connective tissue function: studies on the production of collagen synthesis inhibitory factor by populations of human peripheral blood mononuclear cells. Cell Immunology 74: 126

McCarthy D M, Dorr C A, Mackintosh C F 1969 Unilateral localized gigantism of the extremities with lipomatosis, arthropathy and psoriasis. Journal of Bone and Joint Surgery 51B : 348

Meister P, Konrad E A, Buckmann F W 1979 Nodular fasciitis and proliferative myositis as variants of one disease entity. Investigative Cell Pathology 2: 277–281

Mori Y, Yumoto T 1975 A case of hibernoma. Japanese Journal Cancer Clinic 21: 360

Murphy N G 1974 Ossifying lipoma. British Journal of Radiology 47: 97

Napolitano L 1963 The differentiation of white adipose cells: an electron microscopic study. Journal of Cell Biology 18: 663

Oliver J M, Vuletin J C, Moussouris H F, Gillooley J F 1987 Adult variant of cranial fasciitis of childhood. Laboratory Investigation 56: 57A (Abstract)

Patchefsky A, Enzinger F M 1981 Intravascular fasciitis. American Journal of Surgical Pathology 5: 29-36

Patterson J W, Moran S L, Konerding H 1988 Cranial fasciitis. Journal of Cutaneous Pathology 15: 335 (Abstract)

Postlethwaite A E, Smith G N, Mainardi C L, Seyer J M, Kang A H 1984 Lymphocyte modulation of fibroblast function in vitro: stimulation and inhibition of collagen production by different effector molecules. Journal of Immunology 132: 2470

Postlethwaite A E, Snyderman R, Kang A H 1976 The chemotactic attraction of human fibroblasts to a lymphocyte-derived factor. Journal of Experimental Medicine 114: 1188

Raffeld M, Wright J J, Lipfad E et al 1987 Clonal evaluation of + (14;18) follicular lymphomas demonstrated by immunoglobulin genes and the 18q 21 major breakpoint region. Cancer 47: 2537–2542

Rickwood A M K, Hemalatha V, Zachary R B 1979 Lipoma of the cauda equina (lumbrosacral lipoma): a study of 74 cases operated in childhood. Zeitschrift für Kinderchirurgie 27: 159

Rola-Pleszczynski M, Lieu H, Hamel J, Lemaire I 1982 Stimulated human lymphocytes produce a soluble factor which inhibits fibroblast migration. Cell Immunology 74: 104

Rosai J, Gold J, Landy R 1979 The histocytoid hemangiomas: a unifying concept embracing several previously described entities of skin, soft tissue, large vessels, bone and heart. Human Pathology 10: 707–730

Salmon D J, Boone T C, Seeger R C et al 1986 Identification and characterization of the protein encoded by human N-myc oncogene. Science 232: 768–772

Salmon D J, deKernion J B, Verna I M, Cline M J 1984 Expression of cellular oncogenes in human malignancies. Science 224: 256–262

Schmidt J A, Mizel S B, Cohen D, Green I 1982 Interleukin 1: a potential regulator of fibroblast proliferation. Journal of Immunology 128: 2177

Schrier R W, Melmon K L, Fenster L F 1965 Subcutaneous nodular fat necrosis in pancreatitis. Archives of Internal Medicine 116: 832

Schuler F A III, Graham J K, Horton CHE 1976 Benign symmetrical lipomatosis (Madelung's disease). Journal of Plastic and Reconstructive Surgery 57: 662

Schwab M, Alitulo K, Klenprauer K H et al 1983 Amplified DNA with limited homology to myc cellular oncogene is shared by human neuroblastoma cell lines and a neuroblastoma tumor. Nature 305: 245–248

Schwab M, Ellison J, Busch M et al 1984 Enhanced expression of the human gene N-myc consequent to amplification of DNA may contribute to malignant progression of neuroblastoma. Proceedings of National Academy of Science (USA) 81: 4940–4944

Scott G A, Rosai J 1988 Spindle cell hemangioendothelioma. Report of seven additional cases of a recently described vascular neoplasm. American Journal of Dermatopathology 10: 281–288

Seeger R C, Broden G M, Sather H et al 1985 Association of multiple copies of N-myc oncogene with rapid progression of neuroblastoma. Proceedings of National Academy of Science (USA) 313: 111–116

Seemayer T A, Thelmoa L, Bolande R P et al 1975 Peripheral neuroectodermal tumors. Perspectives in Pediatric Pathology 2: 151–172

Shmookler B M, Enzinger F M 1981 Pleomorphic lipoma: a benign tumor simulating liposarcoma. Cancer 47: 126–133

Shmookler B M, Enzinger F M 1983 Liposarcoma occurring in children: an analysis of 17 cases and review of the literature. Cancer 52: 567–574

Silverman T A, Enzinger F M 1985 Fibrolipomatous hamartoma of nerve, a clinicopathologic analysis of 26 cases. American Journal of Surgical Pathology 9: 7–14

Sklar J 1985 DNA hybridization in diagnostic pathology. Human Pathology 16: 654

Smetana H F, Bernhard W 1950 Sclerosing lipogranuloma. Archives of Pathology 50: 296

Soule E H, Lattes R, Enzinger F M 1986 Pseudosarcomatous (proliferative) fibroblastic lesions. ASCP Classic Teaching Collections, Soft Tissue Series No. 1, American Society of Clinical Pathologists Press, Chicago, p 2

Southern E M 1975 Detection of specific sequences among DNA fragments separated by gel electrophoresis. Journal of Molecular Biology 98: 503

Spielvogel R L, Goltz R W, Kersey J H 1977 Scleroderma-like changes in chronic graft vs. host disease. Archives of Dermatology 113: 1424

Spjut H J, Dorfman H D 1981 Florid reactive periostitis of the tubular bones of the hands and feet. A benign lesion which may simulate osteosarcoma. American Journal of Surgical Pathology 5: 423

Stout A P 1944 Liposarcoma – the malignant tumor of lipoblasts. Annals of Surgery 119: 86–107

Stout A P 1948 Fibrosarcoma: the malignant tumor of fibroblasts. Cancer 1: 30–63

Stout A P 1953 Tumors of the soft tissue. In: Atlas of tumor pathology, 2nd series, fascile 5. Armed Forces Institute of Pathology, Washington D C, Fig. 78, p 125

Strydum D J, Fett J W, Lobb R R et al 1985 Amino acid sequence of human tumor-derived angiogenin. Biochemistry 24(20): 5486–5494

Sullivan C R, Dahlin D C, Bryan R S 1956 Lipoma of the tendon sheath. Journal of Bone and Joint Surgery 38A: 1275

Tsukamoto Y W, Helsel W E, Wahl S M 1981 Macrophage production of fibronectin: a chemoattractant for fibroblasts. Journal of Immunology 127: 673

Tulcinsky D B, Deutsch V, Bubis J J 1970 Myelolipoma of the adrenal gland. British Journal of Surgery 57: 465

Vellios F, Baez J M, Shumacker H B 1958 Lipoblastomatosis: a tumor of fetal fat different from hibernoma. Report of a case with observations on the embryogenesis of human adipose tissue. American Journal of Pathology 34: 1149

Wahl S M, Gately C L 1982 Modulation of fibroblast growth by a lymphokine of human T cell and continuous T cell line of origin. Journal of Immunology 130: 1226

Waldman T W, David M M, Bongiovanni K F et al 1985 Rearrangements of gene for the antigen receptor on T cells as markers of lineage and clonality in human lymphoid neoplasms. New England Journal of Medicine 313: 776

Webb W R 1986 Magnetic resonance imaging of the thorax: review of uses and comparison with computed tomography. In: Proto A V, Greene R (eds) Categorical course on chest radiology. American Roentgen and Radiological Society, Washington D C p 177–184

Weiss S W, Enzinger F M 1986 Spindle cell hemangioendothelioma — a low-grade angiosarcoma resembling a cavenous hemangioma and Kaposi's sarcoma. American Journal of Surgical Pathology 10: 521–530

Weiss S W, Enzinger F M 1982 Epithelioid hemangioendothelioma: a vascular tumor often mistaken for carcinoma. Cancer 50: 970–981

Weiss S W, Ishak K G, Dail D H, Sweet D E, Enzinger F M 1986 Epithelioid hemangioendothelioma and related lesions. Seminars in Diagnostic Pathology 3: 259–287

Weldon-Linne C M, Victor T A, Christ M L 1981 Angiogenic nature of 'intravascular bronchioloalveolar tumor'. Archives of Pathology 105: 628

Woolner L B 1981 Recent advances in pulmonary cytology: early detection and localization of occult lung cancer in symptomless males. In: Koss L G, Coleman D V (eds) Advances in clinical cytology. Butterworth, London p 95–135

World Health Organisation International 1969 Histological classification of tumors, no 3: Histologic typing of soft tissue tumours. World Health Organisation, Geneva

Wrotnowski U, Cooper P H, Shmookler B M 1988 Fibrosarcomatous change in dermatofibrosarcoma protuberans. American Journal of Surgical Pathology 12: 287–293

Young J, Miller R W 1975 Incidence of malignant tumors in US children. Journal of Pediatrics 86: 254

Zavala D C 1975 Diagnostic fiberoptic bronchoscopy; techniques and results of biopsy in 600 patients. Chest 68: 12–19

14. Progress in malignant soft tissue tumours

C. D. M. Fletcher   P. H. McKee

Some of the important aspects in which the diagnosis and management of soft tissue sarcomas has progressed in recent years have been discussed elsewhere in this book, particularly the impact that immunohistochemistry has had on classification (Ch. 8) and the gradual development of readily applied, prognostically useful grading systems (Ch. 11).

This chapter aims to discuss advances in classification and nomenclature, briefly to delineate some of the more recently defined entities and to mention the role of cytogenetic and flow cytometric studies in improving our understanding of the biological nature of some sarcomas. Kaposi's sarcoma, which is probably not a malignant neoplasm anyway, is thoroughly discussed in Chapter 7. Details of all the recent controversial work on malignant fibrous histiocytoma are covered in Chapter 6.

As mentioned in the introductory chapter, while some rather nihilistic individuals might regard the seemingly endless reclassification that goes on in the field of soft tissue tumours as inappropriate and unnecessary, it should be remembered that this simply represents very vital refining of what was once a diagnostic mêlée and that this refining has been telescoped into a relatively short period of time because of the dramatic impact of modern investigative techniques. The importance of this pursuit of accurate categorisation lies in the fact that soft tissue sarcomas are, clinically, one of the worst treated groups of malignant tumours and only by the application of consistent diagnostic criteria can patient management be improved, particularly with regard to determining the sensitivities of a given tumour type to different forms of chemotherapy or radiotherapy.

LIPOSARCOMA

As mentioned briefly in Chapter 13, the most important advance in our attitude to liposarcomas has been the recognition that histologically-pure well differentiated cases, for practical purposes, never metastasise (Evans et al 1979, Kindblom et al 1982). The significance of this finding is that wide excision of a well-differentiated liposarcoma arising in somatic soft tissue (usually a limb) should be curative and tumour-related deaths should not occur. However, this rule does not apply to histologically comparable neoplasms in the retroperitonium because complete excision is rarely possible and relentless local recurrence with involvement of vital structures often leads to the patient's death. For these reasons, Evans et al (1979), proposed the alternative term atypical lipoma for lesions arising in surgically amenable soft tissue, while retaining the name well-differentiated liposarcoma (be it lipoma-like, sclerosing or inflammatory) for such tumours in the retroperitoneum. The value and validity of this change in nomenclature has been borne out by subsequently published large series (Azumi et al 1987).

It should be noted that also encompassed within the term atypical lipoma are adipocytic tumours of somatic, usually deep, soft tissue in which scattered pleomorphic, hyperchromatic and sometimes multinucleate stromal cells are evident (Fig. 14.1) and in which adipocyte nuclei may also appear hyperchromatic. While such lipoma-like lesions often contain occasional multivacuolated lipoblasts, the latter are not a prerequisite for the diagnosis of atypical lipoma (Kindblom et al 1982).

Adoption of the term atypical lipoma has several very important clinico-pathological implications which must be understood if patients are not to be mismanaged. Atypical lipoma of somatic soft tissue, particularly if deeply located, has a local recurrence rate of around 30%, especially if not widely excised. Extensive sampling of both the primary neoplasm and any local recurrences is mandatory to exclude the, albeit uncommon, presence or

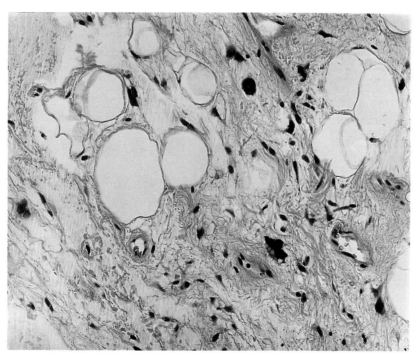

Fig. 14.1 Atypical lipoma. This large tumor from the thigh lacked identifiable lipoblasts but contained hyperchromatic and multinucleate stromal cells. × 250.

development of frankly malignant, cellular pleomorphic or undifferentiated foci which then necessitate the diagnosis of so-called dedifferentiated liposarcoma (Evans 1979, Hashimoto & Enjoji 1982). Dedifferentiated liposarcoma is an aggressive neoplasm which often metastasises and frequently pursues a fatal course. It is therefore vital to appreciate firstly, that such foci must be carefully sought in well-differentiated liposarcomas (irrespective of site or nomenclature) and, secondly, that the phenomenon of so-called dedifferentiation may occur in local recurrences of what had been regarded as an atypical lipoma (Hashimoto & Enjoji 1982), hence dramatically altering the prognosis.

As a consequence, it is also important to distinguish atypical lipoma from infiltrative intramuscular lipoma, since the latter recurs much less often and never behaves in a malignant fashion (Fletcher & Martin-Bates 1988). In our view, in addition, it is inappropriate to lump the clinically characteristic, subcutaneous pleomorphic and spindle cell lipomas with atypical lipoma, as some authors have done (Azumi et al 1987), because the latter lesions almost never recur and also never undergo dedifferentiation (Enzinger & Harvey 1975, Shmookler & Enzinger 1981, Fletcher & Martin-Bates 1987). Perhaps of paramount importance is the necessity of ensuring that clinicians understand the meaning and significance of the term atypical lipoma, in order that patients are adequately treated and properly followed up.

To conclude this section on liposarcoma, a specific chromosomal translocation, t(12;16) (q13;p11), has recently been demonstrated in myxoid liposarcoma (Limon et al 1986, Turc-Carel et al 1986a, Mertens et al 1987). Whether this finding will prove to be of regular differential diagnostic value is arguable, since it is unrealistic to imagine that sophisticated cytogenetic techniques will become routinely available in any but a few laboratories. It will, however, be of interest to see if the same translocation can be found in round cell liposarcoma, which, if present, would provide evidence to support the widely held belief that the latter tumour is simply the poorly differentiated version of myxoid liposarcoma.

RHABDOMYOSARCOMA

Undoubtedly the most significant advance with regard to rhabdomyosarcomas has been the tremendous improvement in cure rate or prolonged survival of childhood cases, particularly of the embryonal type. This is directly attributable to the increasing use of surgery, chemotherapy and radiotherapy in combination, as exemplified by the large, long-term Intergroup Rhabdomyosarcoma Study in the USA. Details of this work are beyond the scope of this chapter and readers are referred to several major papers on the subject (Maurer et al 1977, Raney et al 1978, Raney et al 1982, Sutow et al 1982, Hawkins & Camacho-Velasquez 1987, Raney et al 1987). While embryonal rhabdomyosarcoma was accepted to have about an 80% mortality in the past (Horn & Enterline 1958, Lawrence et al 1964, Soule et al 1978), with most fatalities occurring within a year of diagnosis, 3-year survival figures of anything between 50% and 80% are now widely accepted (Maurer et al 1988). The importance of these results to the pathologist is that every effort should be made to categorise 'small round cell sarcomas' of childhood, often with the implementation of immunohistochemistry and electron microscopy, since there is good evidence that embryonal rhabdomyosarcomas are much more treatable and have a much better prognosis than, for example, unclassifiable small cell sarcomas, extraskeletal Ewing's sarcoma and primitive neuroecto-dermal tumours. Furthermore, clinicians should be encouraged to ensure that patients with embryonal rhabdomyosarcoma are treated in centres with the capability of providing up-to-date multimodal therapy.

There have also been morphological advances in the diagnosis of other variants of rhabdomyosarcoma. Pleomorphic rhabdomyosarcoma, which was formerly thought to be a relatively common sarcoma of adulthood (Linscheid et al 1965, Keyhani & Booher 1968) has been the subject of vigorous culling in recent years, largely because the majority of cases so diagnosed show no evidence of rhabdomyoblastic differentiation, despite being composed of large eosinophilic cells which theoretically represent a more mature stage of muscle differentiation than is seen in the embryonal or alveolar types. In particular, glycogen and cross-striations are absent in the vast majority of cases and less that 10% express immunohistochemical markers of myogenic differentiation (Molenaar et al 1985, De Jong et al 1987). Most neoplasms formerly classified as pleomorphic rhabdomyosarcoma would nowadays be recategorised under the all-embracing term pleomorphic malignant fibrous histiocytoma, which often contains large eosinophilic cells (Weiss 1982).

Nevertheless, there is no doubt that occasional cases of pleomorphic rhabdomyosarcoma, showing identifiable differentiation, do exist both in infancy and adulthood but there are too few data available by which to create a clear-cut clinicopathological picture of such lesions. It should also be remembered that, infrequently, examples of both embryonal and alveolar rhabdomyosarcoma may contain pleomorphic areas.

A further histopathological development has been the recognition of a 'solid' variant of alveolar rhabdomyosarcoma, which may be confused with embryonal rhabdomyosarcoma, and which carries a very poor prognosis (Tsokos et al 1984, Tsokos 1986, Tsokos & Triche 1986). Unfortunately the details of this work by Tsokos and her colleagues have to date only been published in abstract form and it is therefore difficult to be certain of their diagnostic criteria. However, it would appear that their cases are comparable to the solid type of alveolar rhabdomyosarcoma described by Enzinger and Weiss (1983). These lesions are composed predominantly of solid, diffuse sheets of rounded basophilic cells, distinguishable from poorly differentiated embryonal rhabdomyosarcoma by their greater uniformity and rather larger size (Fig. 14.2). Only about 10% of cases seem to show a focally characteristic alveolar pattern, but further evidence that they do represent a variant of alveolar, rather than embryonal, rhabdomyosarcoma has been provided by

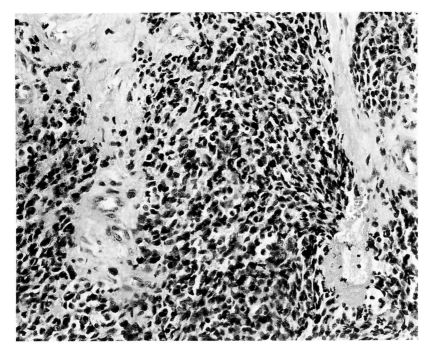

Fig. 14.2 Solid variant of alveolar rhabdomyosarcoma consisting of sheets of uniform rounded cells with small amounts of variably eosinophilic cytoplasm. × 250.

studies in nude mice, in which inoculation of classical alveolar tumours produces solid pattern neoplasms similar to those described above (Kouraklis et al 1987). Further published work on this apparently prognostically important tumour is keenly awaited.

Interestingly, conventional alveolar rhabdomyosarcoma has also proved to be one of the few sarcomas described to date to show a specific chromosomal translocation, repeatedly found to be t(2;13) (q37;q14) (Seidal et al 1982, Turc-Carel et al 1986b, Rowe et al 1987, Sandberg & Turc-Carel 1987). As Rowe et al point out, this finding may be of oncogenetic significance since band q14 on chromosome 13 is thought to represent a tumour-suppressing gene, rearrangement of which might obviously disrupt its function. Demonstration of this same translocation in the solid rhabdomyosarcomas described above would add considerable weight to their suggested relationship with alveolar rhabdomyosarcoma.

SYNOVIAL SARCOMA

The most important fact that has come to light about synovial sarcoma in recent years is the realisation that it is histogenetically totally unrelated to synovium and therefore the only, rather weak justification for retaining the name 'synovial' sarcoma is that these lesions frequently arise in tissues adjacent to large joints. However, this is by no means always the case as this tumour is well recognised to arise at such varied sites as the abdominal wall, pharynx and orofacial region.

Much evidence has accumulated against a true synovial origin, initially from ultrastructural studies which have consistently demonstrated a basal lamina between tumour cells, a feature which has never been described in normal or reactive synovium (Gabbiani et al 1971, Mickelson et al 1980, Fisher 1986). Major enzyme histochemical differences from synovium have also been found (Pisa et al 1982), but the most overwhelming evidence has been derived from immunohistochemistry. Numerous studies have repeatedly demonstrated the presence of cytokeratin and epithelial membrane antigen (EMA) in classical synovial sarcoma, both of which markers are absent from synovium, reactive synovial lesions and known synovial tumours, such as giant cell tumour of tendon sheath (Miettinen et al 1982, Corson et al 1984, Miettinen & Virtanen 1984, Salisbury & Isaacson 1985, Fisher 1986, Leader et al 1987). Miettinen and Virtanen (1984) also demonstrated clear differences in the lectin binding patterns of normal synovium and synovial sarcoma and they were the first authors to propose that these tumours should be reclassified as carcinosarcomas of soft tissue, on the principal grounds that these neoplasms coexpress both epithelial and mesenchymal (vimentin) markers, In fact, synovial sarcoma shows very great histological, histochemical and immunohistochemical similarities to malignant mesothelioma.

While the name 'carcinosarcoma' is both more logical and rather more accurate than synovial sarcoma, it has several drawbacks. Firstly, it sidesteps the problem of histogenesis, however futile pursuit of that question may be, and therefore fails to explain the presence of epithelial differentiation in mesenchymal soft tissue. Secondly, epithelioid sarcoma, the histogenesis of which is also unknown, fulfils all the same criteria to be relabelled carcinosarcoma of soft tissue in so far as electron microscopy and immunohistochemistry go; yet it is obviously clinicopathologically different from synovial sarcoma and it would be foolish to merge the two entities, as some have suggested, on the basis of the technical evidence available to date. Thirdly, and in some ways most importantly, it would be inappropriate to impose a precipitate change in nomenclature which would probably be impermanent and which could well disturb and confuse the fairly clear image that most clinicians and pathologists have of the biological nature of so-called synovial sarcoma. Any future alteration in this tumour's name should be defensible in the long term and should be based on the evident need to provide a clear distinction from epithelioid sarcoma.

While immunohistochemistry and electron microscopy could be held responsible for promoting confusion over the nature of synovial sarcoma, they have, at the same time, played a major role in supporting the existence of monophasic spindle-celled synovial sarcomas, which have been a source of controversy for many years. While careful sampling might sometimes be the easiest way of proving the diagnosis of synovial sarcoma by demonstrating albeit tiny foci of glandular differentiation (Mackenzie 1977), there are undoubtedly lesions in which such differentiation is undetectable but in which the diagnosis of synovial sarcoma is suggested by the typical fibrosarcoma-like appearance associated with a pericytoma-like vascular pattern, a rather hyaline stroma, calcification and/or peripheral ossification and a prominent mast cell infiltrate in the stroma. Convincing evidence has now emerged that the majority of these tumours do belong in the category of synovial sarcoma, as demonstrated by their ultrastructural similarities to ordinary biphasic synovial sarcoma (Krall et al 1981, Miettinen et al 1983, Fisher 1986) and by their same coexpression of epithelial and mesenchymal markers (Corson et al 1984, Abenoza et al 1986, Fisher 1986). There are, therefore, now more reliable means of defending the diagnosis of monophasic synovial sarcoma than simple morphological findings.

Further compelling evidence for the existence of monophasic synovial sarcoma has been the demonstration of a specific chromosomal translocation, t(x;18)(q22.1;q11.2), in both biphasic and monophasic variants of this tumour (Turc-Carel et al 1986c), which has now been demonstrated in over a dozen published cases and efforts have been made to map the precise breakpoint of the X chromosome (Reeves et al 1989). Recent evidence suggests that chromosome 18 may play the more important role in the cytogenetic rearrangements seen in synovial sarcoma (Limon et al 1989).

Another variant of synovial sarcoma has only fairly recently been described and is characterised by extensive calcification — so-called calcifying synovial sarcoma (Varela-Duran & Enzinger 1982). All such tumours are of the biphasic type and predominantly arise in the limbs. They are typified by very widespread calcification, both within hyalinised collagen of the spindle cell component and within glandular spaces (Fig. 14.3), often in association with osseous or chondroid metaplasia. Their importance lies in their much better prognosis than ordinary synovial sarcoma, with a 5-year survival of 82.6%, as opposed to about 50% (Wright et al 1982, Tsuneyoshi et al 1983), and a 10-year survival of 66%. The only obvious problem with this entity is to know where to draw the cut-off point between the not uncommon calcification seen in ordinary synovial sarcomas and the heavy calcification which confers a good prognosis. Currently there is no answer to this question, but it would seem advisable to err on the side of caution when making prognostic predictions.

Cagle et al (1987) have suggested what appears to be a fairly reliable grading system applicable to all types of synovial sarcoma, which is based on the extent of glandular differentiation and mitotic activity. Tumours showing greater than 50% glandular differentiation and less than 15 mitoses per 10 high power fields (HPF) have an excellent prognosis (quoted 3-year survival 100%), whereas those with less than 50% glandularity and more than 15 mitoses per 10 HPF had a 3-year survival of 43% and those falling between the two groups had a 3-year figure of 82%. Other authors have recently confirmed the importance of the mitotic count, but have stressed that tumour size may be the most significant prognostic factor (Rooser et al 1989).

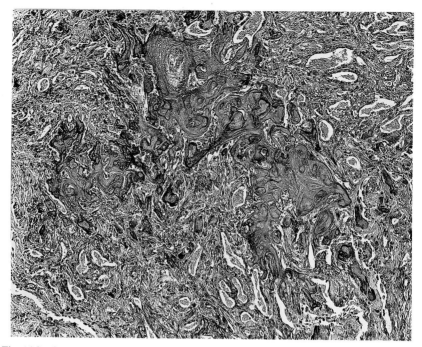

Fig. 14.3   Calcifying synovial sarcoma. This biphasic lesion from the thigh shows massive calcification and ossification. × 100.

MALIGNANT MELANOMA OF SOFT TISSUES

Malignant melanoma of soft tissues (Chung & Enzinger 1983) is now the preferred name for clear cell sarcoma of tendons and aponeuroses, as was first described by Enzinger in 1965. This relatively uncommon neoplasm, which principally arises in the distal portions of the limbs of young adults, has long been noted to contain pigment in many cases (Fig. 14.4), but this was formerly thought to be iron (Enzinger 1965, Angervall & Stener 1969). However, numerous subsequent case studies have shown the pigment to be melanin and irrefutable ultrastructural evidence of melanogenesis within tumour cells (Fig. 14.5) has been provided (Hoffman & Carter 1973, Mackenzie 1974, Bearman et al 1975, Boudreaux & Waisman 1978, Toe & Saw 1978, Ekfors & Rantakokko 1979). Despite a bid to separate clear cell sarcoma into melanotic and synovial types (Tsuneyoshi et al 1978), good evidence that both the melanotic and amelanotic cases represent a common entity, totally unrelated to synovial sarcoma, refutes this proposition (Kindblom et al 1983, Mukai et al 1984). Immunohistochemically this tumour shows the same phenotype as cutaneous malignant melanoma, including expression of melanoma-specific antigens such as HMB-45 (Swanson & Wick 1989), and hence distinction from metastatic melanoma may sometimes depend on clinical features.

Clear cell sarcoma does, nevertheless, show ultrastructural differences from ordinary cutaneous malignant melanoma (Benson et al 1985) and its precise

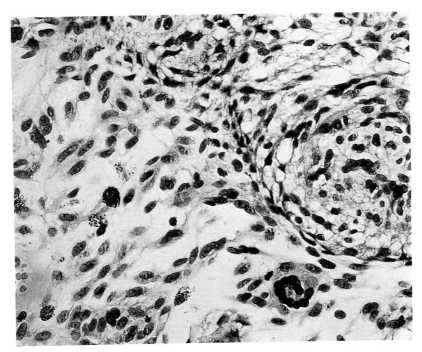

Fig. 14.4 Malignant melanoma of soft tissues. Granular melanin pigment and a typical multinucleate, wreath-like giant cell are evident in this tumor from the ankle region. × 400.

histogenesis remains uncertain. While it is possible that it is derived from melanocytes that migrated to periarticular soft tissue in utero, as proposed by Enzinger and Weiss (1983), it can only be stated with any degreee of certainty that so-called clear cell sarcoma is a neuroectodermal neoplasm and that the evident melanogenesis may simply reflect the pluripotentiality of almost any cell type derived from the neural crest.

PERIPHERAL NEUROEPITHELIOMA, EXTRASKELETAL EWING'S SARCOMA AND ASKIN TUMOURS

Under this heading, recent fascinating revelations of shared patterns of differentiation and proposed histogenetic similarities between the above group of primitive 'small cell' sarcomas (as described briefly in Ch.13) are discussed.

It is, perhaps, easiest to comprehend these recent developments if one takes peripheral neuroepithelioma (primitive neuroectodermal tumour of soft tissue) as the prototype. Peripheral neuroepithelioma (Bolen & Thorning 1980, Harper et al 1981, Hashimoto et al 1983, Voss et al 1984, Coffin & Dehner 1986) may present over a wide range but is commonest in adolescents and young adults, may arise almost anywhere in somatic soft tissue (most often the trunk) and shows demonstrable origin from a nerve in about 20% of cases. The prognosis is generally rather poor. While sometimes being composed almost entirely of small, round basophilic cells, it frequently shows

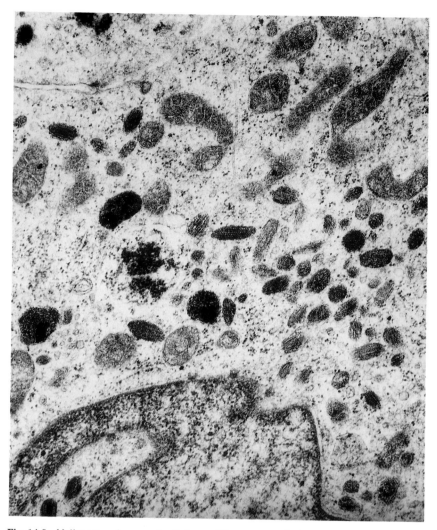

Fig. 14.5 Malignant melanoma of soft tissues. The tumour cells in this lesion from the calf musculature show typical structured melanosomes. × 33 000.

rosettes (of the Homer-Wright type) (Fig. 14.6) or pseudorosettes. Up to one-third of cases contain small amounts of glycogen by the PAS technique, the majority express neuron-specific enolase or neurofilaments immunohistochemically and ultrastructurally their neural nature is confirmed by the invariable presence of two or more of the following features: complex, interdigitating cell processes, neurosecretory-type granules and microtubules. Urinary catecholamine metabolites are only occasionally elevated (Voss et al 1984), but clearly, in most cases (particularly in children), spread from an underlying neuroblastoma must be excluded clinically. Of paramount importance to this discussion is the presence of a specific chromosomal transloca-

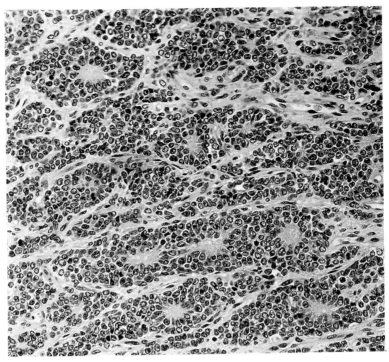

Fig. 14.6 Peripheral neuroepithelioma. Rosettes are particularly prominent in this tumour removed from the pectoral muscles. × 250.

tion, t(11;22) (q24;q12) in peripheral neuroepithelioma (Whang-Peng et al 1984), (Fig. 14.7), which is very different to the chromosomal changes seen in conventional neuroblastoma.

Turning now to extraskeletal Ewing's sarcoma (Angervall & Enzinger 1975, Meister & Gokel 1978, Soule et al 1978, Hashimoto et al 1985, Shimada et al 1988), this uncommon tumour arises most often in adolescents and young adults of either sex and shows a predilection for the trunk, followed by the limbs. As in peripheral neuroepithelioma, the prognosis has usually been poor with many patients dying within a year of diagnosis, although recent evidence suggests that treatment following the IRS rhabdomyosarcoma protocol may be remarkably efficacious (Shimada et al 1988). The tumour cells have scanty cytoplasm and basophilic vesicular nuclei with prominent single, small nucleoli. Mitoses are surprisingly few in number. A reticulin stain often reveals a coarsely lobulated pattern and the tumour cells contain copious glycogen. The latter feature has often been mistakenly employed as evidence against neuroectodermal origin. Ultrastructurally, extraskeletal Ewing's tumours contain few organelles and show little in the way of differentiation other than occasional bundles of intermediate filaments and copious glycogen arranged in rosettes. However, Ewing's sarcoma of bone when grown in tissue culture and incubated with cyclic-AMP or phorbol

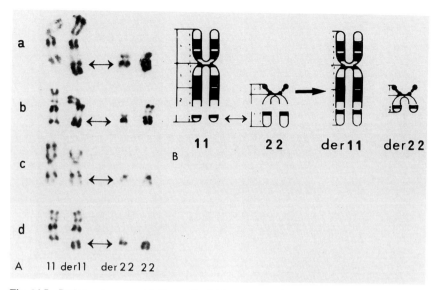

Fig. 14.7 Peripheral neuroepithelioma. Partial karyotype and schematic representation of translocation t(11;22) (q24;q12). (Courtesy of Dr Avery A. Sandberg, The Cancer Center, Arizona, USA.)

12-myristate 13-acetate (TPA) shows full-blown neural differentiation both ultrastructurally and immunocytochemically (Cavazzana et al 1987a). Furthermore, a series of cell lines derived from Ewing's sarcoma have recently been shown to express neuroectodermal antigens, such as ganglioside GD2 and the neural cell adhesion molecule (Lipinski et al 1987).

Yet, in contrast to the latter finding, conventionally studied Ewing's sarcoma of both soft tissue and bone shows immunohistochemical evidence of neural differentiation in only a proportion of cases (Cavazzana et al 1987b, Donner et al 1987, Moll et al 1987, Shimada et al 1988, Ushigome et al 1989) and, in fact, these tumours appear to display a degree of immunohistochemical heterogeneity. Thus far, then, there are only limited data suggestive of a relationship with peripheral neuroepithelioma. However, the overwhelming evidence to support such a relationship has been the demonstration of the identical translocation to neuroepiethelioma, t(11;22) (q24;q12), in repeated cases of Ewing's sarcoma (Aurias et al 1984, Turc-Carel et al 1984, Becroft et al 1984, Whang-Peng et al 1986, Cavazanna et al 1987a).

Then one comes to the so-called Askin tumour (malignant small cell tumour of the thoracopulmonary region), first described by Askin et al in 1979. This neoplasm arises in the pleura, ribs or soft tissue of the chest wall in children or adolescents. Elevated catecholamine levels are not a feature and, like the tumours discussed above, many patients die within a year of diagnosis, although recent results suggest a much improved outlook with multimodality management (Jurgens et al 1988). Histologically, these tumours are composed of sheets or nests of small basophilic cells with little cytoplasm and a coarse nuclear chromatin pattern. Pseudorosettes are a frequent finding and this feature, combined with PAS-negativity and the ultrastructural demonstration of neurosecretory granules, led Askin in his original paper to propose a primitive neuroectodermal original. Since then it has become more generally appreciated that all types of primitve neuroectodermal tumour may, in fact, contain small amounts of glycogen. Other authors (Gonzalez-Crussi et al 1984, Linnoila et al 1986) have gone on to demonstrate convincing neuroectodermal differentiation in Askin tumours, both ultrastructurally and immunohistochemically, and have also shown that these lesions are often PAS positive.

Finally, to further underline the similarities between Askin tumours and peripheral neuroepithelioma, the translocation, t(11;22) (q24;q12), has again been identified in a small number of Askin tumours that have been examined (DeChadarevian et al 1984, Seemayer et al 1985, Whang-Peng et al 1986).

What can one justifiably conclude from these findings? Certainly there is good evidence that peripheral neuroepitheliomas and Askin tumours are of neuroectodermal origin and there is ever increasing reason to believe that at least a significant proportion of what have usually been called extraskeletal Ewing's sarcomas are similarly derived. Should they all be regarded as the same tumour, variants of a single histogenetic entity or simply different tumours all of primitive neuroectodermal origin? This problem has been masterfully reviewed by Dehner (1986) and we would support his contention that these are all phenotypically related neoplasms, which can be grouped under the heading 'peripheral primitive neuroectodermal tumours'. Undoubtedly, ultrastructural similarities and an identical immunohistochemical phenotype are not sufficient grounds to prove a common histogenetic origin and in fact, differences in the lectin binding profile of these three entities have very recently been reported (Swanson et al 1989). Obviously the reproducible, characteristic chromosomal translocation suggests a very close relationship between the three tumour types, but it should be remembered that this finding may only reflect an identical genetic basis for malignant tranasformation in any primitive neuroectodermal cell line and does not of itself prove an identical specific cell of origin. Interestingly, it has been noted that the proto-oncogene C-sis is located on chromosome 22, distal to band q,[11] and that this oncogene is therefore translocated in all these tumour types (Whang-Peng et al 1984): whether this has any significance in terms of malignant transformation as yet remains undecided.

In conclusion, these three tumours, in many cases, appear to be closely related malignant neoplasms of primitive neuroectodermal origin which, while showing minor clinicopathological differences, predominantly affect adolescents and young adults and carry a generally rather poor prognosis. It does seem, however, that there is a case for retaining the term Ewing's sarcoma for those tumours that show no immunohistochemical or ultrastructural evidence of specialised differentiation whatever (Wick et al 1988).

EXTRARENAL RHABDOID TUMOUR

The term rhabdoid tumour was first coined for a group of childhood renal tumours which had originally been thought to represent 'rhabdomyosarcomatoid' variants of Wilm's tumour (Haas et al 1981), but which lacked any evidence of skeletal muscle differentiation. Although Lynch et al (1983) were the first to use this name for lesions arising outside the kidney, previous cases had been described under different guises by Hajdu (1979), who used the term rhabdomyoblastoma, and Gonzalez-Crussi et al (1982). Over the last three years or so, extrarenal rhabdoid tumour has become widely regarded as a diagnostic entity and several small series of the soft tissue variant have been published (Tsuneyoshi et al 1985, Sotelo-Avila et al 1986, Kent et al 1987) along with scattered case reports. It should be noted that extrarenal rhabdoid tumours have now been described to arise at a wide variety of sites, including urinary bladder (Harris et al 1987, Carter et al 1989), liver (Sotelo-Avila et al 1986), brain (Biggs et al 1987) and skin (Dabbs & Park 1988).

Extrarenal rhabdoid tumours, at whatever site, present over a wide age range, extending into middle age as described to date, but are commonest in infants and children. There is an apparent predilection for males. They are characterised clinically by a rapidly growing, infiltrative mass which is frequently inoperable. Despite modern multimodal therapy, the majority of

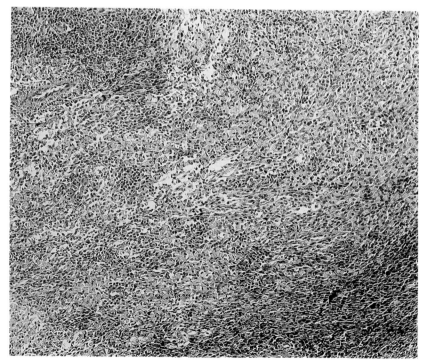

Fig. 14.8   Extrarenal rhabdoid tumour. This tumour from the axillary region of a young woman consists of seemingly undifferentiated round and spindle-shaped cells. × 100.

patients succumb within one or two years with widely disseminated disease. Interestingly, extrarenal rhabdoid tumours do not appear to be as frequently associated with the separate development of a primary intracranial primitive neuroectodermal tumour as are their renal counterparts (Sotelo-Avila et al 1986).

Histologically these tumours are extremely cellular and often show widespread necrosis. In most cases the cells are arranged in diffuse sheets (Fig. 14.8), but a poorly formed trabecular or alveolar pattern is occasionally evident. The majority of the tumour cells are fairly small, of round or polygonal shape and have copious eosinophilic cytoplasm, hence the resemblance to rhabdomyoblasts. The characteristic feature is the presence in many of the cells of a spherical, hyaline, brightly eosinophilic intracytoplasmic inclusion, which often seems to occupy much of the cytoplasm (Fig. 14.9). These inclusions may be weakly PAS-positive, diastase-resistant. The nuclei are ovoid or polygonal with a vesicular appearance and a prominent, large eosinophilic nucleolus, the latter being a useful diagnostic feature. Mitotic figures are generally quite prominent. Focally, the tumour may adopt a more basophilic, spindle-celled appearance.

Ultrastructurally, the diagnostic sine qua non is the presence of prominent paranuclear whorls of 7–10 nm intermediate filaments (Fig. 14.10), which correspond to the hyaline intracytoplasmic inclusions and within which entrapped mitochondria or lipid remnants may be seen. The cells have no

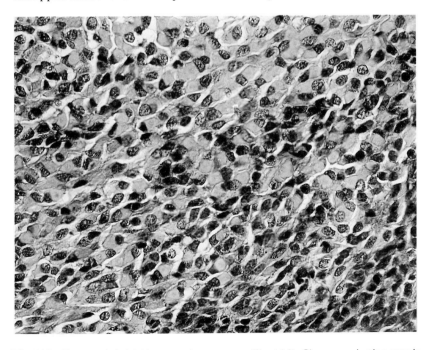

Fig. 14.9 Extrarenal rhabdoid tumour (same case as Fig. 14.8). Closer examination reveals typical hyaline intracytoplasmic inclusions. × 400.

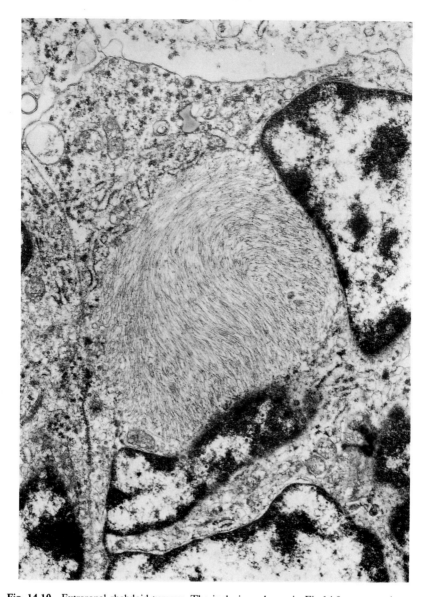

Fig. 14.10   Extrarenal rhabdoid tumour. The inclusions shown in Fig.14.9 correspond to striking paranuclear whorled aggregates of intermediate filaments, as seen in this different case (Courtesy of Dr P Dervan, Mater Misericordiae Hospital, Dublin.) × 16 000.

other distinguishing electron microscopic features, other than that they lack any sarcomeric differentiation or a basal lamina.

Immunohistochemical studies have produced very variable results, other than the consistent striking vimentin positivity of the intracytoplasmic inclusions. These tumours have been variously reported to be positive for epithelial markers (such as EMA and cytokeratin — Tsuneyoshi et al 1985,

Sotelo-Avila et al 1986, Harris et al 1987, Parham et al 1987, Tsokos et al 1987), neural markers (such as S-100 protein, neuron-specific enolase and glial fibrillary acidic protein — Sotelo-Avila et al 1986, Harris et al 1987, Kent et al 1987, Parham et al 1987), and myogenous markers (such as desmin and myoglobin — Parham et al 1987, Tsokos et al 1989). In contrast, some authors have only demonstrated vimentin positivity with a complete absence of all the antigens listed above (Biggs et al 1987, Dervan et al 1987). Since immuno-histochemistry is now a routine, reasonably reliable technique, it is not possible to ignore these varied results on the grounds of shoddy methodology or dubious antisera.

All manner of histogeneses have been proposed for extrarenal rhabdoid tumours, including histiocytic, epithelial, neuroectodermal or primitive mesenchymal. Incontrovertible evidence is not available to support any one of these single hypotheses and the current general concensus would seem to be that these lesions represent the shared morphological appearance of a wide range of high-grade, primitive neoplasms of variable or uncertain histogenetic origin showing phenotypic diversity. Such a suggestion is, to some extent, supported by the recent demonstration of varying numbers of ultrastructurally characteristic rhabdoid cells within a variety of otherwise typical specified sarcomas (Tsuneyoshi et al 1987). In contrast to this uncertain picture, renal rhabdoid tumours appear to be defensible as a discrete entity (Weeks et al 1989).

DNA FLOW CYTOMETRY OF SOFT TISSUE SARCOMAS

Very little work has been published on the possible prognostic or diagnostic use of DNA flow cytometry in soft tissue tumours. Until about five years ago, this was explicable by the relative dearth of suitably prepared fresh material in single centres, but the description of a technique suitable for the examination of paraffin-embedded material (Hedley et al 1983) has allowed a dramatic expansion in the number of cases available for study. Even so, with the exception of a small number of international centres, very few workers are able to collect a sufficiently large number of a given diagnostic entity to allow the necessary degree of statistical analysis to provide prognostically worth-while data, as has been possible with the more common carcinomas and lymphomas.

Several papers have stated that the majority of sarcomas are aneuploid, but there seems to be little agreement as to whether ploidy correlates with histological grade (Barlogie et al 1983, Kreicbergs et al 1987, Xiang et al 1987). While nearly all benign soft tissue tumours studied to date have been diploid (Kreicbergs et al 1987, El-Naggar et al 1988a, Radio et al 1988), with a few notable exceptions (Fletcher & Camplejohn 1987, Koss et al 1989), this finding is of no use in a differential diagnostic sense since a proportion of sarcomas are also diploid. Whether sarcomas with a diploid DNA content have a better prognosis irrespective of histological grade, as has recently been suggested (El-Naggar et al 1988a, Radio et al 1988) remains to be substantiated by larger series. It is of interest to note that in a comparative study of the different types of MFH, the angiomatoid variant was found to be consistently diploid in stark contrast to the other types (El-Naggar et al 1988b).

The possible utility of measuring S-phase fraction as a prognostic indicator is hampered by a certain amount of disagreement over both the validity of calculating S-phase fractions in aneuploid tumours and the technique by which such fractions are calculated. However, Kreicbergs et al (1987) found assessment of the proportion of cells in S-phase to be unhelpful and simply a reflection of ploidy. More depressingly, there do not even seem to be internationally agreed criteria for the recognition of aneuploidy as yet (Xiang et al 1987).

Therefore, at the current time, DNA flow cytometry offers an apparently limited amount of clinically useful information on soft tissue sarcomas. There is, however, scope for a great deal more work in this area and future results may prove to be of considerable interest. In this regard, Molenaar et al (1988) have recently shown that DNA aneuploidy may be a useful means of distinguishing rhabdomyosarcomas from other round cell sarcomas of childhood.

An alternative means of assessing proliferative activity is immunohistochemical staining with the monoclonal antibody Ki-67. Interestingly, in contrast to measurement of S-phase fraction, the extent of nuclear staining with Ki-67 has very recently been shown to correlate fairly well with prognosis in sarcomas (Ueda et al 1989).

STEROID HORMONE RECEPTORS IN SOFT TISSUE SARCOMAS

The possible influence of female sex hormones on desmoid fibromatoses has long been recognised (see recent review by Fletcher et al 1986), and Hayry et al (1982) have demonstrated both oestrogen and progesterone receptors in these lesions. However, a search for the presence of hormone receptors in true soft tissue sarcomas has only been made in recent years.

Based on some evidence that premenopausal females with soft tissue sarcoma have an improved prognosis, Chaudhuri et al (1980, 1981) studied a wide range of sarcomas for the presence of androgen, oestrogen, progesterone and glucocorticoid receptors using steroid receptor binding assays on fresh frozen material. They found that, overall, 55% of 66 sarcomas studied bound at least one steroid hormone, of which glucocorticoid was the commonest. Receptor status was not related to age, but the incidence of oestrogen and glucocorticoid receptors was increased in females. Although these receptors were distributed among a variety of sarcoma types, these authors made the interesting observations, firstly that female sex hormone receptors were totally absent from malignant fibrous histiocytoma and fibrosarcoma and, secondly, that progesterone receptors were only demonstrated in Kaposi's sarcoma.

Weiss et al (1986) have more recently examined a range of sarcomas for oestrogen and progesterone receptors using monoclonal antibodies, steroid-binding assay and enzyme immunoassay techniques. They found the steroid-binding assay to be the most reliable and that only 6 out of 33 cases contained oestrogen receptor protein and that a similar number of tumours carried progesterone receptors, albeit usually in lower concentrations.

As yet there are no convincing data to suggest that steroid receptor status bears any relationship to histological type, grade or prognosis, although oestrogen receptors, not surprisingly, are more common in sarcomas arising in females. Nor is there any evidence to date that soft tissue sarcomas are hormonally dependent.

REFERENCES

Abenoza R, Manivel J C, Swanson P E, Wick M R 1986 Synovial sarcoma: ultrastructural study and immunohistochemical analysis by a combined peroxidase/antiperoxidase/avidin-biotin-peroxidase complex procedure. Human Pathology 17: 1107–1115

Angervall L, Enzinger F M 1975 Extraskeletal neoplasm resembling Ewing's sarcoma. Cancer 36: 240–251

Angervall L, Stener B 1969 Clear cell sarcoma of tendons. A study of 4 cases. Acta Pathologica Microbiologica Scandinavica 77: 589–597

Askin F B, Rosai J, Sibley R K, Dehner L P, McAllister W H 1979 Malignant small cell tumor of the thoracopulmonary region in childhood. A distinctive clinicopathological entity of uncertain histogenesis. Cancer 43: 2438–2451

Aurias A, Rimbaut C, Buffe D, Zucker J-M, Mazabraud A 1984 Translocation involving chromosome 22 in Ewing's sarcoma. A cytogenetic study of four fresh tumours. Cancer Genetics and Cytogenetics 12: 21–25

Azumi N, Curtis J, Kempson R L, Hendrickson M R 1987 Atypical and malignant neoplasms showing lipomatous differentiation. A study of 111 cases. American Journal of Surgical Pathology 11: 161–183

Barlogie B, Raber M N, Schumann J et al 1983 Flow cytometry in clinical cancer research. Cancer Research 43: 3982–3997

Bearman R M, Noe J, Kempson R L 1975 Clear cell sarcoma with melanin pigment. Cancer 36: 977–984

Becroft D M O, Pearson A, Shaw R L, Zwi L J 1984 Chromosome translocation in extraskeletal Ewing's tumour. Lancet 2: 400 (Letter)

Benson J D, Kraemer B, Mackay B 1985 Malignant melanoma of soft parts: an ultrastructural study of four cases. Ultrastructural Pathology 8: 57–70

Biggs P J, Garen P D, Powers J M, Garvin A J 1987 Malignant rhabdoid tumor of the central nervous system. Human Pathology 18: 332–337

Bolen J W, Thorning D 1980 Peripheral neuroepithelioma. A light and electron microscopic study. Cancer 46: 2456–2462

Boudreaux D, Waisman J 1978 Clear cell sarcoma with melanogenesis. Cancer 41: 1387–1394

Cagle L A, Mirra J M, Storm K, Roe D J, Eilber F R 1987 Histologic features relating to prognosis in synovial sarcom. Cancer 59: 1810–1814

Carter R L, McCarthy K P, Al-Sam S Z, Monaghan P, Agrawal M, McElwain T J 1989 Malignant rhabdoid tumour of the bladder with immunohistochemical and ultrastructural evidence suggesting histiocytic origin. Histopathology 14: 179–190

Cavazzana A D, Miser J S, Jefferson J, Triche T J 1987a Experimental evidence for a neural origin of Ewing's sarcoma of bone. American Journal of Pathology 127: 507–518

Cavazzana A D, Navarro S, Triche T J, Llombart-Bosch A 1987b Ewing's sarcoma and neuroepithelioma compared. Laboratory Investigation 56: 12A (abstract)

Chaudhuri P K, Walker M J, Beattie C W, Das Gupta T K 1980 Presence of steroid receptors in human soft tissue sarcomas of diverse histological origin. Cancer Research 40: 861–865

Chaudhuri P K, Walker M J, Beattie C W, Das Gupta T K 1981 Distribution of steroid hormone receptors in human soft tissue sarcomas. Surgery 90: 149–153

Chung E B, Enzinger F M 1983 Malignant melanoma of soft parts. A reassessment of clear cell sarcoma. American Journal of Surgical Pathology 7: 405–413

Coffin C M, Dehner L P 1986 Peripheral neurogenic tumors in children and adolescents. A clinicopathologic study of 134 cases. Laboratory Investigation 54: 12A (Abstract)

Corson J M, Weiss L M, Banks-Schlegel S P, Pinkus G S 1984 Keratin proteins and carcinoembryonic antigen in synovial sarcomas: an immunohistochemical study of 24 cases. Human Pathology 15: 615–621

Dabbs D J, Park H K 1988 Malignant rhabdoid skin tumor: an uncommon primary skin neoplasm. Ultrastructural and immunohistochemical analysis. Journal of Cutaneous Pathology 15: 109–115

De Chadarevian J-P, Vekemans M, Seemayer T 1984 Reciprocal translocation in small cell sarcomas. New England Journal of Medicine 311: 1702 (Letter)

Dehner LP 1986 Peripheral and central primitive neuroectodermal tumors. A nosologic concept seeking a concensus. Archives of Pathology and Laboratory Medicine 110: 997–1005

De Jong A S H, Van Kessel-Van Vark M, Albus-Lutter C E 1987 Pleomorphic rhabdomyosarcoma in adults: immunohistochemistry as a tool for its diagnosis. Human Pathology 18: 298–303

Dervan P A, Cahalane S F, Kneafsey P, Mynes A, McAllister K 1987 Malignant rhabdoid tumour of soft tissue. An ultrastructural and immunohistochemical study of a pelvic tumour. Histopathology 11: 183–190

Donner L R, Ayala A G, Mackay B 1987 Ewing's sarcoma and peripheral neuroepithelioma: a comparative study. Laboratory Investigation 56: 19A (Abstract)

Ekfors T O, Rantakokko Y 1979 Clear cell sarcoma of tendons and aponeuroses: malignant melanoma of soft tissues? Pathology in Research and Practice 165: 422–428

El-Naggar A, Barlogie B, Ro J, Ayala A, Batsakis J G 1988a Flow cytometric analysis of soft tissue neoplasms. Laboratory Investigation 58: 27A (Abstract)

El-Naggar A, Ro J Y, Ayala A G, Hinchey W D, Abdul-Karim F, Batsakis J 1988b Angiomatoid malignant fibrous histiocytoma: a DNA flow cytometric analysis of seven cases. American Journal of Clinical Pathology 90: 502 (Abstract)

Enzinger F M 1965 Clear-cell sarcoma of tendons and aponeuroses. An analysis of 21 cases. Cancer 18: 1163–1174

Enzinger F M, Harvey D A 1975 Spindle cell lipoma. Cancer 36: 1852–1859

Enzinger F M, Weiss S W 1983 Soft Tissue Tumours. CV Mosby, St Louis

Evans H L 1979 Liposarcoma. A study of 55 cases with a reassessment of its classification American Journal of Surgical Pathology 3: 507–523

Evans H L, Soule E H, Winkelmann R K 1979 Atypical lipoma, atypical intramuscular lipoma and well differentiated retroperitoneal liposarcoma. A reappraisal of 30 cases formerly classified as well differentiated liposarcoma. Cancer 43: 574–584

Fisher C 1986 Synovial sarcoma: ultrastructural and immunohistochemical features of epithelial differentiation in monphasic and biphasic tumors. Human Pathology 17: 996–1008

Fletcher C D M, Camplejohn R S 1987 DNA flow cytometry in haemangiopericytomas is of no prognostic value. Journal of Pathology 151: 31A (Abstract)

Fletcher C D M, Martin-Bates E 1987 Spindle cell lipoma: a clinicopathological study with some original observations. Histopathology 11: 803–817

Fletcher C D M, Martin-Bates E 1988 Intramuscular and intermuscular lipoma: neglected diagnoses. Histopathology 12: 275–287

Fletcher C D M, Stirling R W, Smith M A, Pambakian H, McKee P H 1986 Multicentric extra-abdominal 'myofibromatosis': report of a case with ultrastructural findings. Histopathology 10: 713–724

Gabbiani G, Kay G I, Lattes R, Majno G 1971 Synovial sarcoma. Electron microscopic study of a typical case. Cancer 28: 1031–1039

Gonzalez-Crussi F, Goldschmidt R A, Hsueh W, Trujillo Y P 1982 Infantile sarcoma with intracytoplasmic filamentous inclusions. Distinctive tumor of possible histiocytic origin. Cancer 49: 2365–2375

Gonzalez-Crussi F, Wolfson S L, Misugi K, Nakajima T 1984 Peripheral neuroectodermal tumors of the chest wall in childhood. Cancer 54: 2519–2527

Haas J E, Palmer N F, Weinberg A G, Beckwith J B 1981 Ultrastructure of malignant rhabdoid tumor of the kidney. A distinctive renal tumor of children. Human Pathology 12: 646–657

Hajdu S I 1979 Rhabdomyoblastoma. In Pathology of soft tissue tumors. Lea and Febiger, Philadelphia, p 352–356

Harper P G, Pringle J, Souhami R L 1981 Neuroepithelioma — a rare malignant peripheral nerve tumor of primitive origin: report of two new cases and a review of the literature. Cancer 48: 2282–2287

Harris M, Eyden B P, Joglekar V M 1987 Rhabdoid tumor of the bladder: a histological, ultrastructural and immunohistochemical study. Histopathology 11: 1083–1092

Hashimoto H, Enjoji M 1982 Liposarcoma. A clinicopathologic subtyping of 52 cases. Acta Pathologica Japonica 32: 933–948

Hashimoto H, Enjoji M, Nakajima T, Kiryu H, Daimaru Y 1983 Malignant neuroepithelioma (peripheral neuroblastoma). A clinicopathologic study of 15 cases. American Journal of Surgical Pathology 7: 309–318

Hashimoto H, Tsuneyoshi M, Daimaru Y, Enjoji M 1985 Extraskeletal Ewing's sarcoma. A clinicopathologic and electron microscopic analysis of 8 cases. Acta Pathologica Japonica 35: 1087–1098

Hawkins H K, Comacho-Velasquez J V 1987 Rhabdomyosarcoma in children. Correlation of form and prognosis in one institution's experience. American Journal of Surgical Pathology 11: 531–542

Hayry P, Reitamo J J, Vihko R et al 1982 The desmoid tumor. III. A biochemical and genetic analysis. American Journal of Clinical Pathology 77: 681–685

Hedley D W, Friedlander M L, Taylor I W, Rugg C A, Musgrove E A, 1983 Method for analysis of cellular DNA content of paraffin-embedded pathological material using flow cytometry. Journal of Histopathology and Cytochemistry 31: 1333–1335

Hoffman G J, Carter D 1973 Clear cell sarcoma of tendons and aponeuroses with melanin. Archives of Pathology 95: 22–25

Horn R C, Enterline H T, 1958 Rhabdomyosarcoma: a clinicopathologic study and classification of 39 cases. Cancer 11: 181–199

Jurgens H, Bier V, Harms D et al 1988 Malignant peripheral neuroectodermal tumors. A retrospective analysis of 42 patients. Cancer 61: 349–357

Kent A L, Mahoney D H, Gresik M V, Teuber C P, Fernback D J 1987 Malignant rhabdoid tumor of the extremity. Cancer 60: 1056–1059

Keyhani A, Booher R J 1968 Pleomorphic rhabdomyosarcoma. Cancer 22: 956–967

Kindblom L-G, Angervall L, Fassina A S 1982 Atypical lipoma. Acta Pathological Microbiologica Scandinavica A 90: 27–36

Kindblom L-G, Lodding P, Angervall L 1983 Clear-cell sarcoma of tendons and aponeuroses. An immunohistochemical and electron microscopic analysis indicating neural crest origin. Virchows Archiv A Pathological Anatomy 401: 109–128

Koss L G, Czerniak B, Herz F, Wersto R P 1989 Flow cytometric measurements of DNA and other cell components in human tumors: a critical appraisal. Human Pathology 20 528–548

Kouraklis G, Triche T J, Jefferson J, Tsokos M 1987 Study of rhabdomyosarcoma in vitro and in nude mice. Laboratory Investigation 56: 40A (Abstract)

Krall R A, Kostianovsky M, Patchefsky A S, 1981 Synovial sarcoma. A clinical, pathological and ultrastructural study of 26 cases supporting the recognition of a monophasic variant. American Journal of Surgical Pathology 5: 137–151

Kreicbergs A, Tribukait B, Willems J, Bauer H S F 1987 DNA flow analysis of soft tissue tumors. Cancer 59: 128–133

Lawrence W, Jegge G, Foote F W 1964 Embryonal rhabdomyosarcoma. A clinicopathologic study. Cancer 17: 361–376

Leader M, Patel J, Collins M, Henry K 1987 Synovial sarcomas. True carcinosarcomas ? Cancer 59: 2096–2098

Limon J, Turc-Carel C, Dal Cin P, Rao U, Sandberg A A 1986 Recurrent chromosome translocations in liposarcoma. Cancer Genetics and Cytogenetics 22: 92–94

Limon J, Mrozek K, Nedoszytko B et al 1989 Cytogenetic findings in two synovial sarcomas. Cancer Genetics and Cytogenetics 38: 215–222.

Linnoila R I, Tsokos M, Triche T J, Marangos P J, Chandra R S 1986 Evidence for neural origin and PAS-positive variants of the malignant small cell tumour of thoracopulmonary region ('Askin tumor'). American Journal of Surgical Pathology 10: 124–133

Linscheid R L, Soule E H, Henderson E D 1965 Pleomorphic rhabdomyosarcomata on the extremities and limb girdles. A clinicopathologic study. Journal of Bone and Joint Surgery 47A: 715–726

Lipinski M, Braham K, Philip I et al 1987 Neuroectoderm-associated antigens on Ewing's sarcoma cell lines. Cancer Research 47: 183–187

Lynch H T, Shurlin S B, Dahms B B, Izant R J, Lynch J, Danes B S 1983 Paravertebral malignant rhabdoid tumor in infancy. In vitro studies of a familial tumor. Cancer 52: 290–296

Mackenzie D H 1974 Clear cell sarcoma of tendons and aponeuroses with melanin production. Journal of Pathology 114: 231–235

Mackenzie D H 1977 Monophasic synovial sarcoma — a histological entity? Histopathology 1: 151–157

Maurer H M, Moon T, Donaldson M et al 1977 The Intergroup Rhabdomyosarcoma Study; A preliminary report. Cancer 40: 2015–2026

Maurer H M, Beltangady M, Gehan E A et al 1988 The Intergroup Rhabdomyosarcoma Study; I. A final report. Cancer 61: 209–220

Meister P, Gokel J M, 1978 Extraskeletal Ewing's sarcoma. Virchows Archiv A Pathological Anatomy and Histology 378: 173–179

Mertens F, Johannsson B, Mandahl N et al 1987 Clonal chromosome abnormalities in two liposarcomas. Cancer Genetics and Cytogenetics 28: 137–144

Mickelson M R, Brown G A, Maynard J A, Cooper R R, Bonfiglio M 1980 Synovial sarcoma. An electron microscopic study of monophasic and biphasic forms. Cancer 45: 2109–2118

Miettinen M, Virtanen I 1984 Synovial sarcoma — a misnomer. American Journal of Pathology 117: 18–25

Miettinen M, Lehto V-P, Virtanen I 1982 Keratin in the epithelial-like cells of classical biphasic synovial sarcoma. Virchows Archiv B Cellular Pathology 40: 157–161

Miettinen M, Lehto V-P, Virtanen I 1983 Monophasic synovial sarcoma of spindle cell type. Epithelial differentiation as revealed by ultrastructural features, content of prekeratin and binding of peanut agglutinin. Virchows Archiv B Cellular Pathology 44: 187–199

Molenaar W M, Oosterhuis A M, Ramaekers F C S 1985 The rarity of rhabdomyosarcomas in the adult. A morphologic and immunohistochemical study. Pathology in Research and Practice 180: 400–405

Molenaar W M, Dam-Meiring A, Kamps W A, Cornelisse C J 1988 DNA aneuploidy in rhabdomyosarcomas as compared with other sarcomas of childhood and adolescence. Human Pathology 19: 573–579

Moll R, Lee I, Gould V E, Berndt R, Roessner A, Franke W W, 1987 Immunocytochemical analysis of Ewing's tumors. Patterns of expression of intermediate filaments and desmosomal proteins indicate cell type heterogeneity and pluripotential differentiation. American Journal of Pathology 127: 288–304

Mukai M, Torikata C, Iri H et al 1984 Histogenesis of clear cell sarcoma of tendons and aponeuroses. An electron microscopic, biochemical, enzyme histochemical and immunohistochemical study. American Journal of Pathology 114: 264–272

Parham D M, Jenkins J J, Holt H, Calliman T R 1987 Phenotypic diversity in pediatric rhabdoid tumors: a morphologic and immunohistochemical study. Laboratory Investigation 56: 58A (Abstract)

Pisa R, Bonetti F, Chilosi M, Iannucci A, Menestrina F 1982 Synovial sarcoma. Enzyme histochemistry of a typical case. Virchows Archiv A Pathological Anatomy 398: 67–73

Radio S J, Wooldridge T N, Linder J 1988 Flow cytometric DNA analysis of malignant fibrous histiocytoma and related fibrohistiocytic tumors. Human Pathology 19: 74–77

Raney R B, Hays D M, Lawrence W, Soule E H, Tefft M, Donaldson M H 1978 Paratesticular rhabdomyosarcoma in childhood. Cancer 42: 729–736

Raney R B, Ragab A H, Ruymann F B et al 1982 Soft tissue sarcoma of the trunk in childhood. Results of the Intergroup Rhabdomyosarcoma Study. Cancer 49: 2612–2616

Raney R B, Tefft M, Newton W A et al 1987 Improved prognosis with intensive treatment of children with cranial soft tissue sarcomas arising in non-orbital parameningeal sites. A report from the Intergroup Rhabdomyosarcoma Study. Cancer 59: 147–155

Reeves B R, Smith S, Fisher C et al 1989 Characterisation of the translocation between chromosomes X and 18 in human synovial sarcomas. Oncogene 4: 373–378

Rooser B, Willen H, Hugoson A, Rydholm A 1989 Prognostic factors in synovial sarcoma. Cancer 63: 2182–2185

Rowe D, Gerrard M, Gibbons B, Malpas J S 1987 Two further cases of t(2;13) in alveolar rhabdomyosarcoma indicating a review of the published chromosome breakpoints. British Journal of Cancer 56: 379–380 (Letter)

Salisbury J R, Isaacson P G 1985 Synovial sarcoma: an immunohistochemical study. Journal of Pathology 147: 49–57

Sandberg A A, Turc-Carel C 1987 The cytogenetics of solid tumors. Relation to diagnosis, classification and pathology. Cancer 59: 387–395

Seemayer T A, Vekemans M, De Chadarevian J P 1985 Histological and cytogenetic findings in a malignant tumor of the chest wall and lung (Askin tumor). Virchows Archiv A Pathological Anatomy 408: 289–296

Seidal T, Mark J, Hagmar B, Angervall L 1982 Alveolar rhabdomyosarcoma: a cytogenetic and correlated cytological and histological study. Acta Pathologica Microbiologica Immunologica Scandinavica A 90: 345–354

Shimada H, Newton W A, Soule E H et al 1988 Pathologic features of extraosseous Ewing's sarcoma: a report from the Intergroup Rhabdomyosarcoma Study. Human Pathology 19: 442–453

Shmookler B M, Enzinger F M 1981 Pleomorphic lipoma: a benign tumor simulating liposarcoma. A clinicopathological analysis of 48 cases. Cancer 47: 126–133

Sotelo-Avila C, Gonzalez-Crussi F, Demello D et al 1986 Renal and extrarenal rhabdoid tumors in children: a clinicopathologic study of 14 patients. Seminars in Diagnostic Pathology 3: 151–163

Soule E H, Geitz M, Henderson E D 1969 Embryonal rhabdomyosarcoma of the limbs and limb girdles. A clinicopathologic study of 61 cases. Cancer 23: 1336–1346

Soule E H, Newton W, Moon Te, Tefft M 1978 Extraskeletal Ewing's sarcoma. A preliminary review of 26 cases encountered in the Intergroup Rhabdomyosarcoma Study. Cancer 42: 259–264

Sutow W W, Lindberg R D, Geman E A et al 1982 Three-year relapse free survival rates in childhood rhabdomyosarcoma of the head and neck. Report from the Intergroup Rhabdomyosarcoma Study. Cancer 49: 2217–2221

Swanson P E, Wick M R 1989 Clear cell sarcoma. An immunohistochemical analysis of six cases and comparison with other epithelioid neoplasms of soft tissue. Archives of Pathology and Laboratory Medicine 113: 55–60

Swanson P E, Wick M R, Dehner L P 1989 Lectin histochemistry of small round cell tumors. Laboratory Investigation 60:8P (Abstract)

Toe T K, Saw D 1978 Clear cell sarcoma with melanin. Report of two cases. Cancer 41: 235–238

Tsokos M 1986 The role of immunocytochemistry in the diagnosis of rhabdomyosarcoma. Arch Pathol Lab Med 110: 776–778

Tsokos M, Triche T J 1986 Immunocytochemical and ultrastructural study of primitive 'solid variant' rhabdomyosarcoma. Laboratory Investigation 54: 65A (Abstract)

Tsokos M, Miser A, Pizzo P, Triche T 1984 Histologic and cytologic characteristics of poor prognosis childhood rhabdomyosarcoma. Laboratory Investigation 50: 61A (Abstract)

Tsokos M, Kouraklis G, Chandra R S, Bhagavan B S, Triche T J 1989 Malignant rhabdoid tumor of the kidney and soft tissues. Evidence for a diverse morphological and immunocytochemical phenotype. Archives of Pathology and Laboratory Investigation 113: 115–120

Tsuneyoshi M Enjoji M, Kubo T. 1978 Clear cell sarcoma of tendons and aponeuroses. A comparative study of 13 cases with a provisional subgrouping into the melanotic and synovial types. Cancer 42: 243–252

Tsuneyoshi M, Daimaru Y, Hashimoto H, Enjoji M 1985 Malignant soft tissue neoplasms with the histologic features of renal rhabdoid tumors: an ultrastructural and immunohistochemical study. Human Pathology 16: 1235–1242

Tsuneyoshi M, Yokoyama K, Enjoji M 1983 Synovial sarcoma. A clinicopathologic and ultrastructural study of 42 cases. Acta Pathologica Japonica 33: 23–36

Tsuneyoshi M, Daimaru Y, Hashimoto H, Enjoji M 1987 The existence 'of rhabdoid' cells in specified soft tissue sarcomas. Histopathological, ultrastructural and immunohistochemical evidence. Virchows Archiv A Pathological Anatomy and Histology 411: 509–514

Turc-Carel C, Philip I, Berger M-P, Philip T, Lenoir G M 1984 Chromosome study of

Ewing's sarcoma (ES) cell lines. Consistency of a reciprocal translocation (t11;22) (q24;q12). Cancer Genetics and Cytogenetics 12: 1–19

Turc-Carel C, Cytogenetic studies of adipose tissue tumors: II. Recurrent reciprocal translocation t(12;16)(q13;11) in myxoid liposarcomas. Cancer Genetics and Cytogenetics 23: 291–300

Turc-Carel C, Lizard-Nacol S, Justrabo E, Favrot M, Philip T, Tabone E 1986b Consistent chromosomal translocation in alveolar rhabdomyosarcoma. Cancer Genetics and Cytogenetics 19: 361–362

Turc-Carel C, Limon J, Dal Chin P, Rao U, Karakousis C, Sandberg A A 1986c Translocation X;18 in synovial sarcoma. Cancer Genetics and Cytogenetics 23: 93

Ueda T, Aozasa K, Tsujimoto M et al 1989 Prognostic significance of Ki-67 reactivity in soft tissue sarcomas. Cancer 63: 1607–1611

Ushigome S, Shimoda T, Takaki K et al 1989 Immunocytochemical and ultrastructural studies of the histogenesis of Ewing's sarcoma and putatively related tumors. Cancer 64: 52–62

Varela-Duran J, Enzinger F M, 1982 Calcifying synovial sarcoma. Cancer 50: 345–352

Voss B L, Pysher T J, Humphrey G B 1984 Peripheral neuroepithelioma in childhood. Cancer 54: 3059–3064

Weeks D A, Beckwith J B, Mierau G W, Luckey D W 1989 Rhabdoid tumor of kidney. A report of 111 cases from the National Wilms' Tumor Study Pathology Center. American Journal of Surgical Pathology 13: 439–458

Weiss S W 1982 Malignant fibrous histocytoma. A reaffirmation. American Journal of Surgical Pathology 6: 773–784

Weiss S W, Langloss J M, Shmookler B M et al 1986 Estrogen receptor protein in bone and soft tissue tumors. Laboratory Investigation 54: 689–694

Whang-Peng J, Triche T J, Knutsen T, Miser J, Douglass E C, Israel M A 1984 Chromosome translocation in peripheral neuroepithelioma. New England Journal of Medicine 311: 584–585

Whang-Peng J, Triche T J, Knutsen T et al 1986 Cytogenetic characterization of selected small round cell tumors of childhood. Cancer Genetics and Cytogenetics 21: 185–208

Wick M R, Swanson P E, Manivel J C 1988 Immunohistochemical analysis of soft tissue sarcomas. Comparisons with electron microscopy. Applied Pathology 6: 109–115

Wright P H, Sim F H, Soule E H, Taylor W F 1982 Synovial sarcoma. Journal of Bone and Joint Surgery 64A: 112–122

Xiang J, Spanier S S, Beneson N A, Braylan R C 1987 Flow cytometric analysis of DNA in bone and soft tissue tumors using nuclear suspensions. Cancer 59: 1951–1958

15. Current trends in the treatment of soft tissue sarcomas

J. F. Huth   F. R. Eilber

INTRODUCTION

Soft tissue sarcomas are a relatively rare type of primary malignant neoplasm, comprising less than 1% of all malignant tumours. They occur almost equally in males and females and the average age at the time of diagnosis is 43 years. Approximately two-thirds of these tumours arise in the extremities, and, following simple excision, they have a propensity for local recurrence which has often resulted in extremity amputation in order to achieve local control. These neoplasms also tend to develop systemic metastases, primarily to the lung, which is the major cause of mortality.

These tumours arise from mesenchyme, and they represent such a diverse and complex group of neoplasms that for many years a clinical staging system for the entire group was not attemped. Yet it was not until their pathology and biology was better understood that progress in the treatment of these tumours could be achieved. A uniform classification and staging system was important in order 1. to determine prognosis for patients with lesions of varying size, location and histological characteristics, and 2. to compare the results of ongoing clinical trials at various institutions specialising in the treatment of soft tissue sarcomas.

PATHOBIOLOGY

James Ewing, in the early 1900s, made major contributions to understanding the pathology of soft tissue sarcomas by his insistence that classification was dependent upon both histogenesis and structure. Broders et al (1939) added the criteria of mitotic index, the number of cells which were dividing at a given time, and recognized the prognostic significance of this finding. Broders also observed that the apparent capsule surrounding soft tissue sarcomas was not a true capsule, but composed of compressed tumour cells and adjacent normal tissue. Stout (1947) organised the classification to reflect:

1. Histogenesis: the type of cell from which the lesion arose
2. Grade: low grade vs high grade similar to Broder's low and high mitotic index
3. Stroma: myxoid or fibrous

4. Cellular uniformity: pleomorphism and structural characteristics, such as biphasic or monophasic.

Although Stout's system was a major advance in the classification of soft tissue sarcomas, it had some major practical problems, especially with regard to histogenesis since it was difficult for pathologists to agree on the cell of origin in many cases. The American Joint Committee on Staging and End Results (Russell et al 1977) developed a method for assessing the grade and size of the tumour which does not take histogenesis into account (Table 15.1). This system is based on the clinical characteristics of the primary neoplasm (size, extension), the involvement of lymph nodes, the presence of metastases, and the grade of the primary tumour. This system, based on examination of 1215 cases of 13 types of soft tissue sarcoma, uses the TMN system with the addition of grade. The major advantage of this system is that cases can be standardised for comparision of therapy in different series of patients with respect to effects of treatment and survival.

Enneking et al (1980) devised a clinical staging system which reflects the grade and anatomical location of the tumour. However, this system combines grade I and grade II tumours, it does not consider histogenesis, and there is no category for local recurrence (Table 15.2).

Understanding the local growth characteristics of soft tissue sarcomas had an important impact on the evolution of the treatment of these neoplasms. Broders et al (1939) recognised that, although the tumours appeared to be encapsulated, they were really surrounded by a pseudocapsule, composed of tumour cells and compressed normal surrounding tissue. Soft tissue tumours tend to expand and push aside surrounding tissues, and local spread appears to be along the path of least resistence. Major fascial barriers such as the intermuscular septum, and the adventitia of nerves, arteries and veins tend to prevent direct extension. Thus it is uncommon for patients with primary soft tissue sarcomas to present with bone or nerve involvement, unless the tumour has originated in a nerve. Barber et al (1957) from the Mayo Clinic found perineural invasion, but not direct nerve bundle invasion in approximately

Table 15.1 American Joint Committee on Staging and End Results (AJC) Staging Parameters

Stage	Tumour size (T) (CM)	Regional nodes (N)	Distant metastases (M)	Grade of malignancy (G)*
I a,b**	1,2	0	0	I
II a,b	1,2	0	0	II
III a,b	1,2	0	0	III
c	Any	1	0	Any
IV a***	3	0,1	0	Any
b	Any	Any	1	Any

*Mitosis per high power field : I = low
**Ia <5 cm; Ib >5 cm
*** IV a = bone, vessel or nerve invasion : IV b = distant metastases.

Table 15.2   Staging system for bone and soft tissue sarcomas. Modified from Enneking et al (1980)

Descriptor	Description
Stage	
I	Low grade lesion (AJCS — grades I & II) without metastases
II	High grade lesion without metastases
III	Any grade with metastases
Anatomical location	
A	Intracompartmental
B	Extracompartmental (popliteal, antecubital and groin are extracompartmental)

10% of patients in an autopsy study. Lymph node involvement is also uncommon (Mazeron & Suit 1987). Lymphatic invasion is more common in children with rhabdomyosarcoma and adults with synovial sarcoma, occurring in up to 10% of cases. There are occasional anecdotal reports of tumour invasion of veins and of tumour thrombi forming in major draining veins of soft tissue sarcomas. The thrombus most likely has its origin in the small veins of the tumour itself and propagates distally as the lesion enlarges.

Anatomy also has an important impact on the treatment of soft tissue sarcomas (Enneking et al 1981, Mandard et al 1981, Rooser 1987). The subcutaneous space has no distinct borders and tumours arising there have early access to a rich lymphatic network. There are few fascial barriers to limit expansion of such neoplasms. Tumours which arise within muscle compartments encounter barriers such as the intramuscular septa which tend to limit their expansion outside the compartment. Certain areas, such as the groin and popliteal space, have no clearly defined fascial boundaries. In the groin, there is direct anatomical continuity to the retroperitoneum along the psoas muscle as well as direct continuity with the anterior abdominal wall. These boundaries and potential areas of localised spread must be taken into consideration when evaluating and treating patients with soft tissue tumours.

Despite problems with local control of sarcomas, the majority of patients who die from this disease do so because of metastases to the lung, the most common site of metastatic disease. The median time from treatment to identification of metastases is 10.5 months with a range of 0–15 years. Other sites in order of frequency are bone, liver, and other soft tissue sites such as the retroperitoneum (Kavenagh et al 1980). Soft tissue sarcomas of the retroperitoneum have a distinct pattern of spread, with local recurrence within the retroperitoneum as the most common site, followed by metastases to the liver.

DIAGNOSIS

A common problem in the treatment of soft tissue sarcomas is delay in making the diagnosis. The median time from appearance of symptoms to diagnosis in a series of parients seen at the University of California, Los Angeles (UCLA) was 13 months. This was due, in part, to delay by the patient in seeking treatment since the tumours were often painless and slowly growing. There was also a delay on the part of the physician due to failure to consider the diagnosis of malignancy. The most common initial diagnosis of an extremity mass was muscle pull or haematoma, and patients were often treated for 5–6 months before the physician became suspicious that the mass was malignant. Muscle pulls or haematomas that result in a palpable mass in a non-athletic adult are extremely rare, and when a mass does appear, there is a rapid resolution of the mass within 3–4 weeks.

The definitive diagnostic test of a soft tissue mass is histological evaluation of biopsied tissue. An incisional biopsy, directly over tumour that does not disturb the deep margins is the most common procedure. It is important to position the incision in such a way that the scar and all disturbed tissue can be excised at the time of the definitive procedure. Wound seeding of incompletely excised tumours is a recognised phenomenon (Enneking & Maale 1988), so dissection of tissue planes should be kept to a minimum and meticulous haemostasis is required to avoid spreading of tumour cells through an uncontrolled haematoma. A frozen section should be obtained to ensure that the tissue that has been removed is adequate for definitive diagnosis. Transverse incisions in the extremity are inappropriate since all the important structures; arteries, veins and nerves, run longitudinally rather than transversely, and transverse incisions transgress numerous fascial planes.

A needle biopsy, with a Vim-Silverman or similar type of needle, is our preferred method of biopsy. This removes a core of tissue for histological examination, but this requires a pathologist who is very familiar with the histology of soft tissue sarcomas. Sometimes, interpretation of the biopsied tissue requires definition of both the stroma and the cytology of the specimen as well as determining whether or not tumour cells are present in the surrounding tissue. In this instance, the core method may not be adequate and an incisional biopsy will be required.

Recently, needle aspiration cytology has gained popularity for the identification of various malignancies. This technique has the advantages of being less traumatic, many areas of the lesion can be sampled at one time, and the diagnosis of malignancy can be made very quickly. However, this technique requires a great deal of experience with soft tissue tumours on the part of the pathologist, since only individual cells and very little stroma are aspirated from the tumour (Layfield et al 1986).

Excisional biopsy is the final method of diagnosis, and we discourage its use. Most soft tissue sarcomas are large (> 5 cm), and complete excision of a mass this size disturbs many of the fascial planes and is associated with potential complications of haematoma and infection. The subsequent operative procedure is much more involved, because it then becomes necessary completely to excise all areas that were previously entered, including drain tracts. This type of biopsy should never be performed on a tumour that might be a soft tissue sarcoma, i.e. any large, deep-seated neoplasm. Benign soft tissue tumours are most often small (< 2 cm) and are frequently located in the subcutaneous space. Complete excision of a mass in this location is indicated, but large deep-seated masses should never be excisionally biopsied.

CLINICAL EVALUATION

The work-up of a patient with a soft tissue sarcoma should begin with a complete history and physical examination. Important aspects of the history include prior exposure to radiation, a history of other primary tumours, a history of chronic lymphoedema, and a family history of neurofibromatosis. The physical examination should be complete and include routine laboratory studies; a complete blood count, SMA-12, chest X-ray, and either whole lung tomograms or a CT scan of the chest to determine whether or not the tumour has spead to the lungs (Neufeld et al 1977, Muhn & Pritchard 1980).

An arteriogram is sometimes helpful for defining vascular displacement or venous invasion of the primary tumour (Hudson et al 1975). However, tumour blush from the arteriogram is inaccurate in defining the extent of the lesion since these neoplasms are often relatively avascular, and an arteriogram does not give an accurate, three-dimensional view of the local anatomy. Standard bone X-rays are helpful for showing whether or not there is any cortical bone destruction, and whether the mass is a primary bone tumour rather than a soft tissue tumour. More recently, CT scanning of the extremities has proved to be the most reliable method for determining the anatomical extent of the tumour spread (Mueller et al 1979, Davidson et al 1987). The CT scan demonstrates the tissue compartments and actual muscle groups, and it provides good definition of the extent of the lesion, its invasive characteristics, and the involvement of fascial compartments. Recently, Chang et al (1987) have described the use of a magnetic resonance imaging (MRI) for evaluating the extent of local invasion in soft tissue sarcomas, and they concluded that MRI is better than CT scanning in the evaluation of soft tissue tumours of the extremity.

TREATMENT

Over the years, methods for the local treatment of soft tissue sarcomas have been modified as we have become more aware of their local growth characteristics and histological characteristics. These methods are still in a state of evolution as we learn more about the usefulness of various forms of therapy as well as their side effects.

Surgery

The early attempts to surgically treat these tumours were almost always followed by local recurrence, because it was not understood that the apparent capsule around sarcomas was composed of neoplastic cells and normal tissue, which was compressed by the expanding tumour. Since the surgical procedure was enucleation or excision through this pseudocapsule, local recurrence occurred in 90–95% of patients. Several authors (Bowden & Booher 1958, Pack 1954, Brennhoud 1966) suggested that a wider excision of the primary tumour mass including the pseudocapsule was necessary to avoid this problem of local recurrence. This spurred clinicians to devise more radical operations which included 1. resection of the tumour capsule, and 2. because these neoplasms tended to spread up fascial planes, muscle groups containing the tumour were removed from origin to insertion for a much wider margin of apparently normal tissue (Pack 1954). Even with these more complete excisions, the local recurrence rate remained high, approximately 30–35% (Clark et al 1957, Martin & Butler 1965, Shiu et al 1975, Gerner et al 1975, Rantakokko & Ekfors 1970, Markhede et al 1981). Table 15.3 summarises the results of surgery alone for the treatment of soft tissue sarcomas of the extremity. Because of these poor results with surgical excision of soft tissue tumours, amputation became the procedure of choice, until other forms of adjuvant treatment became available (Yang & Rosenberg 1989).

Radiation therapy

The results obtained with radiation therapy alone for the treatment of soft tissue sarcomas have been extremely disappointing, with an overall response rate of 20% and a local control rate in the range of 10–12%. However, patients selected for this type of treatment often had far advanced disease (Tepper & Suit 1985). In order to control gross residual disease, the doses had to be very high, 6000–8000 cGy, and the complications from subcutaneous fibrosis and neural injury were unacceptable (Windeyer et al 1966, McNeer et al 1968).

Recently, the development of high energy transfer (LET) radiation therapy and neutron radiation has led to improved clinical results in the treatment of soft tissue tumours. Schmitt et al (1984), in a series of 122 unselected and not previously irradiated patients, showed improved results in both resectable and non-resectable patients with respect to local control and complications of therapy. Larrimore (1983) recently reviewed the world experience with these new forms of therapy in a retrospective review of over 400 patients. The local

Table 15.3 Published results of surgery alone for extremity soft tissue sarcoma

Study/year	Institution	No. of patients	% Amputation	Local recurrence No. (%)	% 5-year survival
Martin & Butler 1965	MD Anderson	253	32	71 (28)	40
Gerner et al 1975	Roswell Park	155	24	43 (60)	40
Shiu et al 1975	Memorial	297	47	53 (18)	54
Enneking et al 1981	Univ of Florida	40	50	6 (15)	60
Markhede et al 1981	Goteborg	97	13	21 (21)	59
Total		842	33	(23)	50

control rate with bulky tumours was 40% which is a tremendous improvement over the usual 10–15% rate of local control with standard radiation therapy. Although standard radiation therapy has been used successfully when combined with other forms of treatment (as will be discussed below), the results with these newer types of radiation therapy may be even more efficacious in the multimodality treatment of soft tissue sarcomas.

Chemotherapy

For many years there were few, if any, chemotherapeutic agents that were useful in the treatment of soft tissue sarcomas. Cytoxan, Vincristine and Actinomycin D were active for alveolar or embryonal rhabdomyosarcomas in children (Donaldson et al 1973), but the response rate in adults to this regimen was poor. However, the introduction of Adriamycin (doxyrubicin) in 1968 dramatically changed this picture with a response rate in metastatic disease of 30–40% (Gottlieb et al 1975). With experience, investigators have found that soft tissue sarcomas respond to Adriamycin in dose-dependent fashion with doses in the 90 mg/m^2 range consistently producing the 40% response. Although never now used as the sole treatment for primary soft tissue sarcomas, Adriamycin has been used in conjunction with other treatment modalities for the treatment of primary tumours (Elias & Antman, 1989) as will be discussed shortly.

Multidisciplinary therapy

Surgery and radiation therapy

In the early 1970s, Suit et al (1975) treated a series of patients at the MD Anderson hospital with radiation therapy, after complete excision of all gross tumour in the extremity. The local failure rate in this group of patients after 6000–7000 cGy was markedly reduced to 15–20%. Lindberg et al (1981) reported similar results in a series of 300 patients with soft tissue sarcomas with a reduction in the total dose of radiation to 5000–5500 cGy. This experience and that of others has shown that radiation therapy appears to be effective when given postoperatively to control possible microscopic residual disease (Tepper 1989). The local recurrence rate is reduced and the rate of limb salvage has been dramatically improved with relatively few complications (Table 15.4). However, it is important to note that the comparative success of radiotherapy may at least partially reflect the effects of specialist treatment, whereby wide excision is the norm. Radiotherapy following inadequate or marginal excision may not improve local control rates (Bell et al 1989).

Certain principles of treatment have arisen from this experience:

1. A strip of skin is spared on the side of the extremity opposite the primary tumour, thus avoiding the severe subcutaneous fibrosis that occurred when the entire extremity was treated.

Table 15.4 Reported trials of surgery and adjuvant radiation therapy for extremity soft tissue sarcomas

Study, year	Institution	XRT dose (cGy)	No.of patients	% amputation	Local recurrence No. %	% survival
Lindberg 1981	MD Anderson	6000–6500	200	10	40 (20)	70
Suit 1982	Massachusetts General	6000*	36*	9	4 (12)	72
Lattuada 1981	Milan, NCI	5500	146	...	3 (30)	59
Total			382	19	(20)	66

*Preoperative radiation.

2. Radiation therapy was much more effective in reducing local recurrence rates when all gross tumour had been removed by surgery (20%), compared to instances when macroscopic residual disease was left behind (50% recurrence rate).

3. Local control was better for tumours distal to the knee or elbow joint that those which were located on the proximal extremity.

Suit et al (1982) reported on a series of patients treated at the Massachusetts General Hospital who were given 5000–6000 cGy of radiation therapy prior to excision of the primary tumour. Local recurrence rates were low (12–15%), but there tended to be an increase in the incidence of postoperative complications in the healing wound. However, the number of patients who required amputation for treatment of their tumours was low (approximately 2%). Suit et al (1985) cited several theoretical advantages for administration of preoperative radiation therapy :

1. The treatment volume is planned to include only the clinically and radiographically demonstrated sarcoma and the known and expected areas of subclinical extension. This is in contrast to the situation for postoperative radiation therapy, which must include all tissues handled surgically, including the drain tract.

2. Since the radiation therapist and surgeon will both have seen the patient preoperatively, there is a greater opportunity for both to participate in treatment planning including the opportunity for intraoperative radiation as a component of the treatment.

3. Most tumour cells, especially those at the periphery, will have been inactivated at the time of surgery, reducing the likelihood of autotransplantation of the neoplasm into the surgical bed or of the establishment of distant metastases as a consequence of exfoliation of viable tumour cells into the circulation during the manipulation of surgery.

Surgery and radiation brachytherapy techniques have been reported by Shiu et al (1984, 1986) at Memorial Hospital in New York. Tumours were widely excised followed by implantation of afterloading catheters, which were loaded with radioactive iridium 3–5 days following surgery. This has the theoretical advantage of delivering high doses of radiation to the area of the least margin, with less radiation being given to the normal tissue at a distance from the resection margins. In this non-randomised, selected series, Shiu et al reported local control rates of approximately 90%.

Chemotherapy and surgery

McBride et al (1974) at the MD Anderson Hospital, and Stehlin (1975) reported their results obtained by isolated limb perfusion with L-PAM and Actinomycin-D in patients with soft tissue sarcomas. The tumour was excised after the drug treatments. They showed that isolated limb perfusion with these relatively inactive drugs was beneficial. The overall local control rate was 80% and the amputation rate was 10%.

Haskell et al (1974) described a pilot study in which patients with soft tissue sarcoma were treated with continuous intra-arterial Adriamycin infusion 72 hours prior to excision. Pathological examination of the resected specimens revealed approximately 50% necrosis following this therapy. The local control rate was good, but no definitive results could be obtained from this small study. However, this study did show that Adriamycin could be given by continuous infusion in high concentrations with minimal systemic side effects.

Karakousis et al (1979) at Roswell Park reported a series of patients treated by intra-arterial Adriamycin administered by infusion into the extremity while blood flow was interrupted by means of a tourniquet. The purpose was to trap the drug in the extremity in order to obtain a more uniform distribution of blood in the tissue of the extremity. A wide excision of the tumour was carried out in the 15 patients entered into this study, and excellent local control was achieved. The use of preoperative limb perfusion with cytotoxic agents continues to receive support, both in achieving local control and reducing tumour bulk so as to avoid amputation (Hoekstra et al 1987, Di Filippo et al 1988).

Chemotherapy, radiation therapy and surgery

After Haskell's study on the effects of intraarterial Adriamycin, Eilber et al (1977) began a series of trials of preoperative intra-arterial Adriamycin followed by radiation therapy and surgery for the treatment of extremity soft tissue sarcomas. This was designed to deliver Adriamycin, a known radiation sensitiser, by the infusion technique, followed by a high dose of radiation therapy, but less than the 5000–6000 cGy required for control of microscopic disease, before excising the tumour. This was called the concept of shrinking fields, i.e. treatment of the entire extremity with chemotherapy, treatment of the entire compartment with radiation therapy, and treatment of the tumour and the immediately surrounding area by a wide surgical excision (Fig. 15.1). Since experimental evidence had shown that radiation therapy had a shoulder effect, i.e. higher dose fractions were more effective than more frequent lower

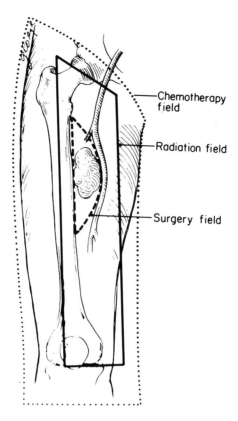

Fig. 15.1   Concept of 'shrinking fields' of preoperative multimodality therapy for soft tissue sarcomas.

dose fractions, the radiation was administered in 350 cGy fractions. The initial series consisted of 86 patients treated by:

1. Intra-arterial Adriamycin, 30 mg/day continuously for 72 hours (total dose 90 mg) followed by
2. Radiation therapy, 350 cGy fractions x 10, followed by
3. Wide local excision with pathologically negative margins.

In the first series of 86 patients, there were 2 local recurrences, for an overall local recurrence rate of 3%. Four patients required amputation with a resulting limb salvage rate of 92%. Five patients with large thigh sarcomas, in whom the periosteum of the underlying bone was stripped off during the wide excision, had a subsequent fracture of the femur. This occurred an average of 14 months following resection of the tumour. These all healed following reoperation and insertion of an intramedullary rod. None of these patients had any evidence of local recurrence at the time of reoperation (Eilber et al 1980). Whether the surgical procedure or the radiation therapy was the cause of these complications is not known. However, to reduce the possibility of this serious complication, and to reduce the fibrosis that occurred in some of the other patients, a second group of 137 patients was treated with the same regimen of intra-arterial Adriamycin, but the radiation therapy dose was reduced to 1750 cGy (Eilber et al 1985). With this lower dose of radiation, there was less tumour necrosis in the resected specimen, an average of 20% necrosis as compared to 80% in the group with the higher radiation dose. The reduced dose of radiation therapy resulted in less complications, but the incidence of local recurrence increased to 12%.

In 1984, the radiation dose was adjusted to 2800 cGy in an attempt to improve the local control rate while avoiding the serious complications encountered with the 3500 cGy dose. This has proven to be a satisfactory compromise. This series now has 75 patients enrolled, and the local recurrence rate has been reduced to 5%. The complication rate has been reduced to 20%, most of which were minor wound healing problems, amenable to conservative management. Only 10% of patients required reoperation for complications of the original surgery, and amputation has only been required in 2 patients (2.6%). The overall survival in the combined group of patients is 79% with a follow-up of 1–12 years (median 3.7 years). A summary of the various trials is shown in Table 15.5.

From these studies, it appears that multimodality therapy combining chemotherapy, radiation and surgery has improved the rate of limb salvage, reduced the incidence of local recurrence, and resulted in excellent long term survival for these patients. Avoidance of destructive radical surgery in difficult cases may be particularly striking (Hoekstra et at 1989). As can be seen from our experience with changing the dosage of radiation therapy, one must assess each modality individually in order to arrive at a compromise with respect to an acceptable complication rate and an acceptable rate of local recurrence. We are currently comparing the route of administration of Adriamycin in order to determine if the intra-arterial route is necessary since this is more cumbersome than giving the chemotherapy intravenously.

Adjuvant chemotheraphy

There is considerable debate regarding the efficacy of adjuvant chemotherapy in the prevention of metastatic disease. Initially it was assumed by the

Table 15.5   Summary of trials at UCLA using preoperative Adriamycin and varying doses of preoperative radiation therapy

Year	Dose of RT (cGy)	No. of patients	Local recurrence No. (%)	Complications No. (%)	Amputations No. (%)	Free of disease No. (%)
1971–81	None	47	13 (27)	7 (15)	18 (38)	34 (72)
1974–81	3500	77	4 (5)	27 (35)	3 (4)	48 (62)
1981–84	1750	137	17 (12)	35 (25)	4 (3)	108 (79)
1984–87	2800	75	4 (5)	15 (20)	1 (1)	71 (94)

Amercian Joint Committee on Staging and End Results that the recurrence rate would approach 70% with a survival rate of 20% or less for patients with grade III soft tissue sarcomas (Russell et al 1977). However, several investigators reported in non-randomised studies that treatment with Adriamycin as a single agent, or Adriamycin plus various drug combinations was beneficial with overall survival rates approaching 60–70%. It was noted that in almost all of these studies the local recurrence rate was reduced. Several investigators began to question whether this improvement in survival was in fact due to better local control as a result of more radical surgical procedures. A randomised prospective trial of CyVADACT following surgical resection and postoperative radiation vs no adjuvant chemotherapy showed no difference in overall survival or local recurrence rate (Lindberg et al 1978). Edmonson et al (1980) at the Mayo Clinic reported a randomised trial of no adjuvant chemotherapy vs Adriamycin/Actinomycin D/Cytoxan in a group of patients who had wide excision as therapy for the primary tumour. Initially, there appeared to be a reduced incidence of systemic metastases in patients treated with adjuvant chemotherapy, but after longer follow-up, there were no differences between the groups, and local recurrence rates were 30%. Rosenberg et al (1983) at the NIH reported a survival advantage in patients receiving adjuvant Adriamycin, Cytoxan and methotrexate. Recently two randomised trials have been reported which showed no difference in survival between patients treated with adjuvant Adriamycin and a control population which did not receive postoperative chemotherapy (Alvegard 1986, Eilber et al 1986). Currently, a new co-operative trials is beginning which will compare Adriamycin and Ifosfamide vs no adjuvant chemotherapy in grade III soft tissue sarcoma.

SUMMARY

The three major factors that must be taken into account in evaluating treatment modalities in soft tissue sarcomas are 1. survival, 2. local recurrence and 3. quality of life. The initial shift in therapy from local excision to amputation was prompted by the recognition that the rate of local recurrence was too high and the survival rate was too low. When amputation became the procedure of choice, there was an improvement in local control and survival at the expense of quality of life. Recent results from many centres using a combination of chemotherapy, radiation therapy and surgery have demonstrated that one can achieve a local control rate of 95%, a 5-year survival rate of 60–70%, with an amputation rate of less than 10%. In the future, one can expect further advances in our ability to deliver effective chemotherapy as newer drugs and dosing schedules are developed. Advances in the delivery of radiation therapy, such as neutrons and other heavy particle radiation, may also alter our approach to treatment at the primary site. The rarity of these tumours, and the complexity of current treatment warrant referral of these patients to facilities specialising in the treatment of soft tissue sarcomas. This will not only improve the care of these patients, but will also allow meaningful evaluation of new treatment modalities as they are developed.

REFERENCE

Alvegard T A 1986 Adjuvant chemotherapy with adriamycin in high grade malignant soft tissue sarcoma – a Scandinavian randomized study. Proceedings of the American Society of Clinical Oncology 5: 125

Barber J R, Coventry M B, McDonald J R 1957 The spread of soft-tissue sarcomata of the extremities along peripheral nerve trunks. Journal of Bone and Joint Surgery 39A: 534–540

Bell R S, O'Sullivan B, Liu F F et al 1989 The surgical margin in soft tissue sarcoma. Journal of Bone and Joint Surgery 71A: 370–375

Bowden L, Booher R J 1958 The principles and technique of resection of soft parts for sarcoma. Cancer 14: 963–977

Brennhoud I O 1966 The treatment of soft tissue sarcomas: A plea for a more urgent and aggressive approach. Acta Chirurgica Scandinavica 131: 438–442

Chang A E, Matory Y L, Dwyer A J 1987 Magnetic resonance imaging versus computed tomography in the evaluation of soft tissue tumors of the extremity. Annals of Surgery 205: 340–348

Clark R L, Martin R G, White E C 1957 Clinical aspects of soft tissue tumors. Archives of Surgery 74: 859–870

Davidson T, Cooke J, Parsons C, Westbury G 1987 Preoperative assessment of soft tissue sarcomas by computed tomography. British Journal of Surgery 74: 474–478

Di Filippo F, Calabro A M, Cavallari A et al 1988 The role of hyperthermic perfusion as a first step in the treatment of soft tissue sarcoma of the extremities. World Journal of Surgery 12: 332–339

Donaldson S, Castro J, Wilbur J et al 1973 Rhadomysarcoma of the head and neck in children: Combination treatment by surgery, irradiation, and chemotherapy. Cancer 31: 26–35

Edmonson J H, Fleming T R, Ivins J C et al 1980 Reduced hematogenous metastasis in patients who received systemic chemotherapy following excision of soft tissue sarcoma. Proceedings of the American Association of Cancer Research 21:192

Eilber F R, Townsend C M, Weisenberger T H et al 1977 A clinicopathologic study: Preoperative intraarterial Adriamycin and radiation therapy for extremity soft tissue sarcomas. In: Management of primary soft tissue tumors: Proceedings of the Annual Clinical Conference on Cancer, M D Anderson Hospital. Year Book Medical Publishers, Chicago, 411–422

Eilber F R, Mirra J J, Grant T T et al 1980 Is amputation necessary for sarcomas? A seven year experience with limb salvage. Annals of Surgery 192: 431–437

Eilber F R, Giuliano A E, Huth J F et al 1985 Limb salvage for high grade soft tissue sarcomas of the extremity: Experience at the University of California, Los Angeles. Cancer Treatment Symposia 3: 49–57

Eilber F R, Giuliano A E, Huth J F et al 1986 Adjuvant Adriamycin in high grade extremity soft-tissue sarcoma – a randomized prospective trial. Proceedings of the American Society of Clinical Oncology 5: 125

Elias A D, Antman K H 1989 Adjuvant chemotherapy for soft tissue sarcoma: an approach in search of an effective regimen. Seminars in Oncology 16: 305–311

Enneking W F, Maale G E 1988 The effect of inadvertent tumour contamination of wounds during the surgical resection of musculoskeletal neoplasms. Cancer 62: 1251–1256

Enneking W F, Spanier S S, Goodman M M 1980 Current concepts review: The surgical staging of musculoskeletal sarcoma. Journal of Bone and Joint Surgery 62A: 1027–1030

Enneking W F, Spanier S S, Malawer M M 1981 The effect of the anatomic setting on the results of surgical procedures for soft-part sarcomas of the thigh. Cancer 47: 1005–1022

Gerner R E, Moore G E, Pickren J W 1975 Soft tissue sarcomas. Annals of Surgery 181: 803–808

Gottlieb J A, Baker L H, O'Bryan R M et al 1975 Adriamycin used alone and in combination for soft tissue and bony sarcomas. Cancer Chemotherapeutic Reports 6: 271–282

Haskell C M, Silverstein M, Rangel D et al 1974 Multimodality cancer therapy in man: A pilot study of adriamycin by arterial infusion. Cancer 33: 1485–1490

Hoekstra H J, Koops H S, Molenaar W M, Oldhoff J 1987 Results of isolated regional perfusion in the treatment of malignant soft tissue tumors of the extremities. Cancer 60: 1703–1707

Hoekstra H J, Koops H S, Molenaar W M et al 1989 A combination of intraarterial chemotherapy, preoperative and postoperative radiotherapy and surgery as limb-saving treatment of primarily unresectable high-grade soft tissue sarcomas of the extremities. Cancer 63: 59–62

Hudson T M, Haas G, Enneking W et al 1975 Angiography in the management of musculoskeletal tumors. Surgery, Gynecology and Obstetrics 141: 11–21

Karakousis C P, Rao U, Holterman O H et al 1979 Tourniquet infusion chemotherapy in extremities with malignant lesions. Surgery, Gynecology and Obstetrics 149: 481–490

Kavenagh T, Yap B, Luna M et al 1980 Metastatic patterns of adult soft-tissue sarcomas. Proceeding of the American Association of Cancer Research 21: 480

Larriemore G E 1983 Experience with fast neutron therapy of sarcoma of soft tissue. Presented at the National Meeting of the American Association of Therapeutic Radiologists, Los Angeles

Lattuada A, Kenda R 1981 Postoperative radiotherapy of soft tissue sarcoma. Tumori 67: 191

Layfield L J, Anders K H, Glasgow B J, Mirra J M 1986 Fine-needle aspiration of primary soft tissue lesions. Archives of Pathology and Laboratory Medicine 110: 420–424

Lindberg R B, Murphy W K, Sincoviks J et al 1987 Adjuvant chemotherapy in the treatment of primary soft tissue sarcomas. In: Management of primary bone and soft tissue tumors. Year Book Medical Publishers, Chicago, p 343–357

Lindberg R, Martin R, Romsdahl M et al 1981 Conservative surgery and postoperative radiotherapy in 300 adults with soft tissue sarcoma. Cancer 47: 2391–2397

Mandard A, Chasle J, Mandard J 1981 The pathologist's role in multidisciplinary approach for soft part sarcoma: A reappraisal (39 cases). Journal of Surgical Oncology 17: 69–81

Markhede G, Angervall L, Stener B 1981 A multivariate analysis of the prognosis after surgical treatment of malignant soft-tissue tumors. Cancer 49: 1721–1733

Martin R, Butler J 1965 Soft tissue tumor: Surgical treatment and results. In: Tumors of bone and soft tissue. Year Book Medical Publishers, Chicago, p 333–347

McBride C M 1974 Sarcoma of the limb: Results of adjuvant chemotherapy using isolated limb perfusion. Archives of Surgery 109: 304–308

McNeer G, Cantin J, Chu F et al 1968 Effectiveness of radiation therapy in the management of sarcoma of the somatic soft tissue. Cancer 22: 391–397

Mazeron J J, Suit H D 1987 Lymph nodes as sites of metastases from sarcomas of soft tissue. Cancer 60: 1800–1808

Mueller P R, Wittenberg J, Ferrucci J 1979 CT scanning in bone and soft tissue tumors. Journal of Computer Assisted Tomography 3: 570–579

Muhn J R, Pritchard D J 1980 Computer tomography for the detection of pulmonary metastasis in patients with sarcoma. Proceedings of the American Association for Cancer Research 71: 148

Neufeld J P, Michallis L, Dopman J 1977 Suspected pulmonary metastases: Correlation of chest X-ray, whole-lung tomograms, and operative findings, Cancer 39: 383–387

Pack G 1954 End results in the treatment of sarcomata of the soft somatic tissue. Journal of Bone and Joint Surgery 36: 241–263

Rantakokko V, Ekfors T O 1970 Sarcomas of the soft tissue in the extremities and limb girdles. Acta Chirurgica Scandinavica 145: 385–394

Rooser B 1987 Prognosis in soft tissue sarcoma. Acta Orthopaedica Scandinavica (Suppl no 285) 58: 1–54

Rosenberg S A, Tepper J, Glatstein E et al 1983 Prospective randomized evaluation of adjuvant chemotherapy in adults with soft tissue sarcomas of the extremity. Cancer 52: 424–434

Russell W O, Cohen J, Enzinger F et al 1977 A clinical and pathological staging system for soft tissue sarcomas. Cancer 40: 1562–1570

Schmitt G, Rassow J, Schnabel K 1984 Radiotherapy of soft tissue sarcomas with neutrons or a neutron boost. The British Journal of Radiology 57: 247–250

Shiu M H, Castro E B, Hajdu S I 1975 Surgical treatment of 297 soft tissue sarcomas of the extremity. Annals of Surgery 182: 597–602

Shiu M H, Turnbull A D, Nori D et al 1984 Control of locally advanced extremity soft tissue sarcomas by function-saving resection and brachytherapy. Cancer 53(6): 385–92

Shiu M N, Collin C, Hilaris B S et al 1986 Limb preservation and tumor control in the treatment of popliteal and ante-cubital soft tissue sarcomas. Cancer 57: 1632–1639

Stehlin J S, de Ipolyi P, Peters D et al 1975 Soft tissue sarcomas of the extremity: Multidisciplinary therapy employing hyperthermic perfusion. American Journal of Surgery 130: 643–646

Stout A P 1974 Sarcomas of soft parts. Journal of the Missouri Medical Association 44: 329–334

Suit H D, Russell W O, Martin R G 1975 Sarcoma of soft tissue: Clinical and histopathologic parameters and response to treatment. Cancer 35: 1478–1483

Suit H D, Propper K H, Mankin N J et al 1982 Radiation therapy and conservative surgery for sarcoma of soft tissue. Progress in Clinical Cancer 8: 311–318

Suit H D, Mankin H J, Wood W C et al 1985 Preoperative, intraoperative and postoperative radiation in the treatment of primary soft tissue sarcoma. Cancer 55: 2659–2667

Tepper J E, Suit H D 1989 Role of radiation therapy in the management of patients with bone and soft tissue sarcomas. Seminars in Oncology 16: 281–288

Tepper J E, Suit H D 1985 Radiation therapy alone for sarcoma of soft tissue. Cancer 56: 475–479

Windeyer S B, Dische S, Mansfield J 1966 The place of radiation therapy in the management of fibrosarcoma of the soft tissue. Clinical Radiology 17: 32–40

Yang J C, Rosenberg S A, 1989 Surgery for adult patients with soft tissue sarcomas. Seminars in Oncology 16: 289–296

16. Future prospects

C. D. M. Fletcher

Despite the enormous advances in the diagnosis, classification and understanding of the biology of soft tissue tumours that have occurred over the last 30 years or so, it remains fairly self evident that the extent of our insight into this group of neoplasms is rather limited when compared to the more common carcinomas or lymphomas. There are perhaps three principal reasons for this root problem.

Firstly, many subtypes of soft tissue tumour are relatively rare, particularly in a non-specialist centre, and therefore both clinicopathological and more esoteric, scientific studies are restricted by the lack of either sufficient case material or suitably prepared fresh tissue. Secondly, as has been pointed out elsewhere in this text, diagnostic criteria are often imprecise and inconsistently applied, leading to very significant interobserver variation in diagnosis at not only hospital but also national and international level. Thirdly, it has to be admitted that this field is probably one of the least popular in diagnostic histopathology, hence attempts at accurate categorisation are often no more than cursory and many cases seem only to be very broadly classified in order to give some indication of future behaviour. This is particularly dangerous since many benign lesions have a deceptively malignant appearance, while, in contrast, some sarcomas have a very indolent and even non-metastasising course, obviating the need for very radical treatment.

How, then, should we look for further advances in the field of soft tissue neoplasia, both at the individual patient management level and at the 'cutting edge' of specialist research?

This question is best addressed by considering these lesions from their inception, through their treatment, to their final outcome. It is painfully obvious from Chapter 2, despite the comprehensive efforts of Professor Enjoji and Dr Tsuneyoshi, that the extent to which we understand the aetiology of most soft tissue tumours is minimal. To this day, the exact role of trauma in the genesis of sarcomas remains uncertain. While many would argue that injury simply brings a pre-existent lesion to the patient's attention, there are many well-substantiated cases in which a significant soft tissue insult, be it accidental or surgical, is subsequently complicated by the isotopic development of a neoplasm. Since minor injuries are almost day-to-day events for many people, it is highly likely that the majority of such incidents are soon forgotten by the patient, particularly if the latent period preceding neoplasia is measured in years (as is likely to be the case). This question is therefore extremely difficult to assess with any degree of accuracy. A possible avenue of exploration might involve a major epidemiological study of a large cohort of sarcoma patients to determine occupational and social class distributions and thence to investigate prospectively any apparently high-risk groups of, as yet, unaffected individuals. This may, however, be rather a simplistic approach, in view of the histological heterogeneity of soft tissue sarcomas.

From the genetic viewpoint, with the obvious exceptions of von Reckling-hausen's disease and Gardner's syndrome, it would seem that the recent spate of specific primary karyotypic events (particularly reciprocal translocations) identified in some lesions (see Chs. 12–14) does not reflect a constitutional abnormality in the patients examined and therefore screening for predisposed individuals is not a likely prospect. Nevertheless, it may be of interest to determine whether or not sporadic patients with malignant peripheral nerve sheath tumours are asymptomatic carriers of the neurofibromatosis gene or perhaps show some similar genetic aberration of limited penetrance.

In some ways perhaps more important than pursuing the massive problem of aetiology, there is a great need to develop a reliable means of making the initial diagnosis prior to definitive surgery. Although such techniques as CAT scanning or magnetic resonance imaging have greatly improved the pre-operative delineation of a given neoplasm, most surgeons prefer to know whether they are about to operate on a benign or malignant lesion, as this will clearly influence the extent of their resection. If such information is not available, then there is an unfortunate tendency to err on the side of conservative resection margins and, should the tumour prove to be a sarcoma, it is not always easy to obtain either surgical enthusiasm or patient consent to an immediate further wide excision. In terms of outcome, this tendency automatically has a deleterious effect since, in nearly all sarcomas, local recurrence (particularly if rapid) correlates with a reduced survival.

Clearly, with small lesions, excision margins are quite often adequate (irrespective of histology), because anxieties about the size of the resultant tissue defect are less. The problem really arises with tumours greater than 5 cm in diameter, under which circumstances surgeons are often keen to preserve adjacent muscle bulk or neurovascular structures, especially if the lesion might be biologically innocuous.

What is the best way of rendering a preoperative histological diagnosis? At present there are four principal means: fine-needle aspiration cytology, needle (core) biopsy, incisional biopsy or intraoperative frozen section. To this author, it seems most important, with any of these techniques, to try and determine whether the tumour is benign or malignant, since, under most circumstances, this is sufficient to determine appropriate surgery. However, as already mentioned, it should be admitted that this distinction is not always easy in the absence of a firm pathological diagnosis.

Despite reports to the contrary (Angervall et al 1986, Kissin et al 1986, Layfield et al 1986, Kissin et al 1987), fine-needle aspiration or needle biopsy are fraught with the problems both of sampling error and of examining cells or tiny fragments of tissue in the absence of their natural architecture or background. Not only may the specimen be obtained from the 'reactive' margins of the lesion (rather than the tumour itself), but also the small sample obtained may often fail to reflect the nature of the neoplasm as a whole. The other very significant problem, which applies particularly to cytology, is that very few centres (and hence very few pathologists) see a sufficiently large number of cases to facilitate any degree of experience or accuracy in reporting such material. Obviously, if one is lucky enough to sample unequivocally malignant tissue then these techniques will be of use. Conversely, however, how is one to distinguish between the mature fat of an intramuscular lipoma, or that obtained from a misguided normal subcutaneous sample? Who would reliably distinguish the central zone of myositis ossificans from a sarcoma?

There probably is a role for these techniques, given a considerable amount of practice, and their use should be encouraged if only to provide that experience, but their dangerous limitation should always be borne in mind both by clinician and pathologist. Perhaps one area of particular use is in the documentation of local recurrence or metastasis in a patient whom one might wish to spare further surgery.

At present, intraoperative frozen section performed on a 1–2 cm fragment of viable tumour is possibly the best means of distinguishing benign from malignant in most non-specialist hospitals. There is no absolute necessity to 'name' the lesion, unless the answer is fairly apparent, but this approach does have two big advantages. Firstly, it ensures that fresh material will be available, both to be suitably prepared for electron microscopy and, if need be, to be fresh frozen for certain immunocytochemical or enzyme histochemical stains. Secondly, it is less dangerous than incisional biopsy (followed by a separate operation perhaps a week or so later) in terms of tumour spillage or seeding into the wound or along tissue planes, since the surgeon is 'in control' of the operative field and is aware, there and then, of how much tissue will need to be excised. Delayed definitive operations are often complicated by the presence of granulation tissue or haematoma which may obscure the extent of the tumour, or the extent of tissue damage from the preceding biopsy. It should, however, be remembered that there remain certain instances in which frozen section distinction of benign from malignant is probably foolhardy, if not impossible. This applies particularly to low-grade neural and adipocytic neoplasms.

In reality and perhaps regrettably, there remain not infrequent cases in which an incisional biopsy is necessary. Obviously, this will include those lesions in which frozen section is not diagnostic, such that firm advice on the type of resection required cannot be provided. In addition, when there is significant preoperative clinical doubt about the nature of a mass, for example a well-circumscribed, asymptomatic tumour of about 5 cm diameter and of apparently prolonged duration, a surgeon understandably may not wish to discuss the full range of frightening diagnostic possibilities with a patient, nor may the patient wish to give the surgeon operative carte blanche without knowing what the lesion is. Given the limitations of needle biopsy or aspiration, open biopsy may therefore become necessary. It is mandatory that such a procedure be confined to one anatomical compartment and that the whole biopsy site is widely excised (subject to a diagnosis of malignancy) at the time of definitive resection, which should not be long delayed.

Accurate diagnosis prior to definitive surgery remains a major problem to which there is, at present, no ideal answer. It should, nevertheless, be borne in mind that a multidisciplinary approach, taking into account clinical history, radiological findings and the experience of an oncologist or pathologist where available, will often considerably improve diagnostic accuracy on clinical grounds alone.

Having got to this stage in patient management, there are two further areas in which we should all hope for improvement in the future — neither of which requires much discussion. Firstly, although untrue of specialist centres, there is still a depressing tendency for many sarcomas to be surgically 'shelled out', often with supporting comments about the obvious and easily defined planes of dissection. The latter finding is, of course, predictable since many sarcomas grow in an expansile, pseudoencapsulated (rather than infiltrative) manner. This technique, however, greatly increases the risk of local recurrence and similarly impairs prognosis. It is therefore encumbent upon pathologists, who may be more aware of the natural history of these tumours, to encourage wider excisions (2 cm margins if possible), either at the outset or as soon as possible after the initial enucleation. At the opposite end of the spectrum, efforts should be made to prevent inappropriate and unnecessarily mutilating amputations which are now widely recognised to confer no survival advantage except when wide excision is impossible, for example due to close proximity to a joint. There is much to be said in favour of treating these relatively uncommon neoplasms in regional or national centres, wherein greater expertise and consistency undoubtedly yield much better survival figures (Rydholm 1983, Bell et al 1989).

Secondly, we as pathologists should all work towards uniform application of diagnostic criteria and hence to reasonably reproducible diagnoses. The superb text of Enzinger and Weiss (1983) has done much to foster and facilitate this aim, but there is no doubt that, for example, malignant fibrous histiocytoma is still often used as a diagnostic dustbin for pleomorphic sarcomas and that many more sarcomas are labelled 'unclassifiable' than is strictly necessary. Such habits are only counterproductive since they make identification of clinicopathological or treatment-orientated subgroups impossible. This, in turn, makes reasoned use of adjunctive radiotherapy or chemotherapy virtually impossible, despite the increasing range of ever more sophisticated treatment regimens that are being developed. Immunohistochemistry and electron microscopy have become not only useful, but relatively commonplace adjuncts to conventional morphological assessment, and it currently appears quite likely that cytogenetic analysis is going to play an increasing role in diagnostic classification (Molenaar et al 1989).

Having now reached a diagnosis, how may we improve our ability to predict a given tumour's behaviour? This is, of course, of particular importance in sarcomas — e.g. which haemangiopericytoma, epithelioid haemangioendothelioma, or smooth muscle tumour will metastasise and which will not? While many soft tissue malignancies are readily divisible into low or high grades, there is still a substantial grey area between the two groups, the outlook of which could perhaps be modified if we could identify those needing additional or more aggressive treatment. Clearly a uniform grading system would be of great help, as explained in Chapter 11, but there is still no real consensus as to the best means of grading a given sarcoma. This problem is compounded by the influence of histological type, as witness such lesions as round cell liposarcoma or alveolar soft part sarcoma, which should always, for practical purposes, be regared as high grade, but in which mitoses are usually very scanty; or, for example, extraskeletal Ewing's sarcoma or mesenchymal chondrosarcoma, which also tend to be very aggressive even in the absence of pleomorphism or necrosis. Conversely, atypical fibroxanthoma fulfils many of the criteria of a high-grade tumour, but is almost invariably benign. It would therefore seem unlikely that a universal grading system, applicable to all histological types, could really be successful, but it is still worth pursuing such systems even if they have to be individualised for each entity.

As yet, it remains unclear whether DNA flow cytometry (see Ch. 14) might provide a more objective assessment of likely behaviour (as has been the case, for example, in lymphomas). Much more work is clearly necessary in this area to determine whether the presence or degree of aneuploidy or growth phase fraction might be of prognostic value. Another technique which may prove of use in determining cellular activity or malignancy is the delineation of nucleolar organiser region-associated proteins by silver staining (Ag-NORs) (Crocker & Nar 1987), which has recently proved accurate in distinguishing fibromatoses from fibrosarcoma in infancy (Egan et al 1988a) and fetal rhabdomyoma from rhabdomyosarcoma (Eusebi et al 1989). This method, however, does not appear to provide prognostic information in embryonal rhabdomyosarcoma (Egan et al 1988b) nor in Ewing's sarcoma of bone (Egan et al 1988c). The monoclonal antibody, Ki-67, which labels proliferating cells, appears to be a useful determinant of prognosis (Ueda et al 1989), but it remains to be seen whether this technique offers reliable information over and above that obtained by careful histological grading.

Looking further to the future, it is possible that some of the sarcomas showing a consistent chromosomal translocation may definitely prove to have aberrant expression of cellular oncogenes located close to the site of the karyotypic alteration. Should this be the case, then the presence (or absence) of amplification of these oncogenes may turn out to be of prognostic value, as in neuroblastoma (see Ch. 13) and other malignant neoplasms (Chan & McGee 1987). It is also possible that oncogene products, or their normal equivalent (e.g. nerve growth factor) and/or their receptors, may be used as a measure of likely biological behaviour (Perosio & Brooks 1989). This, again, is a field in which much research could usefully take place in the coming years. Preliminary findings do suggest that overexpression or aberrant expression of various oncogenes is common in sarcomas (Gupta et al 1988).

Having made reasoned attempts to classify, grade and then treat these tumours, one is still left with a number of theoretical questions, some of which may hopefully be answered in the near future. Such questions revolve principally around the problems of determining histogenetic origin or pattern of differentiation.

It is unfortunately true that the histogenesis of many, if not the majority, of the neoplasms of connective tissue remains entirely unknown. It is exceedingly difficult to postulate anything other than an uncommitted mesenchymal stem cell as the progenitor of such lesions as extraskeletal osteosarcoma, chondrosarcoma or embryonal rhabdomyosarcoma arising at sites devoid of voluntary muscle or liposarcoma arising in a muscle belly. Brooks (1986) has recently postulated an elegant model of mesenchymal differentiation which takes into account this very fact. He has also provided a possible rational explanation for the existence of the ubiquitous MFH, the origin of which may lie in an only partially committed primitive cell.

One really wonders if there is anything to be gained from trying to answer this question of lineage, since, at present, there are no suitable techniques which remotely prove a cell of origin. The bulk of recent work, particularly immunocytochemistry, has really only uncovered fascinating patterns of differentiation, rather than histogenetic origins as has so often been mistakenly suggested. As Gould (1986) astutely pointed out, 'it may prove useful to classify certain groups of neoplasms on the basis of what they in fact are, as defined by a series of appropriate phenotypic-differentiation marker expressions, rather than on the basis of questionable assumptions about their origins'. It is, however, natural to feel that this approach is opting out of a basic biological problem. While it may seem insurmountable at the moment, technical advances are being made at a remarkable rate, especially in the field of molecular biology, and it is possible that these questions may be reapproached in a different manner in the future.

Even if we limit ourselves to determining phenotypic differentiation, there are still major gaps in our knowledge to be filled. Lesions such as alveolar soft part sarcoma, parachordoma and fibrous hamartoma are all fairly easily recognised and have a distinctive, seemingly 'differentiated' appearance, yet we have little or no reproducible evidence to explain what cell type or structure, if any, they are recapitulating. Similarly, we have very great difficulty in accounting for the apparent epithelial differentiation of synovial sarcoma and epithelioid sarcoma which are both regarded as exclusively mesenchymal neoplasms.

In addition, it could be of very great value to discover what factors are responsible for programming, for example, monotypic lipoblastic, smooth muscular or osteoblastic differentiation in separate neoplasms arising in identical clinical settings. What influences determine whether a transformed mesenchymal stem cell gives rise, say, to a liposarcoma or any other sarcoma? At the moment there appear to be no clues to these enigmatic phenomena, but this is perhaps an area in which experimental models may prove to be of use, particularly if trophic or inductive factors and/or their receptors can be identified in mesenchymal cells.

To end on a more pragmatic note, there is no doubt that further new histological entities will continue to be described and some better known lesions will probably be reclassified. This should not be greeted with resentment or irritation, since, in most cases, it will facilitate the recognition of clinicopathologically relevant subgroups which, in the past, have been lost through 'lumping' of lesions. Alternatively, reclassification may simply provide a more accurate reflection of the state of our insight into a given tumour. In this respect, possible candidates for reallocation include dermato-fibrosarcoma protuberans which appears almost certainly to be fibroblastic rather than fibrohistiocytic in nature, synovial sarcoma which clearly in most cases has very little to do with synovium, and angiomatoid MFH which really seems to bear little if any relationship to the more common subtypes of MFH and may yet prove to belong in the spectrum of myoid or epithelioid vascular neoplasms.

While soft tissue tumours so often give rise to sensations of incomprehension or inadequacy, they form a rapidly advancing field of histopathology which merits continued research effort and perhaps rather greater attention at the diagnostic level in the coming years. Although not the case when this book was commissioned, at the time of going to press one could already justifiably devote a chapter to the molecular biology of soft tissue tumours and it may be in this area that many of the desirable and inevitable advances will come. To this end, multidisciplinary collaboration to include the involvement of basic scientists, should further be encouraged and expanded.

REFERENCES

Angervall L, Kindblom L-G, Rydholm A, Stener B 1986 The diagnosis and prognosis of soft tissue tumours. Seminars in Diagnostic Pathology 3: 240–258
Bell R S, O'Sullivan B, Liu F F et al 1989 The surgical margin in soft tissue sarcoma. Journal of Bone and Joint Surgery 71A: 370–375
Brooks J J 1986 The significance of double phenotypic patterns and markers in human sarcomas. A new model of mesenchymal differentiation. American Journal of Pathology 125: 113–123
Chan V T W, McGee J O'D 1987 Cellular oncogenes in neoplasia. Journal of Clinical Pathology 40: 1055–1063
Crocker J, Nar P 1987 Nucleolar organizer regions in lymphomas. Journal of Pathology 151: 111–118
Egan M J, Raafat F, Crocker J, Smith K 1988a Nucleolar organiser regions in fibrous proliferations of childhood and infantile fibrosarcoma. Journal of Clinical Pathology 41: 31–33
Egan M J, Raafat F, Crocker J, Williams D 1988b Prognostic importance of nucleolar organiser regions in embryonal rhabdomyosarcoma. Journal of Clinical Pathology 41: 477 (letter)
Egan M J, Raafat F, Crocker J, Williams D 1988c Prognostic importance of nucleolar

organiser regions in Ewing's sarcoma of childhood. Journal of Clinical Pathology 41: 232 (letter)

Enzinger, F M, Weiss S W 1983 Soft tissue tumors. C V Mosby, St Louis

Eusebi V, Ceccarelli C, Cancellieri A, Derenzine M 1989 Nucleolar organiser regions in normal skeletal muscle and benign and malignant rhabdomyoblastic tumours. Tumori 75: 4–7

Gould V E 1986 Histogenesis and differentiation: a re-evaluation of these concepts as criteria for the classification of tumours. Human Pathology 17: 212–215

Gupta V, Donner L R, Shin D M, Blick M 1988 Oncogene expression in human tumours of soft tissue and bone. Laboratory investigation 58: 36A (Abstract)

Kissin M W, Fisher C, Carter R L, Horton L W L, Westbury G 1986 Value of Tru-cut biopsy in the diagnosis of soft tissue tumours. British Journal of Surgery 73: 742–744

Kissin M W, Fisher C, Webb A J, Westbury G 1987 Value of fine-needle aspiration cytology in the diagnosis of soft tissue tumours: a preliminary study on the excised specimen. British Journal of Surgery 74: 479–480

Layfield L J, Anders K H, Glasgow B J, Mirra J M 1986 Fine-needle aspiration of primary soft tissue lesions. Archives of Pathology and Laboratory Medicine, 110: 420–424

Molenaar W M, De Jong B, Buist J et al 1989 Chromosomal analysis and the classification of soft tissue sarcomas. Laboratory Investigation, 60: 266–274

Perosio P M, Brooks J J 1989 Expression of growth factors and growth factor receptors in soft tissue tumours. Implications for the autocrine hypothesis. Laboratory Investigation 60: 245–253

Rydholm A 1983 Management of patients with soft tissue tumours. Strategy developed at a regional oncology center. Acta Orthopaedica Scandinavica 54, Supplement 203: 1–80

Ueda T, Aozasa M, Tsujimoto M et al 1989 Prognostic significance of Ki-67 reactivity in soft tissue sarcomas. Cancer 63: 1607–1611

Index